John Jebb and the Enlightenment Origins of British Radicalism

John Jebb and the Enlightenment Origins of British Radicalism

Anthony Page

Jeremy Black, Advisory Editor

PRAEGER

Westport, Connecticut
London

Library of Congress Cataloging-in-Publication Data

Page, Anthony, 1969–
John Jebb and the enlightenment origins of British radicalism / Anthony Page.
p. cm.
Includes bibliographical references and index.
ISBN 0–275–97775–7 (alk. paper)
1. Jebb, John 1736–1786 2. Radicalism—Great Britain—History—18th century. 3. Great Britain—Politics and goverment—1760–1789. 4. Great Britain—Intellectual life—18th century. 5. College teachers—England—Cambridge—Biography. 6. Social reformers—Great Britain—Biography. 7. Physicians—Great Britain—Biography. 8. Radicals—Great Britain—Biography. I. Title.
DA506.J66P34 2003
941.07'092—dc21
[B] 2002070887

British Library Cataloguing in Publication Data is available.

Library of Congress Catalog Card Number: 2002070887
ISBN: 0–275–97775–7

First published in 2003

Praeger Publishers, 88 Post Road West, Westport, CT 06881
An imprint of Greenwood Publishing Group, Inc.
www.praeger.com

Printed in the United States of America

The paper used in this book complies with the Permanent Paper Standard issued by the National Information Standards Organization (Z39.48–1984).

10 9 8 7 6 5 4 3 2 1

This book is dedicated to

my parents

Gwen and Dudley Page

Contents

Preface

I decided to write a study of John Jebb because his wide-ranging interests and activities would allow me to explore many aspects of eighteenth-century Britain. The result is, I hope, a book that brings to life Jebb's thought and activities while also providing a view of Britain during the period of the American Revolution.

This book was written in the context of post-modern Australia, where the ranks of those teaching and studying British history are dwindling. It is, in part, a contribution to remembering how our democratic culture has been formed through a long and interesting history of struggle and debate. At La Trobe University I was fortunate to be taught by some outstanding enthographic and revisionist historians. I have, I hope, learned their lessons about the 'otherness' of the past and the dangers of anachronistic and teleological thinking. I remain, however, influenced by the progressive teachers I had at Wendouree High Technical School in Ballarat. In particular, Doug Bradby brought Voltaire and the eighteenth century to life for a small group of rural and working class students – inspiring us to examine how fellow human beings grappled with moral, intellectual and political problems in a period of history that resonates beyond the boundaries of Europe.

This book is dedicated to my hard-working, kind and cheerful parents. I will always be thankful for their love and encouragement and the childhood they provided on our dairy farm. My interest in and ability to understand Jebb's mentality owes much to having a mum and dad who live according to the essential spirit of Christianity. Many thanks to the late John Hinchon, who did much to prepare me for university; Dr Damian Powell for his friendship and stimulating conversations on history and the human condition; and the network of friends that has developed out of my days as an undergraduate at La Trobe University.

My experience of being a postgraduate student was greatly enriched by having Professor Wilfrid Prest as a supervisor. He has provided a great deal of support, advice, encouragement and the opportunity to meet and dine with some distinguished British historians. I count myself extremely fortunate to have met with much kindness, candour and generosity on the part of academics who study Rational Dissent – in particular, Dr Martin Fitzpatrick of the University of Wales and Emeritus Professor R.K. Webb of the University of Maryland. Harry Dickinson, Iain McCalman and Grayson Ditchfield have also provided thoughtful comments on the whole text and John Gascoigne on chapter 6. Bernard Bailyn is owed a debt of gratitude for inviting and paying for me to attend a two-week 'International Seminar on the History of the Atlantic World, 1500-1800' at Harvard University in August 2000. I was working as a secondary school teacher at the time and this experience did much to recharge my academic batteries. John Patterson was a wonderfully supportive principal – allowing me two weeks off in the middle of a busy term is only one example of his kindness. Along with George Dimovski and the other staff at Broadford Secondary College, he provided a memorably rewarding and entertaining experience of school teaching.

Many thanks to Professor Michael Bennett and the School of History and Classics, University of Tasmania for providing the opportunity to work and teach as an historian, and to live with my family in a beautiful part of the world – a dream fulfilled. Thanks also to the University of Adelaide for providing a scholarship to undertake the research that forms the basis of this book and the following institutions for their assistance: Barr Smith Library, University of Adelaide; British Library; Dr Williams's Library; John Ryland's Library; Cambridge University Library; Public Record Office, London; Gloucestershire Record Office; Linen Hall Library, Belfast; National Library of Ireland; Massachusetts Historical Society; and St Deiniol's Library, Hawarden, Wales.

The journals *Enlightenment and Dissent* and *History* have kindly granted permission to reprint material that has appeared in the following articles: '"Liberty has an asylum": John Jebb, British Radicalism and the American Revolution', *History*, 87 (2002), pp. 204-26; and 'Enlightenment and a "Second Reformation": the Religion and Philosophy of John Jebb (1736-86)', *Enlightenment and Dissent*, 17 (1998), pp. 48-82.

Thanks to Heather Staines and the people at GPG for publishing this book, especially Katie Chase who has been a very thorough and helpful copyeditor. Many hours have been spent entering her corrections and in the process further modifications and additions have been made. With much help, I have endeavoured to ensure the text is free of errors. Any that remain are my responsibility – but they are not there through want of trying to find and fix them!

My wonderful wife Carmen has carefully read through the entire text and has cheerfully lived with Dr Jebb being the subject of many conversations. While the bulk of this book was completed before we met, without her unflagging love, good humour and encouragement this text may never have seen the printer. Words cannot express how much I appreciate our partnership, and our little Katherine, who is toddling, babbling, exploring the world, and amazing and amusing her parents more and more each day.

A Note on Sources and Abbreviations

The primary text used in this study is *The Works: Theological, Medical, Political and Miscellaneous of John Jebb, MD. FRS., with a Life of the Author* (3 vols., John Disney ed., 1787). Volume I is divided into two parts with separate pagination. The first part (John Disney's 'Memoirs of the Life of the Author') is cited as: 'Life of Jebb'. The second part is simply cited as: Jebb I. The other two volumes are cited as: Jebb II and Jebb III.

There are five volumes of Jebb's interleaved Greek New Testament and a volume of notes for his Theological Lectures in Dr Williams' Library, London. The pages are not numbered, but most citations of the interleaved Testament are from the first few pages of each volume where Jebb tended to write general notes. These are cited as: DWL Jebb mss. I-VI.

JJ	John Jebb
AJ	Ann Jebb
BDMBR	J.O. Baylen and N.J. Grossman eds., *Biographical Dictionary of Modern British Radicals: volume: 1, 1770-1830* (Salem, New Hampshire, 1979).
DNB	*Dictionary of National Biography*
E&D	*Enlightenment and Dissent*
JHI	*Journal of the History of Ideas*

MP	Member of Parliament
SCI	The Society for Constitutional Information

Throughout the book London is place of publication, unless otherwise stated.

Where individual works are not cited in the bibliography, that work is to be found in the collected works by that author.

When multiple articles have been cited from an edited collection of essays, only a short title for the source book is given. Full details can be found where the source book is cited in the bibliography.

The punctuation and capitalisation in original sources has been retained. While printed and manuscript sources from the eighteenth century generally make heavy use of capital letters, the opposite is true of John Disney's edition of Jebb's *Works*.

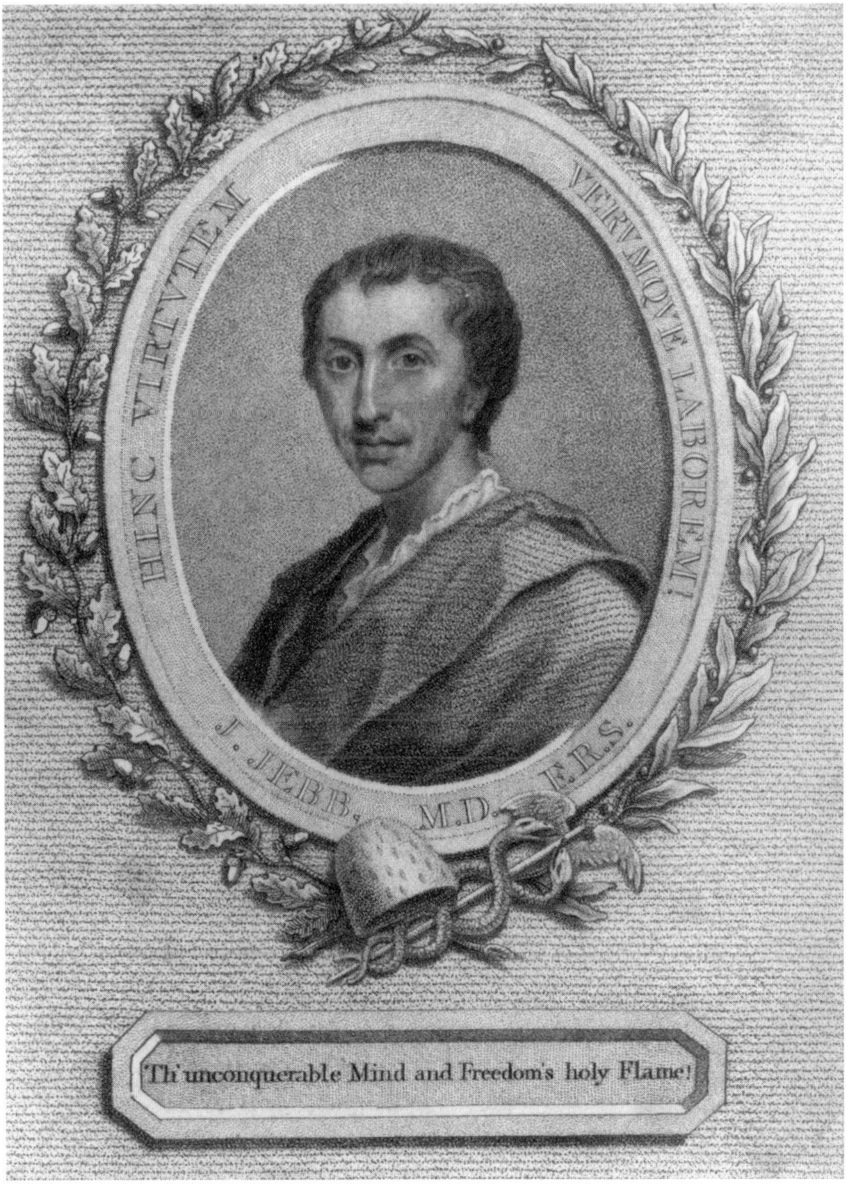
HINC VIRTUTEM
VERUMQUE LABOREM!
J. JEBB, M.D. F.R.S.
Th' unconquerable Mind and Freedom's holy Flame!

John Jebb by Charles Knight after an unknown artist.
By Courtesy of the National Portrait Gallery, London (D10782).

Introduction

This is a study of Enlightenment ideas and their propagation by a man and woman at the forefront of the birth of modern British radicalism. The origins of modern democratic politics lay in the eighteenth century – but exactly where has been open to question. English republicanism was thought to have shot its bolt early, having flourished and failed in the seventeenth century. The origin of nineteenth-century campaigns for democratic reform, according to this view, lay in the inspirational influence of the French Revolution and the republican writings of Thomas Paine.[1] The Industrial Revolution, seen to have been Britain's contribution to the emergence of the modern world, was depicted as having occurred under a relatively unified and uninteresting Hanoverian political establishment. As a result, history courses tended to focus on either the dramatic tumults of the Tudor and Jacobean period or the world-conquering culture of nineteenth-century Britain. Recent research, however, has revealed the profound social, economic, political and intellectual legacy of eighteenth-century Britain. Indeed, Roy Porter has persuasively argued that Enlightenment Britain (rather than revolutionary France) ushered in the modern world.[2] As part of this reassessment, the nature and importance of political dissent has attracted much attention. Historians have demonstrated that modern British radicalism had strong indigenous roots that pre-date 1789 – the War of American Independence being highlighted as a particularly important formative period.[3] It

[1] The classic statement of this view is E.P. Thompson, *The Making of the English Working Class* (1963).
[2] Roy Porter, *Enlightenment: Britain and the creation of the modern world* (2000).
[3] Stephen Conway, *The British Isles and the War of American Independence* (Oxford, 2000), pp. 203-38.

has also been shown that most radicals in this period and throughout the nineteenth century did not reject the political system outright, but rather championed their own versions of an 'ancient constitution' that they claimed had been corrupted.[4]

The traditional division between studies of political action and studies of political thought is being bridged. Those studying eighteenth-century political thought have become increasingly interested in the relationship between political philosophy expounded for a well-educated elite, and its popularisation for a less-educated though broadly literate public.[5] This study adds to our understanding of this process and illuminates the character of the British political radicalism that emerged in the three decades prior to the French Revolution.

While Dr John Jebb (1736-1786) is referred to in studies of the religious, educational and political controversies of his day, extended study of his prominent role in the formative period of British radicalism has been long overdue.[6] Jebb began his career as a clergyman and academic at Cambridge in the 1760s, and died as a doctor and leading figure among political reformers in London. Both friend and foe acknowledged his talents and influence. When the American John Adams arrived in London in 1785 he told Jebb that 'I have long wanted to Communicate with some of the enlightened Friends of Liberty here ... and I know of none who merit the Character better'.[7] This sense of Jebb's important role in the reform movement was echoed over two decades after his death by the conservative critic John Nichols, who wrote: 'No name is better known among the advocates for Parliamentary Reform, than that of Dr Jebb'. Nichols characterised him as 'much celebrated among the violent partisans for unbounded liberty, religious and political; and certainly a man of learning and talents, though they were both so much absorbed in controversy as to leave little among his writings of general use. ... He was an active, enterprising, sincere, good natured man, but of rather too ardent a temper'.[8]

Jebb was committed to reforming all aspects of eighteenth-century British religion, politics and society. At Cambridge he taught mathematics and

---

[4] See, for example, the contributions to James Vernon ed., *Re-Reading the Constitution: new narratives in the political history on England's long nineteenth century* (Cambridge, 1996).

[5] See, for example, the works of H.T. Dickinson, James E. Bradley and Kathleen Wilson cited in the bibliography.

[6] The most substantial treatment until recently was Naomi Miller's entry on Jebb in J.O. Baylen and N.J. Grossman eds., *A Biographical Dictionary of Modern British Radicals: volume 1, 1770-1830* (Salem, N. H., 1979). See also Caroline Robbins, *The Eighteenth Century Commonwealthman: studies in the transmission, development and circumstance of English liberal thought from the Restoration of Charles II until the war with the Thirteen Colonies* (Cambridge, Mass., 1959), pp. 370-73. There have been two recent doctoral dissertations: Kenneth Pearl, 'John Jebb, a British Radical in the Age of the American Revolution' (PhD thesis, City University of New York, 1998); Anthony Page, 'Enlightened Patriot: John Jebb and Dissent in England, 1760-85' (PhD thesis, University of Adelaide, 1999). The latter forms the basis of this book.

[7] John Adams to John Jebb, 21 August 1785, MHS Adams papers.

[8] John Nichols, *Literary Anecdotes of the Eighteenth Century* (1813), II, pp. 711, 571-72.

philosophy, and acted as university examiner on several occasions. Through critical study of the Bible he became a Socinian, and attracted the disapproval of university authorities when he proceeded to deliver lectures on the Greek New Testament. In the early 1770s Jebb became a leading figure in organising the Feathers Tavern petition, which requested that Parliament remove the requirement that Church of England clergy subscribe to the theology and liturgy articulated in the Thirty-Nine Articles. When it became evident that the efforts of the petitioning clergy were to no avail, Jebb turned his attention to educational reform, seeking to broaden the curriculum and introduce annual examinations for all students. Following the narrow failure of his educational proposals, Jebb became increasingly marginalised at Cambridge, a situation exacerbated by his open support for the American colonists. In 1776 he moved to London to undertake the study and practice of medicine. As the American War dragged on with no end in sight, Jebb became a leader in the Association movement that formed to demand parliamentary reform. He worked tirelessly for parliamentary reform in Britain and Ireland until he succumbed to persistent ill health and died in early 1786.

Jebb poured time, energy and ability into promoting the cause of 'liberty'. His uncompromising espousal of deeply held 'rational Christian' principles earned him implacable enemies and devoted friends. William Cole, a Cambridge Tory, described Jebb as a 'thin, spare, pale man, of good Parts, which he applies in a way much to the discredit of the University'. Upon Jebb's resignation from his livings in 1776, Cole observed: 'Thus does this indefatigable man's spirits waste themselves in plans for further Reformation in Religion, and in finding that not likely to succeed, in reforming the University ... I make no doubt but his head is turned: however that be, it is evident that he is a most turbulent, busy Spirit, and the Church is well rid of him.'[9] The ill-disposed radical David Williams claimed that King George III had sneered: '[Jebb] tore off his garments, harassed his friends with reveries, and sunk into the grave in poverty and vexation'.[10]

The praise of Jebb's friends, however, was boundless. John Cartwright, the author of numerous tracts calling for parliamentary reform, declared him the 'friend of my bosom and pattern of my conduct'.[11] According to Capel Lofft, as a preacher Jebb joined great learning with 'simplicity, clearness, peculiar power of persuasion; energy; the advantages of voice and manner; judgement, candour, sincerity, sensibility'. Committed to truth and public duty, Jebb was the 'tenderest and warmest of friends', 'amiable, and even pleasant, in familiar intercourse, to a degree of serene gaiety'. Thomas Brand Hollis remembered the 'feast of reason' he enjoyed in the company of 'this wonderful man'.[12] The poet Anna Seward reflected that 'never were the graces of conciliation, resulting

[9] BL Cole mss. 5378:53.

[10] James Dybikowski, *On Burning Ground: an examination of the ideas, projects, and life of David Williams* (Oxford, 1993), p. 44n.

[11] F.D. Cartwright ed., *The Life and Correspondence of Major Cartwright* (1826), p. 166.

[12] 'Life of Jebb', pp. 240, 243-44, 235.

from warm and ingenious benevolence, more engagingly blended with superior talents, and high-strung virtues, than in that extraordinary man'.[13]

Yet Brand Hollis also reveals why Jebb's opponents found him so irritating: 'Happiness in the present world, he could never have met with; it was not intended by its maker as the mansion of perfection, and nothing that fell short of perfection would have satisfied our honoured friend.'[14] During the political reform agitation of the early 1780s Christopher Wyvill, head of the Yorkshire Association, found the leader of the London radicals to be an impractical idealist. Mutual esteem, however, and 'the incomparable suavity of temper in Dr Jebb' preserved their friendship.[15] Jebb confessed that he would 'grow warm' when addressing fundamental issues of principle – and there was little, if anything, that was not a matter of principle. When offering advice to a former student he wrote: 'Explore with the utmost exertion of your faculties political truth, and having found it, avow it with firmness and perseverance. In the end it must succeed, and your character be stamped with honour. Temporising expedients are always injurious, when contrary to natural right and natural feelings.'[16] While John Cartwright found it an offensive characterisation of his friend, the following seems a fairly accurate assessment:

> Though Dr Jebb's public conduct was in the highest degree upright and consistent, yet he had too much warmth of temper and too little worldly wisdom, to be proposed a model in this respect. His character as a party man was injurious to him professionally, as appeared in the failure of his attempt to obtain the place of an hospital physician, yet he had many warm friends who were ready to serve him, and his practice increased as long as his health permitted him to follow it regularly.[17]

Cartwright responded to this with the following account, which in its own way provides an insight into Jebb's character and the way in which he inspired his students and friends with a radical combination of Christianity and Enlightenment values:

> If [John Jebb's] feelings were acute, and his temperament warm, they served the ends for which the Deity has given us feeling and sympathy, to stimulate to virtuous action; for if any man was a conscientious imitator of the mildness of Jesus, it was my departed friend. Often, indeed, have I seen him agitated ... by the selfish and the criminally ambitious; often have I known him misrepresented and traduced with

---

[13] Anna Seward, *The Letters of Anna Seward* (6 vols., Edinburgh, 1811), I, p. 149.
[14] 'Life of Jebb', pp. 237.
[15] Christopher Wyvill, *Political Papers* (York, 1794), IV, p. 521n.
[16] John Jebb [hereafter 'JJ'] to Archibald Hamilton Rowan, 5 March 1785, in *The Autobiography of Archibald Hamilton Rowan* (Dublin, 1840), 127.
[17] John Aikin ed., *General biography: or Lives, critical and historical, of the most eminent persons of all ages countries conditions and professions* (volume 5, 1804), cited in *Life of Cartwright*, pp. 165-66.

> acrimony; but never did I know him retort, or on such occasions to speak or act otherwise than as the dictates of Christian charity and political wisdom (according to my conceptions of them) dictated to him.[18]

To this we might add the impression of the perceptive young Abigail Adams, daughter of the first American minister to St James's Palace. John Adams enjoyed his conversations with Jebb on politics, and Abigail wrote to her brother: 'the Dr is said to be a very Wise and sensible Man, that he is an agreeable one, I can assure you'.[19] Intelligent and friendly, yet earnest, priggish and unbendingly committed to a particular set of Enlightenment ideals would seem to be a fair summary of Jebb's character.

Jebb did not act alone. At the end of December 1764 he married Ann Torkington (1735-1812), the daughter of a clergyman in Huntingdonshire. We are fortunate that George Meadley published a short *Memoir* of Ann Jebb in which she is depicted as the radical ideal of a wife who was virtuous and politically aware, without behaving in a 'masculine' way. At the Jebb's regular tea parties she actively engaged in religious and political discussion with visitors. In the absence of children, Ann maintained as much interest in politics as her husband, discussed all issues with him and wrote in support of their common causes. Fortunately at least thirty-eight of her letters to the newspapers on clerical subscription (penned under the pseudonym 'Priscilla') have been preserved in John Disney's collection of newspaper clippings.[20] Ann's letters to the newspapers, along with the two tracts she wrote in support of the French Revolution, allow this study of Jebb to become, in part, a study of a partnership. Yet a focus on John is made necessary by the paucity of the remaining sources, which preclude any deep study of Ann's opinions in a manner that would distinguish her from her husband. By all accounts husband and wife were one in their sentiments and ideas. When John was seriously ill in 1782, Theophilus Lindsey observed that 'Mrs Jebb would have been of all women to be pitied if we had lost him – for she lives by him'.[21] Following her husband's death in 1786 Ann felt, according to her friend and biographer George Meadley, that she had lost 'not merely a husband, a partner in a common interest; but her guardian and protector, her guide, philosopher, and friend'.[22]

An understanding of John Jebb's thought and activities helps to illuminate the nature of political radicalism in the first half of George III's reign. While researching his life I found myself asking the question: why did Jebb act in a manner that was so detrimental to his material prosperity? Parental advice

---

[18] John Cartwright cited in F.D. Cartwright ed., *The Life and Correspondence of Major Cartwright* (2 vols., 1826), I, p. 166.

[19] *Adams Family Correspondence* (6 vols., L.H. Butterfield ed., Cambridge, Mass., 1963-93), VI, p. 302.

[20] John Disney, 'A Collection of Letters and Essays on the subject of Religious Liberty published in the Newspapers 1771-74', DWL mss. 87.1-6.

[21] Theophilus Lindsey to William Tayleur, 26 December 1782, JRL Lindsey-Tayleur correspondence.

[22] G.W. Meadley, *Memoir of Mrs Jebb* (1812), p. 24.

and self-interest dictated that he should play the game of patronage politics, and had he been more flexible in his political and religious opinions Jebb could have risen within the Church. Temperament no doubt partly explains his conduct. Some others (most notably William Paley) were exposed to similar influences and took more moderate paths in their thought and conduct. Owing to the potent combination of his religious, philosophical and political convictions, however, Jebb was not prepared to bite his tongue. Instead, he became an inspirational and leading figure among those who sought to reform the Church, Cambridge University and the political system. As a result, a study of his thought and actions brings into sharp relief some of the key aspects of advanced radicalism in the decades prior to the French Revolution.

The nature of radicalism in the eighteenth century has been hotly debated in recent decades. Historians traditionally emphasised the link between radicalism and urbanisation, arguing that political dissent was informed by a developing liberal conception of the autonomous individual.[23] Revisionist historians, however, have demonstrated the pervasive influence of classical republicanism, with its notions of virtue and landed independence underpinning active participatory citizenship. This conservative and backward-looking 'radicalism', they argue, criticised the commercial and state building policies of eighteenth-century governments.[24] To this debate over the relative importance of liberalism and republicanism has been added a recent emphasis on the role of religion. At the end of the 1970s a colloquium of historians agreed that religion was of central importance in the social and political life of eighteenth-century Britain. Yet as John Cannon pointed out, having paid lip service to the importance of religion they largely neglected it in their discussions of politics during the Whig Ascendancy.[25] The years since have witnessed an explosion of research on the period, and the role of religion has received ample attention. In his seminal *English Society 1688-1832* (and a string of subsequent books and articles) Jonathan Clark has argued not only that religious concerns were predominant and pervasive, but that there was broad support for, and deference toward, a 'confessional state' composed of monarchy, aristocracy and the

---

[23] For contemporary statements of this view see: Isaac Kramnick, 'Religion and Radicalism: English political theory in the age of revolutions', *Political Theory,* 5 (1977), pp. 505-34; and *Republicanism and Bourgeois Radicalism: political ideology in late eighteenth-century England and America* (Ithaca, N.Y., 1990); Joyce Appleby, *Liberalism and Republicanism in the Historical Imagination* (Cambridge, Mass., 1992).

[24] The foremost exponent of this view in relation to the British context is J.G.A. Pocock, who authored or edited the following: 'Machiavelli, Harrington, and English Political Ideologies in the Eighteenth Century', *William and Mary Quarterly,* 22 (1965), pp. 549-83; *The Machiavellian Moment: Florentine political thought and the Atlantic republican tradition* (Princeton, N.J., 1975); '*The Machiavellian Moment* Revisited: a study in history and ideology', *Journal of Modern History,* 53 (1981), pp. 49-72; *Virtue, Commerce and History: essays on political thought and history, chiefly in the eighteenth century* (Cambridge, 1985); ed., *The Varieties of British Political Thought 1500-1800* (Cambridge, 1993); see also Bernard Bailyn, *The Ideological Origins of the American Revolution* (Cambridge, Mass., 1967).

[25] John Cannon ed., *The Whig Ascendancy* (1981), pp. 192-95.

Anglican Church.[26] While the important contribution of Rational Dissent to political radicalism has long been recognised, Clark has argued that Anglo-American radicalism was fundamentally rooted in theological dissent from the Anglican confessional state.[27]

In answering Edmund Burke's denigration of the British reformers, Benjamin Bousfield held Jebb up as an example of 'the most disinterested patriot, the most benevolent philosopher, and the most conscientious theologian'.[28] Selectively quoted, Jebb can (and has) been used to support an explanation of political dissent as rooted in liberalism, republicanism or heterodox theology. Such reductionism, however, should be avoided when studying political activists and their thought, and in what follows I endeavour to sketch all aspects of the patriot, philosopher and theologian. Jebb's radicalism needs to be understood in the context of the Enlightenment as it developed in England. The Enlightenment was a trans-national intellectual movement that manifested in different ways in different religious and political contexts. But it can be characterised as reflecting a common attitude of mind, or spirit, that championed reason, scepticism, cosmopolitanism, freedom of expression and the possibility of progress toward greater human happiness.[29] While Enlightenment thinkers differed as to what they regarded as true or important, they shared a common faith that through reason and criticism some things could be shown to be false. This attitude played a role in bringing about the French Revolution and is central to modernity.[30]

John Pocock has characterised England as experiencing a dominant conservative Enlightenment. An angry party of *philosophes* opposed to the state did not develop because the British constitution allowed a degree of political participation and religious toleration. English 'founding fathers' of the Enlightenment such as the scientist Isaac Newton and philosopher John Locke were harnessed as supporters of the established order. Defenders of Church and State used 'enlightened values' such as 'sceptical' philosophy, sound theology, polite letters, science and economic progress to defend civilisation against

---

[26] For J.C.D. Clark's view of the eighteenth century see: 'Eighteenth-Century Social History', *The Historical Journal,* 27 (1984), pp. 773-88; *English Society, 1688-1832* (Cambridge, 1985); *Revolution and Rebellion* (Cambridge, 1986); 'On Hitting the Buffers: the historiography of England's ancien regime. A response', *Past and Present,* 117 (1987), pp. 195-207; 'England's Ancien Regime as a Confessional State', *Albion,* 21 (1989), pp. 450-74; *The Language of Liberty 1660-1832: political discourse and social dynamics in the Anglo-American world* (Cambridge, 1994).

[27] Anthony Lincoln, *Some Political and Social Ideas of English Dissent 1763-1800* (Cambridge, 1938); Clark, *English Society*, chapter 5.

[28] Benjamin Bousfield, *Observations on the Right Hon. Edmund Burke's Pamphlet, On the subject of the French Revolution* (Dublin, 1791), in G. Claeys, *Political Writings of the 1790s* (8 vols., 1995), II, p. 96.

[29] See, for example, the introductory essay and excellent selection of writings in Isaac Kramnick, *The Portable Enlightenment Reader* (Harmondsworth, 1995).

[30] Linda Kirk, 'The Matter of Enlightenment', *The Historical Journal*, 43 (2000), pp. 1129-43.

superstition and sectarian enthusiasm.[31] In the words of another influential historian, 'Enlightenment goals – like criticism, sensibility or faith in progress – throve in England *within* piety'.[32]

There were those, however, who considered themselves enlightened and yet dissented from the conservative Anglican Enlightenment. They were members of the Protestant sects (predominantly the Presbyterians, Congregationalists and Baptists) that began with a refusal to conform to the teachings and episcopal hierarchy of the Church of England following the Act of Uniformity in 1662.[33] Those who, in the course of the eighteenth-century, embraced reason and 'natural religion' as being in harmony with (and the means to accurately understand) the Christian revelation have been labelled 'Rational Dissenters'. Narrowly defined, Rational Dissent is often equated with Unitarianism – which involved a rejection of the theology of original sin and the Trinity. A variety of theological views could be found within the 'Unitarian' traditions. The broad polarities were those of the Arians, who thought that Jesus was not God incarnate, but rather a separate and distinct entity – a son of God who had nevertheless existed in heaven prior to his earthly manifestation; and the Socinians, who rejected the doctrine of atonement, claiming that Jesus was a divinely ordained prophet, sent by God to be the 'saviour' of mankind through precept and example. The late eighteenth-century variant of Socinianism (which Jebb came to espouse) emphasised the simple humanity of Jesus – and it was with this view that Unitarianism was increasingly associated. In a recent important study of *Enlightenment and Religion: Rational Dissent in eighteenth-century Britain* it has been suggested that Rational Dissent needs to be seen as part of a broader commitment to rational religion that included many conservative Dissenters and a wide range of Anglicans. In this view, 'rational religion' encompassed a variety of positions between the extremes of High-Church Anglicanism, orthodox or evangelical Dissent and deism.[34] In light of this, the Rational Dissenters were the advanced elements of those who sought to espouse a Christianity shaped by reason through a process of candid scrutiny and debate. When the ex-Anglican priest Theophilus Lindsey founded the Essex Street Unitarian Church in 1774, it became central to the networks of Rational Dissent and attracted a small number of Anglican dissidents such as Jebb.

---

[31] J.G.A. Pocock, 'Conservative Enlightenment and Democratic Revolutions: the American and French cases in British perspective', *Government and Opposition,* 24 (1989), pp. 81-105; 'History and Sovereignty: the historiographical response to Europeanization in two British Cultures', *Journal of British Studies*, 31 (1992), pp. 358-89.

[32] Roy Porter, 'The Enlightenment in England', in Roy Porter and Mikulas Teich eds., *The Enlightenment in National Context* (Cambridge, 1981), p. 6. 'The religious strength of England's Enlightenment' is demonstrated in B.W. Young, *Religion and Enlightenment in Eighteenth-Century England: theological debate from Locke to Burke* (Oxford, 1998), p. 10.

[33] Michael Watts, *The Dissenters: from the Reformation to the French Revolution* (Oxford, 1978).

[34] Knud Haakonssen, 'Enlightened Dissent: an introduction', in *Enlightenment and Religion: Rational Dissent in eighteenth-century Britain* (Cambridge, 1996), p. 5. This view is presented in RK Webb's essay 'The Emergence of Rational Dissent' in the same volume, pp. 12-41.

The Rational Dissenters were a small proportion of English society, who felt frustrated by the contrasting rapid spread of evangelical Methodism. Their influence, however, greatly outweighed their numerical strength. Rational Dissent included within its ranks many well-connected clergymen, doctors, lawyers, businessmen and even politicians, along with influential writers on science, philosophy, religion and politics. Their prominent role in voicing support for the American Revolution has long been recognised.[35] Rational Dissent was situated in complex ways between the conservative English Enlightenment and the more radical trends on the Continent. As Haakonssen has written, Rational Dissent's 'very success in integrating with the established order ... led to deep ambiguities. On the one hand, it muted democratic, let alone more egalitarian, tendencies and made sure that Rational Dissent on the whole was part of the conservative Enlightenment .... On the other hand, the fact that the legal and political basis for the Rational Dissenters' success was so tenuous tended in the opposite direction, namely toward a search for radical reform'.[36]

Jebb is representative of the link between Rational Dissent and political radicalism in the late eighteenth-century. Thus, his example lends support to Jonathan Clark's emphasis on the link between theology and politics. A close examination of Jebb reveals, however, that there was more to Rational Dissent than heterodox theology. Theology was a key point of confrontation between Jebb and the established order – he was very frustrated with what he saw as a national Church preaching and teaching falsehood. But his radicalism was not simply the result of hot-headed Socinianism. Jebb opposed the established order with a comprehensive and visionary alternative world-view (and thus could be seen to have 'harassed his friends with reveries'). Along with a radical reading of the 'English Constitution', his theology was embedded within an optimistic philosophical system. There were those who were sceptical of orthodox theology, but either lived with or supported the status quo. The relentless enthusiasm and conviction with which Jebb pursued his campaigns against the established constitution in Church and State can be understood only in light of the combined effect of his theological, political and philosophical convictions. It was a combination that he shared in large part with that more famous scourge of Church and State, Joseph Priestley. While theology was undoubtedly a prime motive behind much political dissent, the case of Jebb suggests that we need to look more closely at the way Rational Dissenters espoused, in various forms, an Enlightenment faith in the unity of religion and reason and the inevitability of moral and material progress.

While Jebb's political and religious views have been sketched in previous studies, they have not been adequately set within the context of his philosophical convictions. In providing a comprehensive study of his 'rational dissent', I want to highlight the way Jebb's religious and political thought were profoundly influenced by a philosophical disposition that owed much to David Hartley's seminal *Observations on Man* (1749). Hartley had sought to reconcile

[35] Colin Bonwick, *English Radicals and the American Revolution* (Chapel Hill, N.C., 1977).
[36] Haakonssen, 'Enlightened Dissent: an introduction', in *Enlightenment and Religion*, p. 9.

religion and science by demonstrating that in the mechanism of the human mind was revealed the hand of Providence. To a student schooled in Newtonian Latitudinarianism, Hartley offered a heady blend of unorthodox Christian idealism (including the doctrine of universal salvation) founded on a determinist psychology. This combination of providential optimism with a utilitarian moral philosophy underpinned Jebb's critique of all aspects of eighteenth-century politics and society. It allowed him to employ both utilitarian and natural rights arguments without concern for coherence or consistency; and it gave him the confidence to dismiss prudent concerns as to the prospects for, or consequences of radical reform. Jebb thought the morally autonomous individual had a right and duty to seek and act upon truth – and truth, he believed, was unified and entirely within the reach of reason and scientific scrutiny. This led Jebb to champion free enquiry and argue that Christianity should run with the breeze of enlightenment, or else risk being dashed upon rocks by a rising tide of scepticism. It was this optimistic faith in reason, progress and individual autonomy that led him to be among the earliest advocates for universal manhood suffrage. The dynamic interplay of his ideological development and practical political experience led Jebb to become, in Paul Langford's words, a 'rebel against his church and a reformer at odds with his society'.[37]

Throughout this book I have freely used the terms 'radical' and 'conservative'. They need to be justified and qualified. As James Sack has observed, there is 'difficulty in attempting any type of meaningful historical discourse without using the language of modern politics'.[38] With this in mind I have used these terms to indicate various positions, attitudes and temperaments relative to the status quo.[39] Jebb's reformist activism provoked opposition from various defenders of Church and State and it might be objected that they are too easily branded with the label 'conservative'. The strength, appeal and variety of orthodox Anglicanism in the eighteenth century has been highlighted by a growing body of scholarship.[40] However, while the various intellectual nuances of radical thought are teased out at length, it is not within the scope of this study to do the same for Jebb's opponents. 'Conservative' is at times used as shorthand to describe figures whose opinions ranged from extreme High Church to moderate support for the established religious and political order. This is in line with Samuel Johnson's eighteenth-century definition of 'conservative' as 'having the power of opposing diminution or injury'. This book is primarily concerned with showing how Jebb's thoughts and actions were relatively radical for the times in which he lived and the ways he contributed to developing traditions out of which nineteenth-century radicalism emerged.

---

[37] Paul Langford, *Public Life and the Propertied Englishman, 1689-1798* (Oxford, 1991), p. 1.

[38] James J. Sack, *From Jacobite to Conservative: reaction and orthodoxy in Britain, 1760-1832* (Cambridge, 1993), p. 4.

[39] For similar use of these terms see H.T. Dickinson, *The Politics of the People in Eighteenth-Century Britain* (New York, 1994).

[40] For an overview see P.B. Nockles, *The Oxford Movement in Context: Anglican High Churchmanship, 1760-1857* (Cambridge, 1994), pp. 1-32.

1

A Latitudinarian Education

John Jebb was schooled in the principles of liberal Latitudinarianism. Whig Latitudinarianism emerged out of late seventeenth-century disputes over the location of authority in religion. During the sixteenth century the Church of England sought to define itself as a Protestant church that preserved many Catholic elements in its structure and practice. During the reign of Elizabeth I this compromise was defined in the Thirty-Nine Articles. The English Civil War saw the breakdown of this compromise, with High Churchmen supporting the King and Puritans lining up behind Parliament. While High Churchmen were triumphant with the restoration of the monarchy in 1660, others promoted broad-church notions as a means of avoiding further religious conflict. They argued that a wide latitude of interpretation of the Thirty-Nine Articles should be tolerated. The Latitudinarians adopted the philosophy of John Locke and the science of Newton, and argued that the Anglican Church should occupy a middle ground between the extremes of sectarian enthusiasm and the authoritarian notions of the High Church. Against the enthusiasts they claimed that God had granted humanity reason in order to better understand revelation. They also used the authority of reason to dismiss some of the 'mysteries' grafted onto Christianity by Catholic tradition. They saw the primary role of the Anglican Church as the moral training and policing of society in accordance with the designs of a reasonable God.[1] Advanced Latitudinarians like Benjamin Hoadly (1676-1761) went so far as to argue for an Erastian view of the Church

[1] David A. Pailin, 'Rational Religion in England from Herbert of Cherbury to William Paley', in Sheridan Gilly and W.J. Sheils eds., *A History of Religion in Britain: practice and belief from pre-Roman times to the present* (Oxford, 1994), pp. 210-20; John Spurr, '"Rational Religion" in Restoration England', *JHI,* 49 (1988), pp. 563-85; R.K. Webb, 'The Emergence of Rational Dissent', in Haakonssen, *Enlightenment and Religion*, pp. 12-41.

and government based on contract.[2] In his influential study of the eighteenth-century Church, Norman Sykes wrote of 'the typical Latitudinarian churchmanship dominant in the century'.[3] This view has been somewhat qualified by revisionist historians: Tory and High Church notions survived and evolved throughout the century, and Latitudinarianism was by no means an all-encompassing, uniform and unchanging category.[4] Yet if there was a time when Latitudinarianism was dominant in the Church, it was during the years of Whig supremacy between 1740 and 1760; and if there was a place, it was Cambridge University, to which John Jebb was sent in 1754.[5]

FAMILY BACKGROUND AND EARLY EDUCATION

John Jebb was born in London on 16 February 1736, and attended several schools in England and Ireland. This suggests contact with scattered family members who were making their way in trade and the professions.[6] Jebb's grandfather Samuel Jebb (1670-1743) was a maltster in Woodborough near Mansfield, Nottinghamshire, where his family had lived for some generations. He had nine children with his wife Elizabeth (who hailed from Yorkshire): six sons and three daughters. The most notable of these was the second son Samuel Jebb M.D. (1694-1772) who entered Cambridge as a sizar and became a Non-juror.[7] Unable to take orders he became librarian to Jeremy Collier (1650-1726), the outspoken critic of political and moral corruption. Samuel Jebb became a noted scholar (publishing the first modern edition of Roger Bacon's *Opus Majus* in 1733) before turning to the practice of medicine following Collier's death. While their religious and political views differed, Samuel Jebb set an example for his nephew as a scholar who adhered to principles to the detriment of his career prospects in the Church, turning to medicine as an alternative profession.

Jebb's father and namesake John Jebb D.D. (1705-87) graduated from St John's College Cambridge in 1725, became a fellow of Christ's College, and went to Ireland as a clergyman. Jebb was a Whig and closely associated with John Hoadly, the Archbishop of Dublin (and brother of Benjamin). He also became acquainted with the ageing Jonathan Swift, who wrote:

---

[2] John Gascoigne, 'Anglican Latitudinarianism, Rational Dissent and Political Radicalism in the Late Eighteenth Century', in Haakonssen, *Enlightenment and Religion*, pp. 224-26.

[3] Norman Sykes, *Church and State in England in the Eighteenth Century* (Cambridge, 1934), p. 425.

[4] John Walsh, Colin Haydon and Stephen Taylor eds., *The Church of England, c.1689-c.1833: from toleration to Tractarianism* (Cambridge, 1993), pp. 30-43.

[5] F.C. Mather, *High Church Prophet: Bishop Samuel Horsley (1733-1806) and the Caroline tradition in the later Georgian Church* (Oxford, 1992), p. 9.

[6] John Disney lists the towns of Drogheda, Carlow, and Dublin in Ireland, and Shrewsbury, Stand near Manchester, Leicester and Chesterfield in England as places where Jebb was schooled; 'Life of Jebb', p. 1; Jebb had extended family in Drogheda, Dublin, Manchester and Chesterfield. BL Jebb family papers.

[7] The Non-jurors were those clergymen who refused to swear the oath of allegiance to William and Mary following the Revolution of 1688.

> Mr Jebb hath a very good reputation among us, which I believe he well deserves and hath naturally good principles, but his friends being on the side of power, he is forced to tack the prudence of the serpent to the innocence of the dove. I do not know a more modest, decent, well-behaved person; I see him often, like him very well, and can give allowance for the party he is attached to.[8]

The elder John Jebb was a careerist Anglican clergyman, cultivating patrons on both sides of the Irish Sea.[9] He became chaplain to the Lord Lieutenant of Ireland, Prebend of Ossory and married well. In 1740 he was made Treasurer of Christchurch in Dublin (an office he held until his death in 1787), to which he added the title Doctor of Divinity courtesy of Trinity College Dublin in 1743.[10] The elder John Jebb was clearly an intelligent and politic clergyman concerned only to make friends, to marry well, and raise a family with a comfortable income.

The correspondence between the physician and philosopher David Hartley (1705-57) and the Reverend John Lister reinforces the picture of Jebb as a politically tactful Whig attracted to intellectual company. Hartley became a physician based in London and Bath, and Lister a clergyman at Bury in Lancashire. They had met at school in Yorkshire, and attended Cambridge University together, where they probably met Jebb. Their correspondence is dominated by discussion of the ideas that would compose Hartley's influential *Observations on Man* (1749), but references indicate a close friendship between the elder Jebb and the author whose materialist Christian philosophy was to dominate the intellectual formation of his son.[11] Indeed, Joseph Priestley derived much satisfaction from a meeting with Jebb senior because he had been 'the intimate friend of Dr Hartley'.[12]

In 1769 the elder John Jebb was granted the lucrative Deanery of Cashell in Ireland that enabled him to settle for good in England at Egham Hill near London. The republican Sylas Neville gives the best description of Dean Jebb's philosophical and political opinions.[13] He thought Jebb 'a man of good

---

8 Swift refers to Jebb is in his correspondence with Robert Harley, Second Earl of Oxford (1689-1741). Jonathan Swift, *Correspondence* (6 vols., 1911-13), IV, pp. 437-38.

9 Whilst waiting for a college fellowship in the summer of 1728, Jebb entertained the idea of offering himself for selection to the 'King's list' of twenty scholars to be instructed by the recently established Professor of Modern History and Modern Languages, with an eye to being appointed 'to a secretaryship in England or Ireland or to some envoy or nobleman'. Christopher Wordsworth, *Scholae Academicae: university studies in the eighteenth century* (1910), p. 149n.

10 Swift, *Correspondence,* V, pp. 222-23; *Alumni Cantabrigiensis.*

11 W.B. Trigg, 'The Correspondence of Dr David Hartley and Rev John Lister', *Transactions of the Halifax Antiquarian Society* (1938), p. 263.

12 Joseph Priestley to Theophilus Lindsey, 20 April 1772, in Joseph Priestley, *The Theological and Miscellaneous Works of Joseph Priestley* (J.T. Rutt ed., 25 vols., 1832), I, p. 165.

13 Sylas Neville, *The Diary of Sylas Neville 1767-1788* (Basil Cozens-Hardy ed., Oxford, 1950), p. 79.

sense and most excellent principles. He abhors priestcraft and is an enemy to civil and religious tyranny of every kind'. Jebb spoke with pride of his former association with Jonathan Swift and made it 'clear that Swift was a Deist, if not worse, for he does not think that he had a proper sense even of Natural Religion. He did not believe a word of what he delivers in his sermon on the Trinity'. When the conversation turned to the validity of the orthodox concept of eternal punishment, Jebb observed that 'there are only two texts in Scripture which seem to favour that opinion, and these are only metaphorical expressions common in Eastern languages'. Finally, to characterise the temper of Dean Jebb's opinions, Neville noted that he referred to Joseph Priestley (the scientist and Rational Dissenter) as 'the divine Priestley'.[14] While he prudently courted patronage, it is evident that the elder Jebb was a particularly liberal Latitudinarian with heterodox theological views.

It seems that the young John Jebb was destined to follow his father in a clerical career. The most formative institution in Jebb's schooling seems to have been the Chesterfield Grammar school where he spent 'two or three years'.[15] We can imagine that this would have been the standard grammar school education dominated by Latin and some Greek grammar, learnt by rote under fear of the master's rod.[16] Jebb had the added experience of moving around schools in two kingdoms at an early age. Disney makes note of this, with the observation that it did not disrupt Jebb's attention to his studies.[17] It may however have reinforced a bookish pre-disposition as the young student, unable to form any lasting childhood friendships, retreated into literature as providing a stable and constant companion. It may have also contributed to an interest in national and Anglo-Irish politics, to the extent that in 1785 an American was led to describe Jebb as 'an Irishman for which reason he is so greatly interested in the Present Commercial arrangements with that country'.[18]

Whatever the case with his schooling, when Jebb enrolled as a pensioner at Trinity College Dublin on 4 July 1753, the figure he cut was of a small, slightly built seventeen-year-old, devoted to academic study. While Jebb was to spend only one year at Trinity, it left some impressions on him. When campaigning to introduce annual examinations at Cambridge he often referred to Trinity as the successful model from which he had drawn the idea. In addition, Jebb was keen to note that Trinity did not require students to subscribe to the Thirty-Nine Articles.[19] Trinity College was a cultural bastion of the Anglo-Irish elite. There was a fair degree of social fluidity within the ranks of the Protestant Ascendancy and many of its most prominent figures were self-made men from

[14] Neville, *Diary*, pp. 110-11.
[15] In the Trinity College register Jebb is noted as being referred by 'Mr Saunders, Chesterfield'. *Alumni Dublineses* (Dublin, 1935); 'Life of Jebb', p. 2.
[16] John Lawson and Harold Silver, *A Social History of Education in England* (1973), p. 176.
[17] 'Life of Jebb', p. 4.
[18] Miss Abigail Adams (daughter of John and Abigail Adams) to John Q. Adams, 26 August – 13 September 1785, MHS Adams papers.
[19] Jebb III, p. 15.

professional backgrounds.[20] Thus Jebb began his education in a broad-based social environment that was tinged with the ethic of reward for merit. This provided a contrast with the idle and privileged existence of the sons of the English aristocracy that he would later encounter and combat at Cambridge.

Jebb arrived at Trinity toward the end of the forty-year reign of the old and sickly provost Richard Baldwin. Though Baldwin's power was well on the wane when Jebb arrived, the atmosphere of the College still bore his stamp: Protestant, Whig, and disciplined. It seems that Baldwin, a man of obscure origins, was never promoted to a bishopric because the government valued his 'preoccupation with discipline and political orthodoxy' in an important strategic institution. By the time Jebb went to Trinity, the tradition of riots and drunken brawls involving the Trinity students around Dublin had given way to a more acceptable level of behaviour. In addition to a growing refinement of society, this was owing to 'the reaction which followed an incident in 1734, when the rowdies overreached themselves and killed one of the Fellows'.[21] Jebb was at Trinity College during a transitional phase between the plodding discipline of the first half of the century and the increase in scholarly activity and range of the late eighteenth century.[22]

Jebb's tutor was Thomas Leland, described by one acquaintance as 'the most charitable man alive'. A friend of Edmund Burke, during the American Revolution Leland preached a fast-day sermon in support of the colonists that the Whiggish *Monthly Review* described as 'seasonable and important'.[23] Whig politics aside, Leland's task was to tutor Jebb in academic study. Study for the four-year undergraduate degree at Trinity College was organised under two heads: science and classics. In the science stream logic was read for the first two years, natural science in the third, and ethics in the fourth. The main texts used for the study of logic were the *Institution logicae* of Burgersdicius, and Le Clerc's *Logica, sive ars ratiocinandi* (1692). The first year was devoted entirely to the former, a wearisome, pedantic, broadly Aristotelian text from the early seventeenth century – Edmund Burke referred ironically at the age of fifteen to 'that sprightly Dutchman Burgersdyk'. Le Clerc's *Logica* was used to introduce the second-year students to the principles of Lockean logic. Le Clerc, a French Protestant who befriended John Locke when he was exiled in the Netherlands, produced a number of works that developed the Lockean approach to philosophy and religion. His *Physics* (1700) was used later in the degree at Trinity to present the Newtonian conception of the world.[24] While Jebb's formal

---

[20] R.F. Foster, *Modern Ireland 1600-1972* (Harmondsworth, 1989), pp. 170-73.

[21] R.B. McDowell and D.A. Webb, *Trinity College Dublin 1592-1952: an academic history* (Cambridge, 1982), pp. 49, 38.

[22] Jebb's tutor Thomas Leland is notable for being the first resident fellow to publish a scholarly work for several decades. None of the fellows appointed between 1716 and 1734 published anything. McDowell, *Trinity College Dublin*, p. 40.

[23] Paul Langford, 'The English Clergy and the American Revolution,' in Eckhart Hellmuth ed., *The Transformation of Political Culture: England and Germany in the late eighteenth century* (Oxford, 1990) p. 283.

[24] McDowell, *Trinity College Dublin*, pp. 45-47.

study for the year would have been concerned with coming to grips with the Aristotelian logic, grammar and metaphysics of Burgersdicius, he would have been aware of Le Clerc's and Locke's modern empiricist and mechanistic alternative, and he certainly relied on their writings to a large degree later in life. When it came to the study of classical Greek and Latin authors it appears that Jebb was particularly well taught. During the period 1753-54 Leland only had two students other than Jebb assigned to him,[25] and at this time he published a very well received edition of *The Philippic Orations of Demosthenes* (1754). Jebb was evidently inspired by study of the classics, as he received copies of Horace, Juvenal, Terence and Plato's *Dialogues*, as 'the reward of his diligence and learning'.[26] Along with the idea of annual examinations, the distribution of rewards to encourage study is another practice that Jebb later sought to encourage at Cambridge.

The historians of Trinity College have delineated the principles that the College sought to impress on students as: 'mathematical precision in demonstration, an appreciation of the ordered harmony of the universe, rational empiricism as a habit of thought, liberal oligarchy as the basis of government, [and] the avoidance alike of deism, enthusiasm, and superstition.' There was a single-minded devotion to the works of Locke and Newton that went beyond that of Cambridge. While Locke was not officially included in the undergraduate course until the mid-century, the esteem for him is attested by the radical move of including his *Two Treatises of Government* in the fourth-year ethics course.[27] Though Jebb attended Trinity only for the first year of his degree, it is significant that he did so at an institution even more Whiggish than Cambridge. At Trinity Jebb had the experience of studying in Ireland's bastion of Protestant learning at a time when Enlightenment ideals were beginning to spread. In 1754 Jebb crossed back over the Irish Sea and enrolled at Cambridge University. This began a residence and active academic involvement in Cambridge that would last until he resigned his Church of England livings and moved to London in 1776.

CAMBRIDGE

In comparison to the new Dissenting Academies, the English universities experienced a recession in the eighteenth century. Where in the 1630s total entrants for the two universities had been approximately one thousand per year, this figure had slumped to five hundred in the 1690s, and continued to drop.[28] While Cambridge had an annual average of two hundred and ninety matriculations in the 1660s, this fell to a low point in the 1760s of only one hundred and twelve. This was in part a reflection of the growth of anti-clericalism in the eighteenth century, as the gentry increasingly provided private education for their sons. While in the sixteenth and seventeenth centuries the

---

[25] Trinity College Dublin mss., Catalogue of Students 1725-58.
[26] 'Life of Jebb', p. 3.
[27] McDowell, *Trinity College Dublin*, pp. 72-73.
[28] Lawson, *Social History of Education*, p. 177.

universities were thought to be giving an education for a variety of careers, in the eighteenth century Oxford and Cambridge increasingly reverted to their traditional role of training Anglican clergy.[29] Patronage was the key to clerical and academic advancement. While achieving academic honours would help, to have a future at Cambridge it was more important to be aware of what possible vacancies could arise as academics married or died, and to find the right patrons to ensure advancement.

Life at university reflected the structure of English society. Students entered as noblemen or fellow commoners, pensioners or sizars. The former, as sons of the aristocracy, paid higher fees and were by custom allowed many privileges by university dons eager to cultivate opportunities for future preferment. Fellow commoners were allowed to eat at the high table with the college fellows, and were usually exempt from performing any academic exercises. Most passed their days in extravagance, idleness and contempt for their social inferiors – and many left without taking a degree. The vast majority of students were pensioners and it was among this group that Jebb entered Cambridge. Pensioners were usually the sons of clergy or professionals and would have to earn their own living. Most were destined for a career in the Church, which for all but a talented few meant life spent in a quiet country parish. Below the pensioners, the sizars usually came from poor clergy or farming backgrounds and traditionally paid their way by acting as servants in the college. Not surprisingly, many talented products of the university (Isaac Newton and Samuel Jebb for example) came from this rank of students who had to struggle for their education.[30]

During Jebb's time most of the colleges had only forty or fifty students at best. Choice of a college depended on many factors such as family, region and patronage connections. While Trinity and St John's were the largest and most dominant, other colleges were at various times fashionable. In the middle of the century Peterhouse attracted many young aristocrats because its master, Dr Keene, had a politically influential brother.[31] Perhaps it was the opportunity to meet future Whig patrons that led Jebb to enrol at Peterhouse (his uncle Samuel's old college) rather than either of his father's old colleges. Cambridge University was in many ways an umbrella organisation representing the combined colleges. The course of education varied according to each college, and learning for its own sake was encouraged by tutors, friends and personal interest rather than by the goal of assessment. Many university lecturers never actually gave lectures, and so the students usually relied upon their college tutors for instruction in their studies.[32] William Frend thought his life at

---

[29] John Gascoigne, *Cambridge in the Age of Enlightenment: science, religion and politics from the Restoration to the French Revolution* (Cambridge, 1989), p. 21.

[30] D.A. Winstanley, *Unreformed Cambridge* (Cambridge, 1935), pp. 197-203. That Jebb's father was enrolled as a pensioner some years after his elder brother attended university as a sizar suggests that the fortunes of Jebb's grandfather were rising.

[31] Winstanley, *Unreformed Cambridge*, p. 193.

[32] Wordsworth, *Scholae*, pp. 16, 11. Jebb was enrolled as a pensioner under the tuition of Daniel Longmire (1729-89) and William Oldham (1728-95). Both were active at Cambridge

Cambridge 'resembled that of most other young men who attain to ... the honours of the place'. He 'passed many hours in company', but 'indulged much in solitary walks. When alone my time was dedicated to reading and thinking'.[33] Jebb's experience cannot have been too different.

The content of study at Cambridge was increasingly dominated by mathematics and Newtonian physics, which had been harnessed to Christianity by the Latitudinarians. William Whiston, Newton's successor as Lucasian Professor of mathematics, declared that: 'Mechanical philosophy, which relies chiefly on the Power of Gravity, is, if rightly understood, so far from leading to Atheism, that it solely depends on, supposes and demonstrates the Being and Providence of God; and its study by consequence is the most serviceable to Religion.' Whiston and his colleagues set about teaching a Newtonian philosophy and, after some initial High Church opposition, Newtonianism became the new orthodoxy at Cambridge.[34]

In addition to Latitudinarian encouragement, the rise to dominance of mathematics at Cambridge owed much to the increasing importance and emphasis placed on the Senate House examination at the conclusion of the undergraduate degree. To obtain their degree, students traditionally went through a process of disputations (or 'acts') in their final year that usually involved metaphysical and moral questions.[35] These were performed in front of a moderator who was appointed by the University (a role Jebb would come to perform several times). At the time Jebb graduated, these acts were still considered the main test of a young man's learning. However, while in previous centuries the final examination had been largely ceremonial, during the eighteenth century it evolved to become a real test of the students' abilities, and primarily of their mathematical ability. Just before Jebb arrived the University had begun to print an honour roll that ranked the participants in the final Senate House examination according to merit. As the century wore on this honours list came to supersede the acts as the real measure of ability.[36]

Only the diligent students were subjected to serious examination.[37] Jebb himself has left a detailed account of the Senate House examination that illustrates the dominance of mathematics and natural philosophy at Cambridge. The students were divided into groups of six to ten, of roughly equal ability, and each group would in turn sit around a table with the moderator.

---

into the 1770's. William Cole described Longmire as 'a North Country man, excessively tall, Tutor in the College (Peterhouse) and Vicar of Linton, where he for the most part lives, loving social Company, and has a good Deal of it. His father, I am told, keeps a low ale-house in Cumberland'. BL Cole mss. 5875:144.

[33] Frend writing in 1795, cited in Frida Knight, *University Rebel: the life of William Frend 1757-1841* (1971), p. 28.

[34] Gascoigne, *Cambridge*, pp. 271, 145, 140-84; John Gascoigne, 'From Bentley to the Victorians: the rise and fall of British Newtonian natural theology', *Science in Context*, 2 (1988), pp. 222-30.

[35] Gascoigne, *Cambridge*, p. 23.

[36] Winstanley, *Unreformed Cambridge*, pp. 43-50.

[37] Cited in Winstanley, *Unreformed Cambridge*, p. 49.

> The examination is varied according to the abilities of the students. The moderator generally begins with proposing some questions from the six books of Euclid, plain trigonometry, and the first rules of algebra. If any person fails in an answer, the question goes to the next. From the elements of mathematics, a transition is made to the four branches of philosophy, viz. mechanics, hydrostatics, apparent astronomy, and optics, as explained in the works of Maclaurin, Cotes, Helsham, Hamilton, Rutherforth, Keill, Long, Ferguson, and Smith. If the moderator finds the set of questionists, under examination, capable of answering him, he proceeds to the eleventh and twelfth books of Euclid, conic sections, spherical trigonometry, the higher parts of algebra, and Sir Isaac Newton's *Principia*; more particularly those sections, which treat of the motion of bodies in eccentric and revolving orbits; the mutual action of spheres, composed of particles attracting each other according to various laws; the theory of pulses, propagated through elastic mediums; and the stupendous fabric of the world. Having closed the philosophical examination, he sometimes asks a few questions in Locke's *Essay on the Human Understanding*, Butler's *Analogy*, or Clarke's *Attributes*. But as the highest academical distinctions are invariably given to the best proficients in mathematics and natural philosophy, a very superficial knowledge in morality and metaphysics will suffice.

The highest classes of students were tested with more advanced calculations. Each group was examined twice – once by each of the two moderators. In addition, senior members of the colleges would examine individual students at their own discretion for up to an hour and a half at a time. During the three days of examination, the moderators and tutors representing the various colleges would breakfast and dine together, discussing the relative merits of the students. Twenty-four pupils were settled on, examined again one-on-one, and ranked in a list according to academic proficiency.[38] When Jebb graduated he was ranked 'second wrangler' behind his friend and future Lucasian Professor of mathematics, Edward Waring (1734-98). The mathematical bent to Jebb's Cambridge education culminated in his eventually co-authoring a mathematical textbook that was used extensively in the university.[39]

The increasing emphasis on mathematics does not mean that classical learning was neglected at Cambridge. The mathematical disputations and most textbooks were composed in Latin, and serious students learned to write, speak and even think in Latin.[40] There is ample proof that Jebb devoted much time to study of the classics: in 1758 he won second prize in the university's annual

---

[38] *Remarks ... Upon Education*, Jebb II, pp. 291-96.

[39] Robert Thorpe, George Wollaston and John Jebb, *Excerpta quaedam e Newtoni Principiis philosophiae naturalis, cum notis variorum* (Cambridge, 1765).

[40] Wordsworth, *Scholae*, p. 90.

Latin prose competition, and his proposals for education reform included examination and honours lists that would encourage study of the classics as well as mathematics.[41] Nevertheless, study of the classics or any other branch of knowledge took place within an intellectual context shaped by Newtonianism. Late in the century Edmund Law could claim that Newtonian mathematics 'together with Mr. Locke's *Essay* [and] Dr Clarke's works went hand in hand through our public schools and lectures'.[42]

In early 1756 Jebb fell sick with a fever and was sent by his father to Bath to recover his health. He resided at college during the summer vacation in order to catch up on his studies and graduated B.A. in January 1757.[43] On receiving their degrees Jebb and Edward Waring established the Hyson Club, to which students who obtained honours were invited to drink tea and relax with free ranging 'rational conversation'.[44] A manifestation of the salon culture that was a marked feature of the Enlightenment, in the following years the Hyson Club was attended by some of the most intellectually eminent figures in the University.

With increasing competition for honours in the Senate House examination, there was a corresponding rise in demand for private tutors.[45] On completing his degree Jebb undertook private pupils (a practice he continued throughout his entire time at Cambridge), and instructed as many as 'six or eight young persons, at separate parts of the day', which demonstrates a commitment and ability that, according to Disney, was 'unusual at his early age'.[46] While pecuniary reward was no doubt an important reason, this was also an early manifestation of Jebb's life-long commitment to the promotion of learning. One former student recalled 'with the highest satisfaction' his time with Jebb, as he was taught 'with views much more enlarged than those commonly entertained by the commonality of tutors'.[47] Coaching private pupils was not a familiar practice during Jebb's time, as it would become in the nineteenth century. It was an uncertain field of endeavour both in terms of status and financial reward, but Jebb's success reinforces the picture of him being widely respected for his abilities.[48] He did this work while continuing his own studies, and in 1758 obtained second prize in a competition held annually for best Latin essay in the university. Right from the start Jebb's industrious practice was at variance with the dominant way of life in the eighteenth-century university.

---

[41] 'Life of Jebb', p. 6; See chapter 6.

[42] Cited in Gascoigne, *Cambridge*, p. 174.

[43] 'Life of Jebb', pp. 4-5.

[44] G.W. Meadley, *Memoirs of William Paley* (1809), p. 46; Mary Milner, *The Life of Issac Milner* (1842), p. 9; Christopher Wordsworth, *Social Life at the English Universities in the Eighteenth Century* (1874), p. 334.

[45] Wordsworth, *Scholae*, p. 260.

[46] 'Life of Jebb', p. 6. Private tutors received about 20 pounds a year per pupil. Six to eight students would seem to be the maximum number Jebb tutored at any one time. This would have provided him with a yearly income of at least 120 pounds. Wordsworth, *Social Life*, pp. 112-14.

[47] John Baynes cited in, 'Life of Jebb', p. 16.

[48] M.L. Clarke, *Paley: evidences for the man* (1974), p. 8.

LIBERAL LATITUDINARIANISM

Of the two English universities Cambridge had the better reputation for academic innovation and rigour. It was also considered the 'Whig University', a reputation that was consolidated following the election of the Duke of Newcastle as Chancellor in 1748. Peterhouse was left without a master in the year that Jebb arrived, and remained so until the election of Edmund Law (1703-87) in 1756. With this appointment it can be said that the 'Latitudinarians of an advanced type' reached the high point of their influence.[49]

The writings and personal acquaintance of Edmund Law were to exercise a strong influence over Jebb in the future.[50] Law was one of the most outstanding representatives of Whig Latitudinarianism at Cambridge and on the Episcopal bench in the first half of George III's reign. He published a new edition of John Locke's *Works* in 1775, declaring that 'they have stood the test of time, and in their peculiar tendency to enlarge and improve the mind must continue while a regard to virtue, or religion, science or common sense remains amongst us'.[51] William Paley remembered that Law esteemed John Gay of Sidney Sussex College because 'no man knew the Bible or the works of Locke better',[52] and he published Gay's anonymous tract on materialist psychology which inspired his friend David Hartley to write the *Observations on Man*.[53] William Paley remembered Law as 'a man of great softness of manners, and of the mildest and most tranquil disposition', who had a very large family and lived a 'life of incessant reading and thought'.[54] He presided over a circle at Cambridge that produced many advocates of reform, and among whom Jebb was a prominent representative. Throughout his life Law remained an important friend of those disposed to Unitarianism both within and without the Church, and was still associating with 'my old friend Dr Jebb' in 1783.[55]

As a term Latitudinarianism can be used to denote both a general disposition and a particular intellectual faction within the Church. It is clear that when used to characterise a toleration of differing opinions within the Church, 'Latitudinarian' is a net that gathers a wide variety of Anglican. Yet Latitudinarian can be applied to a specific intellectual faction centred on figures like Newton, Locke, Samuel Clarke, and Benjamin Hoadly. These men were united in their belief that religious doctrine should be arrived at through a combination of faith in the divine origin of the Scriptures, and the ability of rational enquiry to discover theological, moral and natural truth. This led them to hope for a 'Second Reformation' that would see the Anglican Church jettison

---

[49] Mather, *High Church Prophet*, p. 9.

[50] Law and Jebb's father were certainly acquainted. Both graduated from St John's College (Law 1723, Jebb 1725), and they were Fellows of Christ's College at the same time (Law 1723-37, Jebb 1729-34).

[51] Cited in Young, *Religion and Enlightenment*, p. 12.

[52] William Paley, 'Life of Edmund Law', affixed to Edmund Law, *Considerations on the State of the World with regard to the Theory of Religion* (8th ed., 1820, [1745]), p. viii.

[53] Ernest Albee, *A History of English Utilitarianism* (New York, 1962 [1902]), p. 78.

[54] Paley, 'Life of Edmund Law', pp. xii-xiii.

[55] Thomas Belsham, *Memoirs of the Late Theophilus Lindsey* (2nd ed., 1820), p. 121.

its irrational and unscriptural orthodox doctrine and liturgy.[56] The important place of Locke and Newton in Jebb's education has been indicated. In the second half of this chapter I will sketch the main influences and features of the Latitudinarian heritage that constituted Jebb's intellectual starting point.

The eighteenth-century conception of the natural world as a machine governed by rational laws derived largely from the enormous impact of Newton's discoveries in physics. With his work the 'argument from design' as proof of God's existence came into prominence. Surveying his discoveries, Newton reflected that 'this most beautiful system of the sun, planets, and comets could only proceed from the counsel and dominion of an intelligent and powerful being'. It followed that God had designed the universe for a purpose as 'a god without dominion, providence, and final causes is nothing else but Fate and Nature'.[57]

The Bible and Newtonianism were the two rocks upon which Jebb's Christianity rested. A student recalled that Jebb often alluded during his instructions to the points in Newton's system that provided evidence of God's existence.[58] Disney noted that Jebb 'always expressed particular admiration for the last chapter in Maclaurin's *View of Newton's Philosophy*, and often lamented that he had not lived to finish it, as it contained, in his idea, by much the best demonstration of the existence and attributes of the deity'.[59] Jebb would tell his students that 'if the projectile motion shews a forming God, the centripetal force acting incessantly shews a preserving God',[60] and he would try to give them an idea of the strength of God by 'calculating the force with which the planet Saturn must be projected to have its greatest velocity'.[61] He endeavoured to impress that the mind that rejects the Newtonian proof of God 'must reject every other species of proof, and is unable to comprehend any truth whatsoever';[62] and was convinced that 'we have as full an evidence of the Deity's existence as the philosophers have of Phlogiston' (in hindsight, an unfortunate comparison).[63]

While Newtonianism helped shape rational Christianity, the influence was not all one way – Latitudinarianism did much to mute the materialist implications of the new science.[64] The natural world may work according to mechanistic principles, but in Jebb's eyes it was the Christian God who had

---

[56] Larry Stewart, 'Samuel Clarke, Newtonianism and the Factions of Post-Revolutionary England', *JHI*, 42 (1981), pp. 53-72; Stephen Snobelen, 'Caution, Conscience and the Newtonian Reformation: the public and private heresies of Newton, Clarke and Whiston', *E&D*, 16 (1997), pp. 151-84.

[57] Isaac Newton, *Newton's Philosophy of Nature: selections from his writings* (H.S. Thayer ed., New York, 1953), pp. 42, 44.

[58] John Baynes to John Disney, May 4, 1786, 'Life of Jebb', p. 17.

[59] 'Life of Jebb', p. 14.

[60] 'Theological Propositions', Jebb II, p. 162.

[61] 'Life of Jebb', p. 14.

[62] 'Theological Propositions', Jebb II, p. 178.

[63] A loose sheet of note paper; DWL Jebb mss. VI.

[64] M.C. Jacob and B.J.T. Dobbs, *Newton and the Culture of Newtonianism* (Atlantic Highlands, N.J., 1995).

designed it, provided the spark of life, and kept it in motion. Between the late 1750s and early 1770s he taught this view to many students at Cambridge.

John Locke's philosophical and religious writings exerted an enormous influence on the eighteenth century.[65] While he never doubted that some men knew their duty to God, throughout his life Locke struggled to find a clear and easy explanation of how such knowledge (and indeed how any knowledge) was possible.[66] Like his friend Newton, Locke felt confident that the existence of God was beyond reasonable doubt: 'We have knowledge of our own existence by intuition; of the existence of God by demonstration; and of other things by sensation'.[67] This statement is a distillation of Locke's empiricist philosophy. He argued that the traditional philosophical quest for certain knowledge of the essence of things was doomed to failure. Our knowledge of the world derives entirely from the senses and we only perceive the secondary qualities of things. Locke argued that we can be satisfied with a probable knowledge of reality based upon our perception of appearances, because a necessarily all-powerful and just God could not create a system in which his subjects were constantly being deceived.[68] It was left to the less devout David Hume to draw out the sceptical implications of this common sense empiricism.

Locke's was a modest inductive philosophy that dismissed unexplainable religious mysteries as the result of wayward imaginations. Francis Bacon had warned of the tendency to form 'idols of the mind' which led thinkers to spin airy webs out of their own substance.[69] In the same vein, Locke argued that much confusion and conflict in our opinions derives from the loose and ill-defined use of words. A central concern of his approach was the need to clarify our statements and to use plain and simple language as much as possible. Metaphysical disputes stemmed from deductive reasoning and the use of words out of context and away from that to which they were originally meant to correspond. Locke believed that human understanding should rest on induced facts discussed in clear language, and that metaphysical arguments were prone to become a confusing and misleading waste of time.

A commitment to founding ideas upon induced fact pervades Jebb's writings. The primary aim of his theological lectures was to 'banish from the study of divinity, those physical and metaphysical speculations, which have too long disgraced it', and encourage young men to 'strike out a system of faith and practice for themselves' based on independent study.[70] 'Ancient philosophy' had unsuccessfully probed the laws of nature because 'a theory, or an hypothesis,

---

65 Allan P.F. Sell, *John Locke and the Eighteenth-Century Divines* (Cardiff, 1997).

66 John Dunn, *Locke* (Oxford, 1984), p. 61; Richard Ashcraft, 'Faith and knowledge in Locke's philosophy', in John Yolton ed., *John Locke: problems and perspectives* (Cambridge, 1969), pp. 194-223.

67 John Locke, *Essay Concerning Human Understanding* (A.D. Woozley ed., 1964), p. 378.

68 Margaret J. Osler, 'John Locke and the Changing Ideal of Scientific Knowledge', *JHI*, 31 (1970), pp. 3-16.

69 Neal Wood, 'The Baconian Character of Locke's *Essay*', *Studies in the History and Philosophy of Science*, 6 (1975), pp. 42-84.

70 Jebb I, pp. 20, 26.

framed by human fancy, anticipated what ought to have been the result of laborious investigation into fact'.[71] In this spirit, Jebb urged Priestley not to engage in worthless metaphysical dispute with the Scottish sceptics.[72] When seeking information about the origin of a 'printed paper' suggesting the formation of a political association, Jebb wrote to Theophilus Lindsey: 'I do not desire your *opinion* of the paper but only want to be instructed in the *facts*'.[73] His sole medical publication is simply a series of observed cases of paralysis, because 'to describe disorders according to the forms in which they really evidence themselves to the senses, with a careful attention to the patient's feelings, is the most likely method of acquiring both a knowledge of their causes and of their cure'.[74]

While reading Holbach's atheist manifesto *The System of Nature*, Jebb penned a note that gives eloquent expression to his inductive empiricism (and echoes Joseph Butler's *Analogy of Religion and Nature*): 'And how it may be with the minds of others I cannot possibly say. Mine cannot easily contemplate probability in a large number of independent arguments, and form a judgement from the whole. I am too much affected by each subject in its turn, which gets the entire possession of my mind, and leads me into scepticism.' Yet this was clearly not what God intended. 'The best way, therefore, to have conviction on important points, and guard against error' was to 'practice those moralities which are founded upon fact'; to cultivate virtue, fulfil social duties, and promote human happiness; and to read history and 'let opinions rise unbidden to my mind, without those laborious exercises of the brain, of which the produce is aridity and scepticism'.[75]

Locke's philosophy reinforced the humanist distinction between the essential truths of Christianity and those variable external doctrines and practices that were 'things indifferent'. Latitudinarians tended to play down or avoid the mystical aspects of Christianity and focus on the religion of Christ as a body of moral doctrine. Locke argued that while our faculties are not fitted to 'penetrate into the internal fabric and real essences of bodies', the important point is that we can know of God, ourselves, and our duty. It followed from this that 'morality is the proper science and business of mankind in general'.[76]

Casting about for a rational basis for morality, Locke came to rest upon the teaching of Jesus.[77] In the *Reasonableness of Christianity as delivered in the*

---

[71] *Sketch of ... the Society for Promoting Knowledge of the Scriptures*, Jebb II, p. 241.

[72] Priestley, *Works*, I, p. 328.

[73] Jebb to Lindsey, 29 August 1775, in *Illustrated Life of Priestley* DWL mss. 12.79:204.

[74] *Select Cases of the Disorder commonly termed the Paralysis of the Lower Extremities* (1782), Jebb II, p. 399.

[75] Written 12 July 1773 while reading Holbach, Jebb II, pp. 166-67. See Paul Henri Thiry baron d'Holbach, *The System of Nature* (Robert D. Richardson ed., New York, 1984).

[76] Locke, *Essay*, p. 399.

[77] Locke clearly acknowledged that some things are 'above reason', and never rejected 'mystery' outright. Locke's whole philosophy is designed to show that our knowledge is limited, and that we must rely on faith to find meaning in life. He thought that his faith was reasonable because of the external evidence for revelation, such as miracles. Gerard Reedy, *The Bible and Reason: Anglicans and Scripture in late seventeenth-century England*

Scriptures (1695), he argued that a body of ethics conforming to the law of nature, reason, and fitting all duties, was not known prior to Jesus. The 'scattered sayings of wise men, conformable to right reason' were not sufficient, and 'could never make a morality whereof the world could be convinced; could never rise to the force of a law that mankind could with certainty depend on'. A universal morality 'must have its authority either from reason or revelation'. There has always been a law of nature, but before Jesus nobody had outlined it in its entirety. Revelation aided the weakness of reason: 'We have from him a full and sufficient rule for our direction, and conformable to reason. But the truth and obligation of its precepts, have their force, and are put past doubt to us, by the evidence of his mission. He was sent by God: His miracles show it, and the authority of God in his precepts cannot be questioned.'[78] The result was a simple exposition of religion, in the plain language of the people of Jesus' day. Locke argued that this true Christianity 'is a religion suited to vulgar capacities, and the state of mankind in this world, destined to labour and travail'.[79] This was the model that contemporary Christianity should strive to emulate; its simple precepts should be taught to all in plain language, free of complicated doctrines. To this end, Locke argued that Scripture should be read in light of his inductive philosophy in order to draw out its clear and simple message. As will be discussed in chapter 3, Jebb studied the Bible according to Locke's method of making scripture its own interpreter.[80]

An increasing use of reason and empiricism led many liberal Latitudinarians to adopt heterodox theological views. A prime example of this was Samuel Clarke (1675-1729), whom Voltaire described as a 'real reasoning machine'.[81] Styled as Newton's chaplain, Clark's rationalist defence of the existence of God and free will were enormously influential and became the direct target of atheists like Hume and the Baron d'Holbach.[82] In addition to his broad philosophical influence, Clarke became a leading figure among heterodox clergymen and inspired followers like Jebb to scrutinise the Scriptures (see chapter 3). While postmodern theologians are untroubled that orthodox doctrine was largely the product of debates within the early Church, eighteenth-century divines were desperate to clarify its literal scriptural basis. This led to heated debates over what theological doctrines were and were not to be found in the Bible.

Central to orthodox Christianity was the concept of the Trinity, and no doctrine so taxed the minds of critical readers of the Bible. The Trinity became a bitterly contested issue, as the very nature of Christ and his mission was at stake. In the eyes of the orthodox, denying that Jesus was God made flesh undermined such key notions as original sin and atonement. In a valiant attempt to settle the

---

(Philadelphia, 1985), pp. 135-41.

[78] John Locke, *The Reasonableness of Christianity* (I.T. Ramsey ed., 1958 [1705]), pp. 62-63.

[79] Locke, *Reasonableness*, p. 76.

[80] *Short Account of Theological Lectures*, Jebb I, p. 12.

[81] Voltaire, *Letters on England* (L. Tancock trans., Harmondsworth, 1980 [1733]), p. 42.

[82] James Dybikowski, 'Samuel Clarke: Special Issue – Editorial', *E&D*, 16 (1997), p. 1.

issue once and for all, Clarke collated 1,251 texts from the Bible that might touch upon the Trinity. In *The Scripture-Doctrine of the Trinity* (1712) he concluded that while the Bible did not clearly define the relationship between the Father and the Son, it was evident that full divinity belonged only to God. Clarke became the most influential eighteenth-century exponent of Arian theology (the belief that while Jesus was divine, he remained only the Son of God) and was a key influence on the development of Rational Dissent.[83]

The Latitudinarians were distinguished by a belief in Newtonian science, empiricist philosophy and scriptural sufficiency that tended to lead to heterodoxy. This intellectual disposition had profound implications for the relationship between Church and state – implications that were boldly stated by Benjamin Hoadly, who became an inspiration for those Anglicans who wanted greater religious liberty.[84] Hoadly established himself as a leading Whig clergyman in the early decades of the eighteenth century. While his defence of Whig politics and the subordination of the Church to the state made him a hated figure among High Churchmen, 'the stars in their courses seemed on his side, and his cool and acid rationalism was of the very temper of the age'.[85] The Dissenter Andrew Kippis observed that arguments for religious liberty had abounded since the time of the Bangorian Controversy of 1717, when Hoadly was attacked by the lower house of Convocation for declaring that the Church had no real God-given spiritual or moral authority.[86] Edmund Law praised the 'truly candid and judicious' Hoadly for encouraging clergymen to reform a Church less than perfect 'in its Government, Discipline, or Worship'. He thought the Bangorian Controversy and Hoadly's arguments in favour of private judgement had destroyed the High Church case against reform[87] – a view not shared by Archbishop Thomas Secker (1758-68), who responded furiously to the *Confessional* and those 'Low Church controversialists keeping the Hoadliean flag flying'.[88] Hoadly remained the target of High-Church vitriol throughout the century; Samuel Horsley styled him as a republican who 'ventured to espouse the interests of atheism' by denying the divine right of kings.[89] At Cambridge, William Cole saw Jebb as a leading light in 'a restless Generation who will never be contented till they have overturned the Constitution in Church and State'; the inevitable result, he thought, of making 'a Deity' of Hoadly.[90] Hoadly consistently championed the primacy of private judgement in matters of 'conscience and salvation', an Erastian ecclesiology, and a contractual view of government.

---

83 Webb, 'Emergence of Rational Dissent', p. 26.

84 My argument in this chapter follows the work by John Gascoigne which has demonstrated that Cambridge provided the most fertile seed-bed for Hoadly's ideas (see works by Gascoigne in the bibliography); see also Reed Browning, *Political and Constitutional Ideas of the Court Whigs* (Baton Rouge, La., 1982), chapter 2.

85 Ernest Gordon Rupp, *Religion in England 1688-1791* (Oxford, 1986), p. 88.

86 Andrew Kippis, *A Vindication of the Protestant Dissenting Ministers* (1773), p. 42.

87 'A Real Hoadlien' [John Disney], *Whitehall Evening Post*, 20 May 1773.

88 Cited in Mather, *High Church Prophet*, p. 10.

89 Cited in Clark, *English Society*, p. 233.

90 BL Cole mss. 5873:52.

Hoadly drew on the seventeenth-century ultra-Protestant tradition of liberty of conscience. Echoing Milton, he declared that 'in the affairs of Conscience and Eternal Salvation' Christ had 'left behind him no visible, human *Authority*, … no *Interpreters*, upon whom his Subjects are absolutely to depend: no judges over the Consciences or Religion of his people'.[91] The Church of Christ, Hoadly argued, had originally consisted of those who had voluntarily adopted Jesus as their spiritual king. Accordingly, the highest religious authority was the individual conscience. D.O. Thomas has discerned three main themes in Hoadly's moral philosophy: that the main concern of religion is the quest for eternal happiness, the key to eternal life is the practice of virtue, and the chief virtue is sincerity of mind. Hoadly did not believe that the conscience of the individual was infallible, but only that there was no infallible or superior authority in matters of religion. He was not troubled by the fact that the individual may be mistaken when determining and acting upon his or her moral duties, as God would forgive the mistakes of a candid person who acted with '*real sincerity*' and according to his conscience. But this did not mean merely acting as one saw fit. To qualify as truly sincere the individual had to display candour in examining his or her duties. This involved 'enquiry, thoughtfulness, comparing things together, studying the *New Testament*, endeavouring to find out the laws of God and the laws of Christ, and all the like dispositions and habitudes'.[92]

As I will demonstrate in chapter 4, Jebb was in entire agreement with Hoadly's espousal of sincerity and candour as central to fulfilling one's duty to God. His writings are peppered with passages warmly defending private judgement as a right and duty that defined Protestantism – a right that it would be 'treason and rebellion against the majesty of heaven to renounce'.[93] Hoadly shook the pillars of priestcraft from within the Anglican fold. He rejected the notion of the Church visible, and denied that priests represented God's authority on earth. Likewise, Jebb viewed the clergy as teachers, and the Church as merely 'the creature and servant of the state'.[94] Frustrated with the failure of the Feathers Tavern petition, he wrote of the Bishops: 'I must lament that an attachment to the interests of a pitiful corporation, should … render them adverse or inattentive to a question, which so materially concerns the nobler interests of the community, the cause of universal Christianity, and their own emolument and glory, as the constitutional guardians of a Protestant church'.[95]

Hoadly defended the need for an established church, but argued that religion (including Catholicism) should entail no civil disability provided an oath of allegiance to the king were sworn (an opinion with which Jebb

---

[91] Benjamin Hoadly, *The Nature of the Kingdom, or Church of Christ* (1717), cited in Rupp, *Religion in England*, p. 92.

[92] D.O. Thomas, 'Benjamin Hoadly: the ethics of sincerity', *E&D,* 15 (1996), pp. 71-88, Hoadly cited at pp. 82, 84.

[93] *EveryMan His Own Priest*, Jebb III, p. 179.

[94] Jebb I, p. 229.

[95] Jebb III, p. 104.

wholeheartedly agreed).[96] Hoadly argued eloquently in favour of repealing the Test and Corporation Acts, and for this he was greatly respected by the Dissenters.[97] He was careful however not to advocate unlimited private judgement. Hoadly defended the existence of the established Church and its right to exercise authority in 'things indifferent', such as its liturgy and speculative doctrine (provided they agreed with scripture). Yet the Church could not direct an individual's judgement in matters of 'conscience and salvation'.[98] It was dissatisfaction with this compromise that drove the campaign against subscription which flared up following the publication of Francis Blackburne's *Confessional* (1766) (see chapters 3 and 5). Blackburne acknowledged that Hoadly's arguments had inspired the campaign against subscription to the Thirty-Nine Articles, but lamented that the bishop had not actively worked to reform the Church.[99] Blackburne himself was particularly sensitive to the need to show '*Sincerity* in professing the faith'.[100]

Hoadly was first and foremost a pamphleteer for the Whig cause whose views on Church government were influenced by his political stance. His theological development was linked with his attempt to defend an Erastian ecclesiology, as he set about reinterpreting the scripture evidence for passive obedience, and claimed that there was no scriptural support for absolute monarchy or indefeasible hereditary succession. Hoadly did more than anyone to popularise the contractual theory of government.[101] In the American Colonies he was considered one of the more notable figures in the history of political thought, and he 'came to physically embody the continuity of the conglomerate tradition of English radical thought'.[102] Hoadly argued that the 'public good' was superior to the sovereign's right to rule, and that the people were justified in resisting a king who went against their communal interests. While Tories labelled such a view as republican, this mainstream defence of the Glorious Revolution envisaged popular intervention only in times of constitutional crisis. Yet in acknowledging that the people were the ultimate source of political authority, the mainstream Whigs established a political context that fostered the development of radical interpretations of the constitution.[103]

Many of the leading lights of Rational Dissent made a painful journey from orthodoxy to Arianism or Socinianism. Theophilus Lindsey drifted close to

---

[96] Benjamin Hoadly, *The Objections against the Repeal of the Test and Corporation Acts Considered* (1739); Jebb II, pp. 121-22.
[97] Richard Price to Benjamin Rush, 1 January 1783, *The Correspondence of Richard Price* (Bernard Peach and D.O. Thomas eds., 3 vols., Chapel Hill, N.C. and Cardiff, Wales, 1983-94), II, p. 162.
[98] Rupp, *Religion in England*, p. 100.
[99] Francis Blackburne, *The Confessional* (1766), pp. liv-lv.
[100] Francis Blackburne to Theophilus Lindsey, August 1770, DWL Blackburne correspondence 12.52.98.
[101] Benjamin Hoadly, *The Original Institution of Civil Government, discuss'd* (1710); H.T. Dickinson, 'Benjamin Hoadly', *History Today*, 25 (1975), pp. 348-55.
[102] Bailyn, *Ideological Origins*, pp. 37-38.
[103] H.T. Dickinson, *The Politics of the People in Eighteenth-Century Britain* (New York, 1994), p. 198.

Methodism at an early age, and Richard Price and Joseph Priestley both reacted against the oppressive influence of Calvinism. In contrast, Dean Jebb seems to have followed Samuel Clark and Benjamin Hoadly in espousing liberal Latitudinarian views; and sent his son to educational institutions that would inculcate them. The profound and transforming affect David Hartley's philosophy had upon the young Joseph Priestley is well documented. Jebb developed at the very heart of the liberal Latitudinarian tradition, in an environment where David Hartley was a personal acquaintance and his ideas familiar. With the example of Edmund Law before him, the young scholar no doubt looked forward to a successful and perhaps significant career in the Church and Cambridge University.

Britain's political climate, however, was changing. In the years following the accession of George III, Latitudinarians with suspect theological and philosophical views found themselves increasingly out of favour at the highest levels of Church and State. At the same time, Jebb was becoming a Unitarian. In light of the growing difference between his beliefs and the views of the religious and political establishment, it is not surprising that Jebb became caught up in the rising tide of popular radical patriotism.

2

Cambridge Patriot

Jebb became a fellow of Peterhouse in July 1761, was examined and ordained at Buckden a year later, and became a priest in September 1763. A young man ordained at Buckden ten years later has left an account of the proceedings that cannot have been too different from Jebb's experience. Thomas Scott, a largely self-educated son of a farmer, had developed a Socinian bent and approached the examination with some anxiety. Luckily enough, he was examined on the one topic he had studied in depth: the nature of miracles and their truth as proof of the Christian doctrine. Thus, he was able to pass without Gordon perceiving his Socinian views. Of the other candidates during his ordination, Scott wrote that most 'are Oxonian and Cantabrigian bucks, who know more of the wine and the girls of their respective universities, and of setting-dogs, racehorses, and guns in the country, than of Latin and Greek, or divinity. The archdeacon sweated two of them pretty well: but I believe they must pass muster'.[1]

On the recommendation of Edmund Law, in August 1764 Jebb was granted the small vicarage of Gamlingay in Bedfordshire, and in October he was elected by the University Senate to the Rectory of Ovington in Norfolk, defeating a candidate from St John's College. With an income secured, Jebb resigned his fellowship and on 29 December married Ann Torkington (whose father was Rector of Little Stukley near Huntingdon, and mother the daughter of the second Earl of Harborough). The two met at a ball and decided they were perfectly suited.[2] Ann Jebb was twenty-six, small, pale, well read and talkative – one friend thought her the thinnest person he had ever beheld.[3] Writing in 1785 the young Abigail Adams observed that Ann Jebb was 'a great Politicianess,

[1] John Scott, *The Life of Reverend Thomas Scott* (1823), pp. 33-36.
[2] Meadley, *Memoir of Ann Jebb*, p. 6.
[3] Theophilus Lindsey to William Tayleur, 28 July 1778, JRL Lindsey-Tayleur correspondence.

which consequently pleased Mamma. The American War, [and] Present dispute with Ireland ... furnished this woman with subject of conversation'. While her mother found Ann's company engaging, the young Abigail seems to have been less impressed: 'Were I to attempt a description of Mrs Jebb, I should find myself unequal to the business. Perhaps you never saw such a looking Woman. If you have seen Miss Polly Palmer you have seen good Nature, softness, and sweetness of Countenance when compared to this Lady.' (A gun had been discharged near Polly Palmer's head at a young age and she had developed a permanent 'nervous condition').[4] Meadley concedes that Ann was 'of a nervous temperament' and often sick.[5] It would appear that the droll Miss Adams (who loved Parisian society) did not quite take to the earnest and opinionated English 'politicianess'. Assessment of Ann needs to be considered relative to the morally rigorous Rational Dissenting circles in which she moved, where she was respected for 'her ardour and firmness ... tempered with gentleness and urbanity'.[6] It was in contrast with such friends that Ann could depict herself as loving 'fun and wit' and having 'high spirits' and a 'weak body' – a description borne out by her correspondence with the waggish clergyman Henry Taylor.[7]

John and Ann Jebb shared a loving marriage for two decades. After nearly nine years of marriage John hinted at a resignation to childlessness when he reflected that 'the situation which is most agreeable to nature' was 'a country life, if not with children, yet with pupils'.[8] Elsewhere he wrote that there were 'two ways of co-operating' with God: 'one, in giving happiness to those already in existence; the other, in contriving to give being to numerous tribes of rational and irrational animals, and to make them happy'.[9] With this view in mind, and in the absence of children, John and Ann Jebb devoted their energies to improving their nation through intellectual and activist pursuits.

ACADEMIC ASPIRATIONS

Through the mid-1760s Jebb continued to work with an eye to a future academic position in the University. In the summer of 1764 he began to study Hebrew and early in 1765 co-authored a commentary in Latin on Newton's *Principia* that became a standard text at Cambridge.[10] During the summer and autumn of 1765 Jebb applied himself to study while living in rented accommodation at Potton in Bedfordshire near his vicarage. He resigned this living in August after less than twelve months' incumbency, and moved back to Cambridge. The reason is unclear: perhaps there was friction with his congregation, or maybe he saw no

---

[4] Abigail 'Nabby' Adams to John Q. Adams, 31 July and 14 August 1785, *Adams Family Correspondence,* VI, pp. 216, 302.
[5] Meadley, *Memoir of Ann Jebb*, p. 52.
[6] Meadley *Memoir of Ann Jebb*, p. 55.
[7] Henry Taylor to Ann Jebb, 7 April 1777, CUL Taylor papers.
[8] 'Theological Propositions', Jebb II, p. 167.
[9] 'Theological Propositions', Jebb II, p. 139.
[10] R. Thorpe, G. Wollaston and J. Jebb, *Excerpta quaedam e Newtoni Principiis philosophiae naturalis, cum notis variorum* (Cambridge, 1765); Wordsworth, *Scholae Academicae*, p. 71.

chance for clerical promotion in the area. The former is a distinct possibility when we consider what Jebb was studying at this time. He recorded in his notebook that he had 'read through the Pentateuch, harmonised the Gospels, read about five hundred verses of the Koran, and some other things in Arabic, and studied geography'.[11] It has been observed that the growing gap between elite and popular culture led many Anglican parish clergy to become frustrated in the attempt to reform their flocks and promote a literate understanding of the Bible.[12] The only direct reference to Jebb's move comes from the pen of the ill-disposed William Cole, who wrote that when Jebb 'married he had the vicarage of Gamlingay, and hired a house at Potton, but being of a restless turn he soon quitted it'.[13]

Whatever the reason, the end result was that Jebb returned to Cambridge and continued grooming himself for the expected vacancy of the Professorship of Arabic. He was appointed as curate in the parish of St Andrew in March 1766, gave lectures on Butler's *Analogy* on Sunday evenings, and lectured on Cicero's *De Officiis* at Trinity Hall.[14] In October of 1762 Jebb had been elected along with Richard Watson as moderator of disputations in the Sophs' School.[15] He held this office a number of times and the experience encouraged the formulation of his academic reform proposals. In 1767 he also began to give lectures on the Greek New Testament to students in his own house, and spent much time with Edmund Law.[16]

Jebb's predisposition to things academic is illustrated by his co-founding (with Edward Waring) of the Hyson Club. This club became a centre of intellectual activity at the university, providing those who had obtained academic honours with a regular gathering at which they could drink tea and engage in rational conversation. As A.M.C. Waterman has observed, the Hyson Club was 'wedded to no particular theological or political programme', but reflected the atmosphere of 'the high summer of the English Enlightenment, a time when all men of taste and letters however disparate in faith or morals could meet in urbane society'.[17]

The nature of this club is best depicted by a review of some prominent members. The son of a wealthy farmer, Edward Waring was a shy and retiring student who gained such a reputation that he was appointed Lucasian Professor of Mathematics only three years after gaining his BA.[18] Though he did not give

[11] 'Life of Jebb', p. 18.

[12] Jeremy Gregory, 'The Eighteenth-Century Reformation: the pastoral task of Anglican clergy after 1689', in Walsh, Haydon and Taylor, *The Church of England c.1649-c.1833*, p. 79.

[13] Cole mss., BL Add. Mss. 5873:70b.

[14] Wordsworth, *Scholae*, p. 116.

[15] 'Life of Jebb', p. 7.

[16] George Dyer, *History of the University and Colleges of Cambridge* (1814), p. 124; 'Life of Jebb', p. 20.

[17] A.M.C. Waterman, 'A Cambridge "Via Media" in Late Georgian Anglicanism', *Journal of Ecclesiastical History*, 42 (1991), p. 421.

[18] His fitness for the position was vigorously attacked by William Samuel Powell, *Observations on the first chapter of a book called Miscellanea Anylitica* (Cambridge, 1760).

lectures, his examinations came to be seen as one of the most rigorous tests of mathematical skill in Europe. Waring married and retired to live on his rural estate in the same year that the Jebbs left Cambridge, but they remained friends.[19]

Another member was Richard Watson, a characteristic representative of the English Enlightenment whose interests encompassed politics, chemistry, Christian apologetics and religious and educational reform. Though he remained within the Church and became Bishop of Llandaff, he respected Jebb and supported his proposals for academic reform. Watson offended the king when he gave a sermon at Cambridge on 'Revolution Principles' and the right of resistance in 1776, which Cole thought 'distasteful to everyone who wished well to civil government, and would not see the Common People cut the throats of their superiors'.[20] The most detailed study of Watson, however, has styled him as a genuine Whig who was in all things a moderate.[21]

The bright and witty William Paley was Senior Wrangler when Jebb was moderator in 1763, and went on to become an active member of the Hyson Club whilst at Cambridge. Paley was chastised by Jebb for not signing the Feathers Tavern petition on the grounds that (as he said) he 'could not afford to keep a conscience', and his *Moral and Political Philosophy* (1783) angered many Unitarians because of its chapter justifying the imposition of religious tests for an established clergy. Nevertheless, at meetings of the Hyson Club Paley 'joined freely on subjects of scientific and speculative inquiry', and in later life he spoke of his 'pleasant intercourse with Jebb and Waring'.[22] Ann Jebb recalled the very high regard in which Paley was held at Cambridge, particularly among 'the liberal party'. 'I remember', she wrote,

> that Paley used to be looked upon as the life of every party he frequented; and yet I can with truth assert that no one could be a more attentive hearer. In the early part of our acquaintance, when Paley, in company with other of our friends, was drinking tea with us, Mr Jebb as usual spoke his own sentiments very freely; and, after they left us, remarked that he did not know what to make of Paley, for that he said nothing: upon which I observed that he had been very attentive, and gave it as my firm opinion that he would be very liberal. After further acquaintance Mr Jebb told me I was right, for that Paley, he now saw, from the course of his studies, was endeavouring to explore the truth for himself.

---

[19] *DNB*. In 1777 Jebb wrote to Richard Watson that Ann worried that he may come to be considered a greater mathematician than 'her friend Waring', and the signature of the latter appears fourth on Jebb's election certificate to the Royal Society in 1779. Watson, *Anecdotes*, p. 102; Royal Society Mss. IV.6.

[20] Watson, *Anecdotes*, pp. 101, 95; BL Cole mss. 5883:185.

[21] T.J. Brain, 'Some aspects of the Life and Works of Richard Watson, Bishop of Llandaff 1737-1816' (University of Wales PhD., 1982), pp. 311-14.

[22] Edmund Paley, 'The Life of William Paley' in *The Works of William Paley* (6 vols., 1825), I, p. 70.

Perhaps Paley learnt from Jebb the consequences of becoming too readily identified with radical opinions. Ann concluded with the observation that Paley not being made a bishop was 'proof that merit is very far from being the direct road to preferment'.[23]

Members of the Hyson Club were not exclusively of a liberal Whig persuasion. Meadley recounts a debate one evening on the ecclesiastical constitution. Dr John Gordon, 'an avowed Tory in religion and politics, when vehemently opposing the arguments of Mr Jebb ... exclaimed with his usual heat, "you mean, Sir, to impose upon us a new Church government". "You are mistaken, Sir", said Paley, "Jebb only wants to ride his own horse, not to force you to get up behind him"'.[24] Likewise, while the young Isaac Milner was admitted to the club in 1774, and contributed to the 'interest and hilarity of this brilliant company', he was no enemy to conservatives, having been the only student in his college not to sign the student petition against subscription.[25]

Dr Johnson's famous literary 'Club' found it necessary to ban the discussion of politics in order to avoid heated confrontation (particularly between Johnson and Edmund Burke). This was not necessary for the Hyson Club as it was essentially a gathering of Cambridge Whigs. The arguments that did occur reflect the increase in intellectual tensions that forced Whigs to choose between a conservative or reformist stance. If Gordon was a 'Tory', it would seem that he was one out of social fear rather than a re-appraisal of conventional Whig political philosophy. He preached a commencement sermon rejecting the Lockean state of nature, the concept of power deriving from the people, and lamented that 'Clubs of the lowest artificers have been formed to dispute and decide upon the most abstruse questions of Religion and Government'. But he also rejected the 'exploded' Filmerian doctrine of 'Government being founded in parental authority'. John Gascoigne has rightly assessed this sermon as a reflection of

> the intellectual confusion of many in Cambridge who were increasingly concerned at the growing assertiveness of 'the lower orders' and who recoiled from the radical conclusions that self proclaimed custodians of whiggery like Watson drew from the familiar contractual view of government, and yet were still too influenced by Cambridge's whig traditions to return to Filmerite views of government and society.[26]

Gordon was remembered by the young Socinian clergyman Thomas Scott as 'a far more reasonable and candid man, in respect to those who differed from him

[23] Meadley, *Memoirs of Paley*, pp. 35, 54.

[24] Meadley, *Memoirs of Paley*, p. 46; Perhaps Paley had recently read Laurence Sterne's enormously popular *The Life and Opinions of Tristram Shandy*: 'and so long as a man rides his HOBBY-HORSE peaceably and quietly along the King's highway, and neither compels you or me to get up behind him – pray, Sir, what have either you or I to do with it?' (Graham Petrie ed., Harmondsworth, 1967 [1759-67]), I, chapter 7, p. 43.

[25] Milner, *Life of Isaac Milner*, pp. 8, 9.

[26] John Gordon, *The Causes and Consequences of evil speaking against the Government considered* (1771), cited in Gascoigne, *Cambridge*, p. 210.

... than is commonly met with'.[27] Indeed, Gordon was to prove one of those who supported Jebb's academic reform motions, and the proposal to remove subscription for students taking non-clerical degrees.

In short, the Hyson Club was composed of Whigs who responded with varying degrees of enthusiasm or fear to the new developments in religion and politics. In the 1770s debates over religious reform and conflict with the American Colonies forced people to decide and declare their positions. Jebb's free and open expression of his sentiments over cups of china tea must have fuelled his reputation for radicalism and contributed to the redefining of political alignments at Cambridge. For moderates like William Paley and John Hey, debates at the Hyson Club began a process of intellectual development whereby they were 'inexorably drawn toward theological orthodoxy and political conservatism during the last quarter of the century'.[28]

In the 1760s these new intellectual and political divisions at Cambridge were only starting to emerge. Jebb, looking forward to a career in both the Church and University, was preparing to apply for the position of Professor of Arabic upon the expected death of the incumbent, who obliged by departing this world in January 1768. Jebb applied for the professorship but was defeated by his cousin Samuel Hallifax. In order to understand his loss in this academic contest, which he considered 'of the utmost importance for my happiness',[29] we must first consider Jebb's position in the broader political context.

HIGH POLITICS UNDER GEORGE III

Following breakfast on the 25 October 1760, George II went to the toilet, had a massive heart attack, and died in a manner far from majestic. This sudden death encouraged a reconfiguration of British politics. The young George III announced that 'I glory in the name of Briton' and offered to embrace anyone who would loyally serve the crown. Since 1715 the traditional Whig-Tory polarity had gradually been superseded in importance by a Court-Country divide.[30] With the accession of George III high politics became openly factionalised. Any remnant of a Tory party effectively disintegrated and the Whigs stood clearly exposed as a loose body of Members of Parliament clustered around several aristocratic leaders.[31] William Pitt and the old Whig magnate the Duke of Newcastle eventually resigned and left government in the hands of George III's ambitious Scottish favourite Lord Bute. With a young King on the throne (and no alternative ruler to gather around) opposition Whigs attacked what they styled as George III's successive 'Tory' administrations, and appealed to the electorate for support. In reality most of George III's supporters

---

[27] Scott, *Life of Thomas Scott*, p. 34.
[28] Waterman, 'A Cambridge "Via Media"', p. 422.
[29] John Jebb [JJ] to Lord Hardwicke, 18 January 1768, BL Add. Mss. 35,657:f.295.
[30] William Speck, 'Whigs and Tories dim their glories: English political parties under the first two Georges', in Cannon, *Whig Ascendancy*, pp. 51-76.
[31] Frank O'Gorman, *The Long Eighteenth Century: British political and social history, 1688-1832* (1997), p. 201.

were from Whig backgrounds and the traditional Tory party had all but ceased to exist.[32] Thus, to understand politics in the 1760s we need to look at the evolution of the Whigs.

The Whigs were united by the principles of the Glorious Revolution: government based upon contract, the defence of Protestantism, repudiation of Jacobitism and support for religious toleration. Yet a range of opinion and personalities gathered behind the 'old corps' of aristocratic Whigs who held the reins of government following 1715.[33] A broad distinction can be made between Court Whigs and 'True' or 'Real' Whigs. It was during the heated controversy over a standing army in the late 1690s that a deep 'fissure between Cabinet and coffee-house' took shape.[34] This divide became more entrenched following the accession of George I. As John Kenyon has demonstrated, when the aristocratic Whigs came to power they proceeded to distance themselves from, dilute and even reject many traditional Whig principles. They took the support of the Dissenters for granted, and failed to remove their civil disabilities. They instituted the Septennial Act, confined the doctrine of resistance to only the most extreme cases, preached parliamentary sovereignty and manipulated the House of Commons by stacking it with government place-men. Pointing to the spectre of Jacobitism muted any criticism by Real Whigs.[35]

From 1720 to 1760 British politics became divided between three basic dispositions: 'Court Whigs' and their 'Country Tory' and 'Real Whig' opponents. During this period, Tory politicians proved a source of defiant 'patriotic' opposition to the Whig oligarchy; and 'in their encouragement of and co-operation with extra-parliamentary lobbies and voter societies' they 'pioneered or fostered much of the content and many of the methods of subsequent protest'.[36] With the accession of George III and the eclipse of the Jacobites complete, a popular expression of radical Whiggism became possible – adopting many of the tactics developed by extra-parliamentary Tories. The maverick William Pitt prepared the ground for this potential development when he continued to court popular patriotic sentiment as prime minister. While the aristocratic factions jostled for position in the new reign, Real Whig sentiment burst forth in response to several key political developments. First, in response to the more hands-on style of George III, some of the leading Whig magnates left the administration and proceeded to criticise the new 'Toryism'. This was followed by public outcry at what were perceived to be over-generous terms granted to France at the end of the Seven Years War. Then there was the

---

[32] Ian R. Christie, 'Was there a "New Toryism" in the earlier part of George III's reign', in *Myth and Reality in Late Eighteenth Century Politics* (1970), pp. 196-214. See also his *Wars and Revolutions: Britain 1760-1815* (1982), pp. 281-84.

[33] H.T. Dickinson, 'Whiggism in the Eighteenth Century', in Cannon, *Whig Ascendancy*, pp. 28-50.

[34] J.G.A Pocock, 'Radical Criticisms of the Whig Order in the Age between Revolutions', in Margaret C. and James R. Jacob, *The Origins of Anglo-American Radicalism* (1984), p. 37.

[35] John Kenyon, *Revolution Principles: the politics of party 1689-1720* (Cambridge, 1977), pp. 170-241.

[36] Linda Colley, *In Defiance of Oligarchy: the Tory Party 1714-60* (Cambridge, 1982), p. 292.

prosecution of John Wilkes for libel after he subjected the government to severe satire in *The North Briton*. Finally, the American colonies began to resist efforts to impose tax measures by the British Parliament. In light of these developments, we can best understand the post-1760 political landscape if we divide it into three broad categories: a series of Court Whig administrations that drew on old Tory support; aristocratic Court Whig opposition factions; and a largely extra-parliamentary popular radicalism that drew on Real Whig and patriot sentiment.

Agreed that the resurgence of the Tory party was a myth, historians have debated the extent to which governments following 1760 (other than the Rockingham ministry) were characterised by 'Tory' and 'authoritarian' attitudes. Ian Christie has argued that those Court Whigs that composed most of George III's administrations can properly be styled 'conservative' rather than 'Tory'. They followed traditional government practice and were far from promoting the arbitrary despotism that their opponents alleged; indeed, on the domestic front 'liberty was not waning but broadening in the years after 1760'.[37] This assertion is supported by G.M. Ditchfield, who has described Lord North's ecclesiastical policy as reflecting a 'broader tolerance than many of its predecessors'.[38] In this view, it was not a case of government becoming more authoritarian, but rather of opposition demands becoming more innovative. The likes of Jebb wanted progress toward greater religious and political liberty, and became frustrated when the establishment would not move in their favoured direction. Nevertheless, the opposition rhetoric was not entirely unfounded: if domestic policy was not actively oppressive, we can say that government came to rest more comfortably upon a conservative social base and ideology. The impression of a 'Tory resurgence' was encouraged by the fact that George III's successive administrations governed with the support of the old Tory country gentlemen in Parliament. According to Langford, after decades in opposition these men found themselves 'part of a unified ruling class', with access to patronage at a local level and able to defend the 'divine right of properly constituted authority'. The instinctive paternalism of the old Tories provided the parliamentary and popular support that made war against the American colonies possible.[39]

The preaching of deference to the institutions of the 'confessional state' was nothing new. But this alliance between Court Whigs and country squires was accompanied by an increasing emphasis on authority, order, and the bond between Church and State.[40] The tone of Anglican sermons in particular became increasingly strident in response to Wilkite agitation, the challenge posed by the American colonies and attempts to undermine the orthodoxy of the established

---

[37] Christie, 'New Toryism?', in *Myth and Reality*, p. 203.

[38] G.M. Ditchfield, 'Ecclesiastical Policy under Lord North', in Walsh, Haydon and Taylor, *The Church of England c.1649-c.1833*, p. 246.

[39] Paul Langford, 'Old Whigs, Old Tories, and the American Revolution', *Journal of Imperial and Commonwealth History*, 8 (1980), pp. 106-30, esp. pp. 124, 126, 127.

[40] Clark, *English Society*, pp. 199-235.

Church.[41] As James Sack has observed, the debate over Toryism has 'obscured the very real post-1760 authoritarian, anti-Enlightenment, right-wing patronage and factional networks which grew up about ostensibly Whig politicians'. An ascendant neo-Toryism represented the 'survival of basic Tory tendencies as opposed to concrete personalities'. Those tendencies centred on and rallied behind the Anglican Church as the first line of defence of the political establishment against a re-run of the seventeenth-century experience of sectarianism and civil war.[42] This evolution of the composition and ideology of the political establishment does not necessarily add up to an increase in the implementation of 'authoritarian' policies (or at least of 'authoritarian' policy different to that practiced by the Whigs prior to 1760). But if people of progressive religious and political principles were not actively oppressed, they at least found themselves frozen out of official favour as a coherent conservative ideology solidified around the establishment. This change was perceptible at the top of the Church during the reign of Archbishop Secker (1758-68). Respected by High Churchmen, Secker was a determined enemy of those he styled as 'Low Church controversialists keeping the Hoadlien flag flying'.[43] While outspoken heterodox clergy such as Samuel Clarke had not been particularly well favoured during the reigns of George I and II, at least the government was on their side of the religious debate and anti-clerical ministers such as Lord Hardwicke appreciated their work. Following 1760 it became increasingly difficult for those who were progressive in theology and politics to gain advancement to the highest levels within the Church.

In a sense the main parliamentary distinction that developed was between those Whigs who would ultimately listen to the King's wishes (however much influenced by his courtiers), and those Whigs who expected the King to follow their instructions. In the eyes of George III, the Duke of Newcastle represented a system by which the Whig aristocrats had effectively eroded royal power. Newcastle for his part, in the words of one historian, was possessed by the 'neurotic conviction that a king not prepared to accept the shackles of the Pelham family must be an enemy to Revolution principles'.[44] When the young George III sought to reassert the proper constitutional role of the monarch, Newcastle and his allies resigned. After decades of controlling government and its vast system of patronage they began to harangue the Crown's ministers from the opposition benches, styling those who remained in government as Tories intent upon increasing the influence of the Crown over

---

[41] James E. Bradley, 'The Anglican Pulpit, the Social Order, and the Resurgence of Toryism during the American Revolution', *Albion,* 21 (1989), pp. 361-88; G.M Ditchfield, 'The Subscription Issue in British Parliamentary Politics, 1772-79', *Parliamentary History,* 7 (1988), pp. 65-66.

[42] James Sack, *From Jacobite to Conservative: reaction and orthodoxy in Britain, 1760-1832* (Cambridge, 1993), pp. 74, 48, 33.

[43] Mather, *High Church Prophet*, p. 10.

[44] Paul Langford, *A Polite and Commercial People: England 1727-1783* (Oxford, 1989), p. 345.

Parliament.[45] While this may have been a myth, it was a myth that captivated the minds of many, including John Jebb.

Toward the end of 1763, a few months after Jebb had been ordained (and was no doubt looking for preferment), a contest erupted for the position of High Steward of Cambridge. This came to be seen as a significant clash between the government and the opposition. Lord Hardwicke, a celebrated lawyer, and staple member of successive Whig ministries, had held the position for well over twenty years. Lord Sandwich, an ambitious minister, began canvassing for votes in the University when he realised that Hardwicke was dying, and became confident of success. Sandwich's approach was both efficient and tactless, and in the aftermath of his prosecution of John Wilkes, this 'contributed to the impression of ministerial power being deployed rather too forcefully and nakedly'.[46] As Chancellor of the University and close friend of Hardwicke, Newcastle felt that Sandwich had intruded upon his home ground, and saw an opportunity to inflict a defeat upon the ministry outside of Parliament. To this end he encouraged the uninspiring young Lord Hardwicke to stand for his father's position. The election fell on 30 March 1764, but was so close that the issue remained undecided until the question went before King's Bench in May 1765, where Hardwicke was declared successful.[47] This contest split the university, and one Newcastle supporter observed early on that 'nobody has now any character in this place, but that of Sandwichian or Anti-Sandwichian'.[48] Newcastle sent some of his best political agents to Cambridge during the campaign, scenting the opportunity for a significant, if symbolic victory over the ministry.[49]

Jebb's conduct in the election provided ample evidence of both his commitment to the Whig cause, and his inflexible attachment to principle. Despite a dubious reputation Sandwich was backed by most of the clergy, as they 'preferred his political principles to those of Lord Hardwicke, who was supported by the faculties of Law and Medicine'.[50] Sandwich also drew support because there was obviously more to gain by backing a member of the government, than the client of a Chancellor who was now cut off from access to Crown patronage. Jebb, however, remained loyal to the 'Whig interest' and several years later reminded Hardwicke of his conduct in the election:

> It is well known that I engaged as a volunteer in what appeared to me the cause of virtue. I opposed Lord Sandwich from a persuasion that his success and the ruin of the university were inseparably connected.... I therefore engaged with zeal in the service. My conduct was applauded as truly

---

[45] Reed Browning, *The Duke of Newcastle* (New Haven, Conn., 1975), p. 298.
[46] N.A.M. Rogers, *The Insatiable Earl: a life of John Montagu, 4th Earl of Sandwich* (1993), p. 109.
[47] See C.H. Cooper, *Annals of Cambridge* (5 vols, 1842-1908), IV, pp. 334-5.
[48] Gascoigne, *Cambridge*, p. 110.
[49] Browning, *Duke of Newcastle*, p. 303.
[50] Wordsworth, *Social Life at the English Universities*, p. 78.

> disinterested by the party I opposed, and my zeal appeared preposterous in the eyes even of the party which I served.[51]

Jebb would pay dearly for his open opposition to Sandwich in 1780, when the latter helped ensure that he lost an election to be physician at St Bartholomew's Hospital. At the turn of the century, Ann Jebb thanked Hardwicke for recollecting 'the Dr's exertions at so great a distance of time', reminding him that her husband's 'exertions were entirely voluntary'.

> His love of virtue, the great regard he had for your family, and his wish to preserve the honour of the University could not permit him to act otherwise. Therefore, although Lord S[andwiche's] persecution and opposition in every situation, after the contest, ended but with his life: yet the Dr having acted on virtuous principles, he always reviewed his exertions upon that occasion with satisfaction.[52]

1764 was John Disney's first year at Peterhouse, and he remembered that 'Mr Jebb voted for Lord Hardwicke, from the most disinterested motives, notwithstanding the most complicated and pointed solicitations, on the one hand; and the most trying menaces, and threats, on the other. In consequence of his inflexible integrity on this occasion, he suffered much at the time.'[53] Throughout that year (and perhaps for some time earlier) Jebb was courting his future wife. During the election, according to Jebb's 1769 letter to Hardwicke: 'I disregarded the welfare of a father which seemed to be immediately concerned, and was deaf to the entreaties of a mother rather than go back on my engagements'.[54] Perhaps his opposition to the ministerial candidate was detrimental to his father's prospects for further promotion within the Church. At the very least he must have damaged his own interests: what 'complicated and pointed solicitations' did he turn down? Jebb supported Hardwicke 'at a season when it was in my interest to stand well with [my parents] – when I was soliciting their assistance and consent to my marriage, and when I was assured that no indulgence should be shown to me in case I persevered. I have not yet recovered from the consequences of my conduct'.[55]

Theophilus Lindsey observed in September 1776 that Jebb's 'father has one thousand a year, no other child but a son well provided for, yet allows his eldest nothing, approving his principles but disapproving his conduct'.[56] As Jonathan Swift observed, the young Dean Jebb had been careful not to offend anyone on account of politics, and he collected enough preferments to be described as 'a Man of Fortune'.[57] Patronage remained the means of rising within the Church, and Dean Jebb was right to warn his son against offending those in power. But the latter evidently thought it his duty to align with those

---

[51] JJ to Lord Hardwicke, 22 January 1769, BL Add. Mss. 35,658; 1.
[52] AJ to Lord Hardwicke, 10 January 1805, BL Add. Mss. 35,755:182.
[53] 'Life of Jebb', p. 9.
[54] JJ to Lord Hardwicke, 22 Jan. 1769, BL Add. Mss. 35,658; 1.
[55] JJ to Lord Hardwicke, 22 Jan. 1769, BL Add. Mss. 35,658; 1.
[56] H. McLachlan, *Letters of Theophilus Lindsey* (Manchester, 1920), p. 102.
[57] Swift, *Correspondence* IV, pp. 437-38; William Cole mss., BL Add. Mss. 5873:53.

whom he saw as carrying the Whig banner forward. In doing so Jebb provided an early example of the inflexible attachment to principle that would characterise his mature political conduct.

Newcastle handed the leadership of his faction to the Marquis of Rockingham, who, with the aid of Edmund Burke, presided over the formation of a relatively coherent parliamentary party. The Rockinghamites sought to offer a moderate Whig platform in response to the issues of the day. While briefly in power in 1765-66 ('a ministry of boys' in the King's words) they repealed the Stamp Act, but at the same time passed a Declaratory Act which reaffirmed parliamentary sovereignty. Yet as the imperial debate unfolded the Americans denied the authority of the British Parliament, and appealed to the King to grant their provincial assemblies full autonomy under the Crown. As the argument became centred on the demand for 'no taxation without representation' the pragmatic old Whig stance of the opposition became increasingly inadequate. The Rockingham Whigs were in a similar position with respect to parliamentary reform. They constantly tried to ride the waves of popular protest, while at the same time attempting to limit radical proposals and guide the activities of extra-parliamentary organisations. Paul Langford has argued that, while they had allies on the radical fringe, 'the great body of the Rockingham Whigs ... before their leadership passed into the hands of Fox in 1782, feebly criticised the conduct of Parliament without ever demanding fundamental change'.[58] This assessment is, however, probably too harsh. As financially and socially secure country gentlemen, the Rockingham Whigs became relatively indifferent to being in power compared to 'the sense of fulfilment they derived from carrying on the battle against the undue influence of the crown.'[59] In the process they developed into an opposition party that sought systemic change, espousing a moderate programme of 'economical reform' aimed at limiting the government's ability to manipulate Parliament through the use of patronage. In doing so, they preserved and developed the tradition of party politics during a period of factional confusion.

During the Feathers Tavern campaign and his involvement in the parliamentary reform movement Jebb associated with various liberal-minded Whig politicians such as George Saville, William Meredith and the Duke of Richmond. Yet he always remained suspicious of the leading Rockinghamites. Jebb was ready to applaud their speeches against the 'influence of the Crown' and in defence of the Americans. But he felt betrayed by their opposition to the Feathers Tavern petition and vigorously opposed their attempts to guide the deliberations and tactics of the extra-parliamentary reform movement. At base was a difference of opinion as to the proper relationship between the Member of Parliament and the 'voice of the people'. Burke argued that the integrity and independence of a Member of Parliament was compromised by slavishly following the dictates of his electors. Jebb flatly rejected this, asserting that the

[58] Langford, 'Old Whigs, Old Tories, and the American Revolution', p. 119.

[59] W.M. Elofson, *The Rockingham Connection and the Second Founding of the Whig Party, 1768-1773* (Montreal, 1996), p. 8.

representative was only a proxy for his constituents – a political puppet who should dance to the will of his electorate.[60]

Jebb's father, with his old Whig attitudes and experience of tactfully navigating the avenues of patronage in the days of Walpole, urged caution on the new political climate. But filled with youthful enthusiasm, Jebb became openly committed to what he identified as the true Whig cause. It was later observed that throughout his life his 'character as a party man was injurious to him professionally'.[61] That he engaged with a 'zeal' that 'appeared preposterous' to those he served in the election for High Steward at Cambridge suggests that Jebb was motivated by much more than an attachment out of 'interest' to the parliamentary Whig opposition.

WILKES AND LIBERTY

Most Englishmen believed that their constitution allowed the greatest degree of liberty possible without undermining social and political stability, yet there was great disagreement as to exactly what form of liberty it sanctioned. For Court Whigs the eighteenth-century constitution had evolved to a point where it prudently balanced the needs of government, the rights of property, and the civil liberties of the subject. They defended the Septennial Act, unequal electorates and the presence of government placemen in the House of Commons as necessary oil for the wheels government; and throughout the century war and trade drove an expansion in the size of the state. This growth of government and the perceived 'corruption of the constitution' by the Crown's ministers was subjected to sustained criticism by those who argued that English liberties were being subverted. The origin of this opposition ideology lay in the Commonwealth tradition of the seventeenth century, the ideals of classical republicanism and in appeals to natural rights.[62] As the following chapters will demonstrate, Jebb's positive definition of natural political rights was encouraged by his religious dissent and philosophical development. In the first two-thirds of the century, however, most criticisms of the political system were couched as appeals to historical precedent.

The Glorious Revolution had been a conservative affair in which the elite replaced a Catholic with a Protestant king. Yet this precedent in which the Country changed the Court enabled future radicals to argue that 'the people' (variously defined) should increase their participation in the political process. Real Whigs condemned the eighteenth-century political system as a corruption of the principles of the ancient constitution in which, they claimed, the House of Commons had been more representative and independent of Crown influence.

---

[60] Lucy Sutherland, 'Edmund Burke and the Relations between Members of Parliament and their Constituents', *Studies in Burke and His Time,* 10 (1968), pp. 1005-21; Edmund Burke, *The Writings and Speeches of Edmund Burke* (Paul Langford ed., Oxford, 1981), I, pp. 256-60; John Jebb, *Address to the Freeholders of Middlesex* (1779), Jebb II, pp. 453-90.

[61] Cited in F.D. Cartwright ed., *The Life and Correspondence of Major Cartwright* (1826), pp. 165-66.

[62] The way these traditions exerted a joint influence upon Jebb will be examined in chapter 9.

The cause of political corruption was thought to lie in a lack of patriotism. According to the classical republican tradition laws and institutions alone could not sustain liberty. The maintenance of a free constitution, it was argued, depended upon the virtue and patriotism of a nation's citizens. Thus concerns about political corruption were tied to a belief that the moral fabric of English society was being eaten away by an increasing indulgence in luxury and vice.[63]

By far the most popular expression of this view was John Brown's *Estimate of the Manners of the Times* (1757), which launched a withering attack upon the corruption, indolence and Francophilia of the governing class. At the root of the nation's ills lay 'the luxurious and effeminate Manners in the higher Ranks, together with a general Defect of *Principle*'. A general reform of 'Manners and Principles' was necessary, as the ruling powers would only wake 'from their fatal Dream' when 'either the Voice of an abused People rouse them into Fear; or the State itself totter thro' the general Incapacity, Cowardice, and Disunion of those who should support it'.[64] That Jebb shared Brown's concerns is suggested by his ordination sermon on 'this adulterous and sinful generation'.[65] Ten years later he was lamenting the 'deplorable state of morals in this country', and describing the 'present times' as 'depraved beyond the example of all former ages'.[66]

While the unprecedented successes of the Seven Years War swelled chauvinistic English pride, it also fuelled fears that England, like Rome, was about to succumb to imperial decadence and decline. The fears of those Englishmen who worried about the future of their country were aggravated by the increasing importance of the Scottish component of the British nation. The Seven Year's War had been won with the help of soldiers from the Highlands, and under George III ambitious Scots were infiltrating administrative positions; government was no longer the preserve of English Whigs. While these developments eventually led to a strong sense of British identity in the nineteenth century, the initial reaction of many Englishmen to this expansion of the British Empire was a xenophobic and chauvinistic championing of *Englishness*. In this vein, John Horne warned Scots in high office such as Bute and Mansfield against melting 'the English name ... down to Briton'.[67]

---

[63] Linda Colley, *Britons: forging the nation, 1707-1837* (1992), p. 85; see also Linda Colley, 'Radical Patriotism in Eighteenth-Century England', in Raphael Samuel ed., *Patriotism: the making and unmaking of British national identity* (1989), I, pp. 167-87.

[64] Gerald Newman, *The Rise of English Nationalism: a cultural history* (1987), pp. 63-122, cited at 81, 84; Joanna Innes, 'Politics and Morals: the reformation of manners movement in later eighteenth-century England', in Hellmuth, *Transformation of Political Culture*, pp. 57-118.

[65] The text he chose for the sermon was Mark 8:38: 'Whosoever, therefore, shall be ashamed of me, and of my words, in this adulterous and sinful generation, to him also shall the Son of Man be ashamed, when he cometh in the glory of his father, with the holy angels'. Unfortunately we do not have a copy of the sermon itself. 'Life of Jebb', p. 7. Jebb actually opened his *Address to the Members of the Senate of Cambridge* (1775) with an extract from John Brown urging improvements in education. Jebb II, pp. 341, 357-59, 372.

[66] Jebb letters to the newspapers, 28 May 1772 and 27 February 1773, Jebb III, pp. 64, 138.

[67] Cited in Colley, *Britons*, p. 116.

Such popular patriotic concerns found flamboyant expression in the figure of John Wilkes. In his occasional publication *The North Briton*, Wilkes anonymously gave voice to popular dissatisfaction with the terms of the Peace of Paris and the general conduct of government. His increasingly virulent attacks led to expulsion from Parliament for libel following the publication of no. 45 in late 1763, which expressed a violent hatred of the 'Scottish influence' at court, and called on the people to make their discontent known to the Parliament. Wilkes held up to his audience the possibility of a reformed, revitalised and powerful France, and claimed that England's economic supremacy was under threat. Thus, the *English* constitution,

> *That* beautiful and wondrous fabric, the work of ages, the pride and glory of *Britain*, as well as the jealousy of her most powerful neighbours, which has survived two desperate *Scottish* rebellions, seems at last doomed to fall a sacrifice to the incapacity and treachery of a set of men, formerly the objects of the contempt and ridicule and now the abhorrence and hatred of their country.[68]

Wilkes' arrest under a General Warrant caused a storm in Parliament, and was branded by many as an attack upon the rights of Englishmen. Ironically, Pitt and other Whig leaders had themselves used General Warrants against Jacobites. But with the absence of any threat to Hanoverian legitimacy, some Whigs declared General Warrants unnecessary and authoritarian. Following his arrest, Wilkes defended himself in court by claiming that 'the author' of the *North Briton* was not attacking a king who was 'deservedly the idol of his people'. Rather, he argued, what was being claimed by government ministers as abuse of the King, was really only directed at themselves.[69]

Lord Sandwich was one of those ministers, and won notoriety for his enthusiastic prosecution of Wilkes. This included reading, 'with evident relish', Wilkes' pornographic *Essay on Woman* to a shocked House of Lords. To some extent Sandwich's attempt to destroy Wilkes' reputation backfired, as he became the object of patriotic scorn. Wilkes, on the other hand, attained a 'totem-like value as the personification of a certain version of English freedom and liberty'.[70] The cause of 'Wilkes and Liberty' became a conduit for the expression of dissatisfaction by Dissenters, the American Colonists, republicans, heterodox clergy, opposition MPs, and anyone unhappy with the government.[71]

While Wilkes championed traditional English patriotic prejudices in the face of new political realities, he also dramatically helped stimulate debate over representation. Found guilty of libel by the Court of King's Bench in 1764, Wilkes avoided a sentence by fleeing to the Continent, where he increased his worldly experience and debts. In 1768 he returned to London, was elected to

---

[68] John Wilkes, *The North Briton* (2 vols., 1769-71), pp. 162-64.
[69] Langford, *Polite and Commercial People*, pp. 357-58.
[70] Colley, *Britons*, p. 112.
[71] George Rude, *Wilkes and Liberty* (1983 [1962]); Dickinson, *Politics of the People*; Kathleen Wilson, *The Sense of the People: politics, culture and imperialism in England, 1715-1785* (Cambridge, 1995).

Parliament by the freeholders of Middlesex and went to prison for his earlier libel. In December troops fired upon a crowd of demonstrators in St George's Fields, opposite the prison in which Wilkes was comfortably resident. Wilkes condemned this in a letter to the *St James's Chronicle*, which the government used as a pretext to again expel him from Parliament.[72] Wilkes was subsequently re-elected and expelled three times. In April the House of Commons declared him incapable of becoming an MP, and seated his opponent who 'ought to have been returned'.[73] This election controversy can be described as a 'landmark in English political history'.[74] A flood of pamphlets and petitions followed, declaring that the constitution was being corrupted by the influence of the Crown.[75] Perhaps with the exception of Edmund Burke's influential defence of political parties, the most significant product of this controversy was the growth of organised urban radicalism. Most notably, the 'Society of the Supporters of the Bill of Rights' (1769-71) campaigned for 'a more fair and equal representation' and the freedom to publish parliamentary debates.

On 17 March 1769, Jebb illustrated the extent of his radical sympathies when he was one of only two dons openly to vote against a loyal address by the university to the Crown. The 'Address' was drafted by the Duke of Grafton's client, John Hinchcliffe (Master of Trinity 1768-88), and expressed support for the ministry's efforts to prevent Wilkes from taking his seat in the Parliament. It stated that the University was 'fully convinced that this, nor any other nation, never enjoyed the valuable blessings of civil and religious liberty in a greater degree', and condemned those 'bad men' who were 'labouring to seduce the ignorant and unwary from their duty, by infusing into their minds needless fears and jealousies, as if the constitution were in danger'.[76] Jebb's inability to endorse a statement so contrary to his own sentiments is understandable, yet he could have absented himself from the vote. That he openly voted against the 'Address' reveals the depth of Jebb's support for Wilkes and the Americans. Thomas Rutherforth referred to him as 'a professed and eager defender of Mr Wilkes'.[77] When Wilkes visited Cambridge, he told his daughter that he had attracted many interested onlookers as he was shown around the colleges.[78] William Cole recorded for posterity that 'when Wilkes was at Cambridge this Winter 1771, [Jebb] was the only person almost that took any notice of him, and

---

[72] See *St James's Chronicle*, 10 December 1768.

[73] Rude, *Wilkes and Liberty*, pp. 37-73.

[74] Carl B. Cone, *The English Jacobins: reformers in late eighteenth-century England* (New York, 1968), p. 43.

[75] In particular see Edmund Burke, *Thoughts on the Cause of the Present Discontents* (1770); and Obadiah Hulme, *An Historical Essay on the English Constitution* (1771).

[76] 'Life of Jebb', pp. 24-25.

[77] Thomas Rutherforth to Lord Hardwicke, March 1769, BL Add. Mss. 35,640.

[78] 'Mr Dixon's nephew, a young Academic of Cambridge, and two other gentleman of the University, accompanied me in the tour I made to see the curiosities and buildings. The people followed us in great crowds, with prodigious acclamations'. John to Mary Wilkes, 13 February 1771, 'John Wilkes Correspondence with Mary Wilkes 1759-97', BL Add. Mss. 30,879.

who walked about with him to show him the Colleges &c'.[79] From the late 1760s Jebb's open identification with the cause of 'Wilkes and Liberty' identified him as a radical at the University.

It is hard to determine precisely when Jebb struck up his various friendships, however it is significant that Thomas Brand Hollis (1719-1804) claimed to have been acquainted with Jebb since 1767.[80] Thomas Brand was a close friend of Thomas Hollis (1720-74), the republican antiquarian whose name Brand adopted when he inherited Hollis's estate. A quiet and abstemious man, Hollis played an important role as a propagandist for the 'Cause of Liberty'. Having inherited wealth, he spent it in printing, ornamenting and disseminating 'Commonwealthman' literature by the likes of Milton, Harrington, Locke, Sidney, Molesworth and Trenchard. Both Brand and Hollis had been raised as Dissenters, and they spent time together during two visits to the Continent between 1748 and 1753, where they met philosophes such as Voltaire, D'Alembert and Rousseau. These travels only strengthened their intense patriotism and reverence for the English libertarian heritage.[81] Thomas Brand was very much a follower and joiner, and after Hollis's death he seems to have looked to Jebb as his political guide.[82] Their acquaintance in the late 1760s is further evidence of Jebb's early republican sympathies.

The widespread extra-parliamentary nature of agitation in the 1760s marks it out as new departure in English politics.[83] According to H.T. Dickinson, while the essential 'ideology, platform, organisation and popular support' for radicalism was developed in the early eighteenth century, 'a large scale and sustained radical movement failed to appear'. Such a development would have required full application of the notion of universal political rights, the growth of a middle class culture and widespread extra-parliamentary organisations. These elements came together around the charismatic figure of Wilkes, in response to the atmosphere of political crisis in the early part of George III's reign. The new radicalism made a broad and vocal appeal to 'the people' (many of whom could not vote) to join in forcing reform of a corrupted system of government.[84] Wilkite radicalism provided an outlet for the ideology and enthusiasm of Dissent, was adopted as an ally by the Americans and drew support from merchants in London who were annoyed with government corruption. As John Brewer has put it, the reformers of the 1760s were united by the premise that 'government was a trust consigned by the people to their rulers for the good of the public and for their protection'.[85] Jebb came to play an active

---

[79] Cole mss., BL Add. Mss. 5873:52.

[80] Thomas Brand Hollis to John Disney, 12 March 1786, 'Life of Jebb', p. 235.

[81] Caroline Robbins, 'The Strenuous Whig: Thomas Hollis of Lincoln's Inn', *William and Mary Quarterly,* 7 (1950), pp. 406-53.

[82] Colin Bonwick, 'Thomas Brand Hollis (1719-1804)', *BDMBR*, I, p. 61.

[83] Nicholas Rogers, 'Urban Opposition to Whig Oligarchy, 1720-60', in Jacob, *The Origins of Anglo-American Radicalism*, p. 165.

[84] Dickinson, *Politics of the People*, chapters 6 and 7, at pp. 191, 220; H.T. Dickinson, *Liberty and Property: political ideology in eighteenth-century Britain* (1977), pp. 195-97.

[85] John Brewer, 'English Radicalism in the Age of George III', in J.G.A. Pocock ed., *Three British Revolutions: 1641,1688, 1776* (Baltimore, 1979), p. 343.

role in the organisational and ideological development of this political radicalism during the period of the American Revolution.

THE PRICE OF RADICAL TENDENCIES

Jebb's religious and political opinions had a damaging effect upon his career prospects. John Disney greatly exaggerated when he wrote, 'I remember to have heard the general voice of the University decidedly in favour of Mr Jebb' as the next Professor of Arabic. The Professorship drew on two funds: Sir Thomas Adam's foundation of the chair in 1632, and Lord Almoner's readership of 1724.[86] Jebb sought the endorsement of Newcastle, who had helped Edmund Law obtain a prebend in Durham worth five hundred pounds in 1767.[87] But another candidate came forward who was clearly preferred by most of the heads of colleges, who were charged with electing the lecturer.[88] This candidate was Jebb's cousin Samuel Hallifax, who no doubt ran in the knowledge that he would attract the support of those who feared Jebb's radical tendency.[89]

On 14 January Jebb requested the support of the ailing Newcastle and assured him that 'I shall employ my whole attention upon the duties of the office'.[90] Four days later he wrote again to Newcastle thanking him for his promise of support (as he had been informed by Dr Carlyle).[91] While Newcastle seems to have preferred Jebb as the most academically qualified for the position, he was both physically sick and politically weak. And, as John Gascoigne has observed, even at the height of his power the Duke 'was content to allow appointments to chairs to be decided without his intervention'.[92] Jebb also wrote to Lord Hardwicke, whom he had so strongly supported in 1764, requesting his support in the contest. He stressed that he had been studying Arabic for some years and that the fate of the election 'will be of the utmost importance for my happiness'.[93] As both candidates had voted for him in the High Steward election, Hardwicke either remained aloof from the contest or supported Hallifax.[94]

A notable difference in the two pleas is that Jebb referred to having prepared himself through study, while Hallifax merely requested a 'favourable reception from your lordship'.[95] It was acceptable for university lecturers to not deliver lectures – and in this case that would have been expected as there was a lack of student interest in Arabic. Perhaps it was Jebb's commitment to employ his 'whole attention upon the duties of the office' that warned off any solid

---

[86] 'Life of Jebb', p. 21; Wordsworth, *Scholae*, p. 163.

[87] Sykes, *Church and State*, p. 180.

[88] 'Life of Jebb', p. 21.

[89] In the 1770's Hallifax earned the approval of William Cole for his defence of subscription as 'very ingenious ... an universal scholar and good disciplinarian'. Cole mss., BL Add. Mss. 5871:192.

[90] JJ to Duke of Newcastle 14 January 1768, BL Add. Mss. 32,979;228.

[91] JJ to Duke of Newcastle, 18 January 1768, BL Add. Mss. 32,988;42.

[92] Sykes, *Church and State*, p. 336; Gascoigne, *Cambridge in the Enlightenment*, p. 109.

[93] JJ to Lord Hardwicke, 18 January 1768, Add. Mss. 35,657:295.

[94] See Jebb to Lord Hardwicke, 22 January 1769, BL Add. Mss. 35,658:1.

[95] Samuel Hallifax to Lord Hardwicke 15 January 1768, Add. Mss. 35,6257:297.

support. For some, the idea of students being encouraged to study the Koran in Arabic by a lecturer of suspect theological opinions would have been of great concern. Realising he was going to lose the election, Jebb tried to have the two funds that underpinned the position uncoupled. He wrote to Newcastle requesting that he influence Lord Almoner, 'to whom I have written requesting the appointment of Lecturer in the Arabic language; provided the future Professor shall not himself think proper to give lectures'.[96] But, not surprisingly, nothing came of this. While some encouraged Jebb to politely withdraw from the contest, he persisted. The Master of Queens', Robert Plumptre, remembered that one of the fellows of his college advised Jebb to go through with the election against Hallifax 'be the votes ever so few ... and in consequence Mr Jebb stood it out, with the Master of Clare Hall's single vote against nine or ten others'.[97] With this breach of polite manners Jebb did lasting damage to his reputation in the University. One opponent observed: 'Mr Jebb has contrived to give great offence in the course of the late competition, and now excites no small resentment in the University by his attempt to separate Lord Almoner's Bounty from the Arabic Professorship. But he is a warm man and will not be advised by his sedator friends.'[98]

This was the first and most significant rebuff of Jebb's career – one that exerted a profound influence on his future direction. As cousins who shared a scholarly disposition, Jebb and Hallifax had been on friendly terms in the 1750s, however their religious and political views developed in very different directions. An entrenched mutual animosity resulted from the contest over the Arabic Professorship. The outcome of the election was particularly galling for Jebb, because his cousin was already earmarked to succeed as Professor of Civil Law when the incumbent passed on – which he did in 1769. Until then Hallifax, who in true eighteenth-century style neither knew Arabic nor had any intention of giving lectures, held the position as a sinecure and proceeded to publish *Two Sermons delivered before the University in 1768, in Praise of Benefactors*. In the year that he became Professor of Civil Law Hallifax preached a sermon before the House of Commons on January 30, declaring that contemporary reformers were like the 'filthy brood of Enthusiasts' who had had managed 'to overturn the monarchy of Charles' in the seventeenth century.[99] As Richard Watson observed, Hallifax was not above the 'ordinary means of ingratiating himself with great men'.[100]

A year later another opportunity to gain a Cambridge post arose, with the resignation of Edmund Law as University Librarian. While Law proposed Jebb as his successor, Dr John Barnardiston stood forward with the backing of Hardwicke and Thomas Rutherforth, the Professor of Divinity.[101] Jebb asked

---

[96] JJ to Duke of Newcastle, 22 January 1768, BL Add. Mss. 32,988:60.
[97] Robert Plumptre to Lord Hardwicke, 3 January 1769, BL Add. Mss. 35,640:342.
[98] William Talbot to Duke of Newcastle, 29 January 1768, BL Add. Mss. 32,988:109.
[99] Cited in Peter Searby, *A History of the University of Cambridge: volume III, 1750-1870* (Cambridge, 1997), pp. 406-07.
[100] Watson, *Anecdotes*, I, p. 115.
[101] Dr Barnardiston to Lord Hardwicke, 25 January 1769, BL Add. Mss. 35,640:347.

Hardwicke to remain neutral in the affair, though he acknowledged that Barnardiston had a claim 'to the support of your respectable family on account of College connections'. He claimed that Hardwicke's support for Barnardiston had drained away his own support at Queens' College. After reminding Hardwicke at length of his service in 1764, he pleaded somewhat pathetically: 'I only request that I may not feel the whole weight of that influence exerted against me, which if no common friend were concerned, I might have hoped would have been exerted in my support.'[102] But once again, Jebb was defeated.

He retired to spend the summer of 1769 at Bungay, where he read widely in the Latin classics.[103] Why did he retreat to this corner of Suffolk? While he may have been using the spa waters there, the answer seems to lie in his being made vicar of the nearby parish of Flixton in July. Jebb was granted this living by William Adair (b.1741), along with the adjoining rectories of Homersfield and St Cross. Adair had been a student at Peterhouse, as had his relation James Adair (1743-98), the radical MP.[104] Jebb had found a like-minded family able to provide him some modest patronage. At Bungay during the summer of 1770, Jebb busied himself with clerical duties and studies, and acted as guardian of a recently established workhouse. At this time he was also nominated as chaplain to Ann's cousin Robert Sherrard, who succeeded as fourth Earl of Harborough upon his father's death that year. The accumulation of these preferments allowed him to resign the Rectory of Ovington in Norfolk, rather than possess scattered livings.[105]

The career structure of the Georgian Church has been described as like a pyramid with a wide base consisting of several thousand of curates and a distant apex occupied by a few wealthy prelates.[106] Standing somewhere in the middle, with his mixed sources of income Jebb would have been comfortable by the standards of the day. Yet it was becoming increasingly unlikely that he would further ascend the Anglican pyramid. In addition to his outspoken political sentiments, Jebb was gaining a reputation for religious radicalism. While Francis Blackburne's *Confessional* (1766) was causing controversy over reform of Anglican doctrine, Jebb had commenced a series of public theological lectures in November 1768 which led William Warburton, the Bishop of Gloucester, to brand him a heretic.[107]

---

[102] JJ to Lord Hardwicke, 22 January 1769, BL Add. Mss. 35,658:1.
[103] 'Life of Jebb', p. 25.
[104] William Adair was a fellow commoner in 1763, and James was a pensioner in 1759 and fellow in 1765. Sylas Neville refers to how 'Mr Adair, a Member of Parliament, near whose estate [Jebb] has a living', exerted his interest in favour of the Feathers Tavern petition. *Diary of Sylas Neville*, p. 111.
[105] 'Life of Jebb', p. 26.
[106] Peter Virgin, *The Church in an Age of Negligence: ecclesiastical structure and problems of Church reform 1700-1840* (Cambridge, 1989), p. 215.
[107] Jebb I, p. 17.

3

Science, Scripture and Socinianism

It can be said that the Enlightenment consisted of all those who believed two propositions: that 'the present age is more enlightened than the past', and that 'we understand nature and man best through the use of our natural faculties'.[1] It is generally accepted that the Enlightenment began early in England and that it was comparatively conservative. The eighteenth-century British elite confidently saw themselves as governing an enlightened society in an enlightened age.[2] The British constitution allowed a degree of participation that took the sting out of claims for political involvement and prevented the formation of an opposition of excluded *philosophes*. In addition, many of the Anglican clergy saw the rational thought and polite manners of the Enlightenment as useful for combating Methodism. Yet the values and scope of the Enlightenment did not go uncontested, and it is possible to see the English as experiencing a two-phase Enlightenment. The early Enlightenment witnessed the rise of Newtonianism and culminated in a fully-fledged attack on the Anglican establishment by English deists. Then, following a lull in the 1740s, a long 'late Enlightenment' assault on orthodox religion emerged within a wider British dimension.[3]

While the French Enlightenment rapidly developed into a secular phenomenon, critics in Britain (with some notable exceptions) tended to remain within the pale of Christianity. In England, Rational Dissent increasingly challenged the moderate Enlightenment of the aristocratic and clerical establishment.[4] While the Rational Dissenters never formed a unified movement,

---

[1] Henry F. May, *The Enlightenment in America* (Oxford, 1976), p. xiv.

[2] Porter, 'The Enlightenment in England'; John Gascoigne, *Joseph Banks and the English Enlightenment: useful knowledge and polite culture* (Cambridge, 1994), pp. 28-30.

[3] Nigel Aston, 'Horne and Heterodoxy: the defence of Anglican beliefs in the late Enlightenment', *English Historical Review*, 108 (1993), pp. 895-919, at 896.

[4] Pocock, 'Conservative Enlightenment', pp. 97-8.

they were characterised by a shared belief in progress through unrestrained free enquiry and the candid exchange of ideas. The radical implications of their approach encouraged conservatives from various political and religious positions to close ranks in a 'Counter-Enlightenment'.[5]

In his writings in favour of greater liberty Jebb appealed to both natural rights and utilitarian arguments. His failure to see any contradiction between natural rights and utility was rooted in the nature of his rational Christianity. On the one hand Jebb's rejection of orthodox theology strengthened his commitment to individual rights. On the other, his impulse to reform was encouraged by a philosophical disposition that combined Christianity and a utilitarian psychology. In what follows I will outline Jebb's attack upon orthodox theology before examining (in chapter 4) the alternative religious and philosophical stance that underpinned his reform efforts.

THE DEIST CHALLENGE

Peter Harrison has argued that rationalists of the early English Enlightenment were the first to attempt an 'objective' anthropological study of 'the religions'. The origin of the comparative study of religion has traditionally been located in early nineteenth-century Germany. Yet one hundred years earlier in England, '"religion" was cut to fit the new and much-vaunted scientific method. In this manner "religion" entered the realm of the intelligible. It lay open to rational investigation while its specific forms – 'the religions' – could be measured against each other, or against some intellectualist criterion.' Religion came to be seen as having a natural rather than a sacred history.[6] This led to intense debate over the rational basis of revealed religion. The deist Matthew Tindal declared that there is 'a Religion of Nature and Reason written in the hearts of every one of us from the first Creation', and it was in relation to this that any established religion should be judged.[7] The key question was: taking the basics of natural religion (God and morality) as given, what warranted rational assent to the allegedly revealed doctrines and precepts of Christianity? There were three main issues: the degree of need for revealed insights, the historical accuracy of the Scriptures and how to authenticate that the alleged revelations came from God. Jebb's stance on these issues reveals the confidence in rational Christianity that he derived from his Newtonian education.

Jebb saw the difference between deism and Christianity as one of quality rather than kind. In a discussion of the attitudes of Rational Dissenters toward 'truth', Martin Fitzpatrick has suggested that 'perhaps for John Jebb alone was human reason unaided able to reveal the same truths as revelation, although natural religion remained for him a pale reflection of Christianity'.[8]

---

[5] Martin Fitzpatrick, 'Enlightenment in Britain', in Iain McCalman ed., *The Oxford Companion to the Age of Revolutions and Romanticism* (Oxford, 1999), pp. 299-311.

[6] Peter Harrison, *'Religion' and the Religions in the English Enlightenment* (Cambridge, 1990), pp. 2-3.

[7] Pailin, 'Rational Religion in England', pp. 221-22.

[8] Martin Fitzpatrick, 'Toleration and Truth', *E&D*, 1 (1982), p. 29n.

Jebb wrote in his notebook that 'Reason is analogous to the naked eye; revelation to the sight, assisted by the telescope.'[9] The Christian revelation allowed one to clearly perceive the four main elements of true religion: 'sins forgiven, resurrection, love of God, [and] love of man'. Jebb thought that a deist received the latter two from nature, and thus thought deism perfectly compatible with sound moral conduct and reverence for God. A Christian knew this through 'express revelations from the author of nature', who also revealed that sins would be forgiven and there would be eternal life. However, 'Reason leads us, from the knowledge of our Creator, to hope for an hereafter'; revelation only 'confirms that hope beyond the possibility of disappointment'.[10] For Jebb the fundamentals of religion were discoverable by reason, and revelation only gave a more perfect knowledge of them.

A favourite tactic of freethinkers was to cast doubt upon the reliability of biblical reports. The clergymen stood their ground, declaring that the Gospel narratives were accurate eyewitness accounts, verified by the vast number of people who became convinced of Christ's mission. Trying to drive a line between scepticism and uncritical belief, rational Christians often came to doubt the received interpretation of specific biblical accounts. Bishop Francis Hare had ironically suggested that study of the Bible was the best way to become a heretic! While some freethinkers nodded in agreement, Hare's intention was to satirise the retreat from reason and the maintenance of a fixed orthodox doctrine.[11] This is certainly the way Jebb read him, as he recommended Hare's text to those students who had 'the courage' to undertake study of the Scriptures.[12] Rational Christians did not doubt that the Bible contained the word of God. Jebb declared that he had commenced his studies with the assumption that 'every relation in the scripture history is strictly true'.[13] Yet this did not mean that the orthodox interpretation of particular events in Scripture could not be doubted.

This is the attitude that lay behind the criticism Joseph Priestley (among others) levelled at David Hume's views on miracles. As Robert Webb has observed, the arguments of Hume's critics were 'substantially similar and splendidly confident ... whatever problem there was lay with Hume, not with miracles'.[14] Where Hume saw a limited number of ignorant superstitious Hebrews, Priestley saw countless convinced eyewitnesses and converts providing reliable testimony. From this assumption that the Bible was historically accurate and true, the likes of Priestley and Jebb could criticise

---

[9] 'Theological Propositions', Jebb II, p. 137.

[10] 'Theological Propositions', Jebb II, p. 180.

[11] Francis Hare, *The Difficulties and Discouragement which attend the Study of the Scriptures* (1736); R.N. Stromberg, *Religious Liberalism in Eighteenth-Century England* (Oxford, 1954), p. 97.

[12] *Short Account of Theological Lectures*, Jebb I, p. 61.

[13] *Short Account of Theological Lectures*, Jebb I, p. 19.

[14] R.K. Webb, 'Miracles in English Unitarian Thought', in Mark S. Micale and Robert L Dietle eds., *Enlightenment Passion and Modernity: historical essays in European thought and culture* (Stanford, California, 2000), p. 118; R.H., Popkin, 'Joseph Priestley's Criticism of David Hume's Philosophy', *Journal of the History of Philosophy*, 15 (1977), pp. 437-47.

received interpretation. To this end Priestley's *Theological Repository* and the 'Society for Promoting Knowledge of the Scriptures' (for which Jebb wrote the outline of intention) were designed to clarify interpretation of the sacred texts.[15] Confident of the broad literal truth of the Bible, Jebb focused upon the application of a sound critical method in order to gain an accurate understanding of revelation.

Freethinkers also delighted in pointing out the similarities between Christianity and 'false religions', to which Jebb answered that a religion revealed by God must 'be adapted to human nature: and copy after such revelations as had been successful'. Yet when compared closely, the resemblance between Christianity and false religion becomes 'fainter and fainter' in the way that 'two faces may be mistaken for each other when they are seen separately and little attended, between which scarce any resemblance can be perceived when they are deliberately viewed together'.[16] At base this was the long running debate over the 'evidences of Christianity': how can we be certain that the Bible contains the word of God? The 'internal' evidence for Christianity was the unblemished character of Jesus, and the supposedly unsurpassed moral quality of his teachings. As Jebb put it, without divine inspiration, how 'could Galilean fishermen see so deeply?'[17] There were two primary questions for which every person desired an answer: is there an afterlife, and how can one expect to be happy in it? 'A religion which settles both these points, must be from God. Christ's does so, and is supported by proper evidence, therefore, Christ's religion is divine'.[18]

But it was increasingly the 'external' evidence that Christians relied upon: the prophesies predicting Christ, and most of all, the miracles Jesus performed in front of numerous witnesses. Jebb referred students to the work of Nathanial Lardner on 'the truth of those historical facts, which form the foundation of the Christian institution', and Hugh Farmer's 'incomparable treatise upon miracles'.[19] (The latter, according to Alexander Gordon, 'was long the evidential textbook of Rational Dissenters'.)[20] On Sunday evenings in 1766 Jebb lectured on Joseph Butler's influential *Analogy of Religion* (1736). With the deists in his sights, Butler argued that it was 'unreasonable' for those who accepted the existence of God to doubt the truth of revelation, as objections could equally be raised against natural religion – in both cases 'Probability is the very Guide of Life'. While this argument collapses in the face of a sceptical stance on natural religion, it was very much in the English empiricist tradition of settling for probable, as opposed to certain knowledge of reality. Butler was appealing to the confident rationalism of the age, and only addressed those who

[15] *Sketch of ... the Society for Promoting Knowledge of the Scriptures*, Jebb II, pp. 249-50.
[16] DWL Jebb mss. IV.
[17] DWL Jebb mss. I.
[18] 'Theological Propositions', Jebb II, p. 137.
[19] *Short Account of Theological Lectures*, Jebb I, p. 38; Nathaniel Lardner, *The Credibility of Gospel History* (1727-57); Hugh Farmer, *Dissertation on Miracles* (1771). Lardner's text provided the main authority for William Paley in his *Evidences of Christianity* (1794).
[20] Alexander Gordon, *Heads of Unitarian History* (1895), p. 36.

already believed in a God.[21] Jebb's writings reveal a mind in no doubt as to the essential truth of revelation. The essential difference was that whereas Butler stressed the limitations of reason and the need for faith, Jebb called for more reason.[22]

Matthew Tindal presented one of the strongest deist arguments. He claimed that Christianity could not be true because its belated, partial and still imperfect revelation to humanity was inconsistent with the notion of a universally just and kind God.[23] Most of the clergymen who responded to Tindal's book jettisoned the principle of universality, and declared that God could be as partial in his revelation as he was in dishing out natural abilities and blessings.[24] In doing so they drew upon the Enlightenment philosophy of 'optimism', which maintained that despite apparent inequality and hardship all was ultimately for the best in the best of possible worlds.

Jebb's mentor Edmund Law made an important (if belated) contribution to this Anglican polemic with his *Theory of Religion*.[25] Law had become a convinced 'optimist' as a result of his work on William King's *Essay on the Origin of Evil*: the only way to understand God's creation was to appreciate that not one natural defect or inconvenience 'could possibly have been prevented without a greater'.[26] To this Law added the associationist psychology espoused by John Gay and later developed by David Hartley, which held out the possibility of continued moral improvement through education. Law claimed that the real issue was a lack of universally equal comprehension of either revealed or natural religion. Everyone may grasp the basic principles of both, but there was a difference in the quality and refinement of that understanding across various times, places and stations in life. Reaffirming that revelation is essentially an extension of natural religion with the added assurance of an afterlife, Law advanced the original thesis that our comprehension of Christianity was constantly improving.[27] 'Mankind are not',

---

[21] Henry G. van Leeuen, *The Problem of Certainty in English Thought: 1630-1690* (The Hague, 1963); 'Life of Jebb', p. 19; Basil Willey, *The Eighteenth-Century Background* (Harmondsworth, 1972 [1940]), pp. 79-85.

[22] R.K. Webb, 'The Faith of Nineteenth-Century Unitarians: a curious incident', in Richard J. Helmstadter and Bernard Lightman eds., *Victorian Faith in Crisis: essays on continuity and change in nineteenth-century religious belief* (1990), p. 128.

[23] Matthew Tindal, *Christianity as Old as the Creation* (1730).

[24] This was given its classic statement in Joseph Butler's *Analogy of Religion and Nature* (1736).

[25] This went through seven editions between 1745 and 1784, was translated into German in 1771, and appeared in an eighth edition in 1820.

[26] William King, *An Essay on the Origin of Evil* (Edmund Law ed., 3rd ed., 1739), p. 224n; see John Stephens, 'Edmund Law and his circle at Cambridge: some philosophical activity of the 1730s', in G.A.J. Rogers and Sylvana Tomaselli eds., *The Philosophical Canon in the 17th and 18th Centuries. Essays in Honour of John W. Yolton* (Rochester, New York, 1996), pp. 163–73. In his dialogue with King's text, Law was concerned to outline a utilitarian system of ethics.

[27] Leslie Stephen, *History of English Thought in the Eighteenth Century* (Crane Brinton ed., New York, 1962 [1876]), p. 344.

he observed, 'nor ever have been, capable of entering into the Depths of Knowledge at once, of receiving a whole System of Natural or Moral Truths together; but must be let into them by degrees'. Thus, Christianity could never have been 'as old as the creation', because it could only arise when the human mind was appropriately developed. Drawing an analogy with the growth of an individual human being, he claimed that our knowledge as a whole was growing from an original state of barbarism and ignorance to an increasingly true understanding of God's word and works. He pointed to the incredible advances made in the natural sciences and argued that the same progress was possible in regard to understanding the Christian revelation.[28] The reason religious knowledge had not kept pace with natural philosophy, Law suggested, was because the principles of empirical science had not been fully applied to theology. 'I believe', he wrote, 'that as all Arts and Sciences, every improvement in natural and civil life are still drawing near to perfection ... so it is probable that the Knowledge of Religion alone is not at a stand; but on the contrary, that as we continually advance in the study of God's Works, so we will come to a proportionally better understanding of his *Word*'.[29]

To achieve this Law advocated close, critical and uninhibited study of the Scriptures in their original languages, combined with a free and candid exchange of ideas between students. This, he believed, would lead to agreement on the meaning of particular words, doctrinal disputes would come to an end, and a simple rational Christianity would stand revealed to all willing to look. Confident that he had answered the main deist objection, Law thought the way remained open toward an increasingly enlightened Christianity.[30]

THE THIRTY-NINE ARTICLES

If deism had been substantially defeated on English soil, that did not see an end to religious dispute. During the 1750s debate revived over subscription to the Thirty-Nine Articles of the Anglican Church, a controversy in which Jebb would eventually become an active participant and that resulted in the fracture and weakening of the Latitudinarian position.[31] In the year that Jebb graduated, William Samuel Powell (1717-75) preached a Commencement Sunday sermon, which was subsequently published as *A Defence of the Subscriptions required in the Church of England* (1757). Powell (fellow of St John's since 1740 and master since 1765) was to lead those conservatives who opposed Jebb's education reform proposals in the 1770s. His sermon sought to address concern over subscription, which had died down after 1720 following the debate sparked by Samuel Clarke, but had revived in 1749 when an Anglican clergyman

---

[28] Law, *Theory of Religion*, pp. 51-3, 233.

[29] Law, *Theory of Religion*, pp. 182-84.

[30] Richard Brinkley, 'A Liberal Churchman: Edmund Law (1703-87)', *E&D*, 6 (1987), pp. 6-11; R.S. Crane, *The Idea of the Humanities* (Chicago, 1967), pp. 251-287.

[31] Martin Fitzpatrick, 'Latitudinarianism at the Parting of the Ways', in Walsh, Haydon and Taylor, *The Church of England c.1649-c.1833*, pp. 209-227.

suggested a new translation of the Bible and amendments to the liturgy.[32] More immediately, Powell was responding to the heretical outbursts of an Anglo-Irish bishop.

Robert Clayton (1695-1758) became Bishop of Clougher in 1745, and was known for his unbounded generosity. An intimate friend of Samuel Clarke, he wrote a number of pamphlets vindicating the chronology of the Bible and answering the deists. In 1751 he published a tract full of Arian theology, which drew many attacks from across the theological spectrum.[33] William Jones later dated the resurgence of the High Church party from the response to Clayton's tract.[34] This work went through a number of editions, and if Jebb did not read it himself in Dublin, he can scarcely have been ignorant of the controversy that raged and cost Clayton the chance to become Archbishop of Tuam. A speech by Clayton in the House of Lords in 1756 arguing that the Nicene and Athanasian Creeds should be removed from the liturgy caused a stir, and went through many published editions into the nineteenth century. He followed this with his *Vindication of the Old and New Testament* (1757), which contained so many heretical criticisms that the government decided to order his prosecution – but Clayton died before they could proceed. Observing the scorn and condemnation that High Churchmen were capable of pouring on a morally admirable ecclesiastic who deviated from theological orthodoxy must have made an impact on Jebb. When later writing in support of the clerical petition against subscription, he declared that 'the time is come when the injured Clayton shall again be heard … and the heroes of a second reformation will arise'.[35]

Powell dismissed Clayton's arguments and asserted that it was necessary to retain an official standard of orthodoxy for the Church. He also claimed, however, that the Articles were general, indeterminate and 'left room for improvements in theology'. In traditional Latitudinarian style, Powell argued that the Articles were not being subscribed to as entirely true and infallible, but rather as a useful instrument for ensuring religious harmony. In B.W. Young's words, 'Powell declared that the legacy of history (understood as a progressive, Protestant dynamic) had procured a doctrinal ease for believers which was best shaped by adherence to the Thirty-Nine Articles. His peroration took the form of an appeal to latitude and experience, explicitly countering the claims of experiment and perfectionism.'[36] Powell's sermon reflected a conservative Latitudinarianism developed by clergymen associated with St John's College. Republished at the height of the Feathers Tavern controversy (discussed in

---

[32] John Jones, *Free and Candid Disquisitions relating to the Church of England*, (1749); Jones was defended by Francis Blackburne, *An Apology for the Author of the Free and Candid Disquisitions*, (1751); Jebb also referred to the *Candid Disquisitions* in his writings on behalf of the Feathers Tavern petition, see Jebb III, pp. 12, 48.

[33] Robert Clayton, *Essay on Spirit ... with some remarks on the Athanasian and Nicene Creeds* (Dublin, 1751). On the importance of this controversy see Nigel Aston, 'The Limits of Latitudinarianism: English reactions to Bishop Clayton's *An Essay on Spirit*', *Journal of Ecclesiastical History*, 49 (1998), pp. 407-33.

[34] George Horne, *The Works of George Horne* (William Jones ed., 1809), I, p. 9.

[35] Jebb III, p. 8.

[36] Young, *Religion and Enlightenment*, p. 46.

chapter 5), its argument was echoed in the works of Thomas Balguy and Samuel Hallifax. Its publication in 1757 (the year of Jebb's graduation) inaugurated a new round of religious controversy that would develop into a 'competition between Enlightenment and Counter-Enlightenment'.[37]

Foremost among the Hoadlieans who answered Powell was Archdeacon Francis Blackburne (1705-87) who declared that Clayton was a 'good Bishop upon whose grave every lover of truth and liberty will drop a friendly tear'.[38] He appealed to the students of Cambridge and Oxford universities to seriously consider the contents of the Articles, to which they would be asked, before God, to swear belief. He warned those intending to undertake a career in the Church to avoid the mistake made by many older clergymen who had subscribed in youthful ignorance, but subsequently came to hold grave doubts regarding the truth of orthodox doctrine. Men such as himself were now in the position of having to practice and defend a creed in which they did not fully believe, unable to abandon without great hardship their means of living, or to leave a calling to which they had been drawn by God. Thus, they tended to endorse the *use* rather than the *truth* of the liturgy, and to live in hope of reform.[39] But young men like Jebb intent on a career in the Church need not trap themselves in such a morally compromising position. 'To be ingenious with you', Blackburne wrote, 'I apprehend that such of you as have the best capacities of understanding, and the deepest impressions of religion on your minds, will upon a serious and impartial examination of this important case, find the greatest reluctance in yourselves to comply with these terms of ministerial conformity.' He urged such young men to choose an alternative career for which their mathematical studies made them suited, such as 'military, naval, mercantile, and mechanical employments'. Blackburne speculated that if many talented young men turned away from the Church, and publicly owned their reason for doing so, the Anglican hierarchy might be forced to make those reforms 'which so many good men have been so long pleading and sighing for in vain'.[40]

Francis Blackburne became a significant intellectual influence on Jebb, and it is possible that the young graduate would have read a tract so relevant to his own position. Closely associated with Edmund Law, Blackburne was to become the leading advocate of reform of the Church. While Blackburne noted in 1770 that 'he did not have the honour to be personally acquainted with [Jebb]',[41] his influence is evident. While John Disney had been a student of

---

[37] Young, *Religion and Enlightenment*, p. 47.

[38] Francis Blackburne, *Remarks on the Rev. Dr Powell's Sermon in defence of Subscriptions* (1758), p. xiv.

[39] Blackburne, *Remarks on Dr Powell's Sermon*, pp. xiv-xix.

[40] Blackburne, *Remarks on Dr Powell's sermon*, pp. ix, xx.

[41] This is extracted from a letter signed 'Cantabrigiensis, E Claustris, Oct 4'. It was probably the work of Blackburne, the initials 'ADB' are pencilled into the copy in Dr Williams' Library, as is 'Dr Jebb' when the 'lecturer at Cambridge' is mentioned. in [Francis Blackburne ed.], *A Collection of Letters and Essays in Favour of Public Liberty, 1764-70* (1774), III, pp. 245, 259.

Jebb's at Cambridge, their mature friendship ripened 'under the auspices of Archdeacon Blackburne'.[42] When Jebb went out of his way to visit Blackburne in 1775 he was 'pleased to find that I stood high in the Archdeacon's estimation, which I look upon as one of the most favourable testimonies I could receive'.[43]

It is of course possible that Jebb did not read Blackburne's tract. But if he did, it is understandable that he continued on his path toward a career in the Church. We must make allowance for the rhetorical aim of Blackburne's work: a committed Anglican, he lived in hope of reform, and he expressed his arguments and predictions in the most forceful way possible. At the completion of his education, Jebb was committed to academic life and the Church in which his father was a comfortable clergyman. Significant theological and ecclesiological debates were gaining momentum during Jebb's early days at Cambridge and the prospects for reform must have appeared promising.

Driven by veneration for Milton and Luther and their insistence on the primacy of private judgement,[44] Blackburne owed 'his principles to a very accidental piece of advice given him at the age of seventeen, by a worthy old lay gentleman, who said, "young man, let the first book thou readest at Cambridge be Locke upon government"'. He followed this advice, and as a result of conversation with 'liberal minded friends' and 'the reading of Locke, Hoadly, &c. [he] acquired a strong attachment to the principles of ecclesiastical and civil liberty'. In the event, he was denied a college fellowship because he 'disclosed his sentiments too freely' in a speech on the 5th of November, and offended the 'High Royalists' who dominated Catherine Hall.[45]

Blackburne settled at Richmond in Yorkshire, and over the years his thoughts on religion were influenced by his regular correspondence and frequent conversations with Edmund Law.[46] After much coaxing and encouragement by Law, Blackburne finally published his magnum opus *The Confessional: or, a full and free inquiry into the Right, Utility, Edification, and Success of establishing systematical confessions of faith and doctrine in Protestant Churches* (1766).[47] At the outset he boldly declared that

> JESUS CHRIST hath, by his gospel, called all men unto liberty, that glorious liberty of the sons of God, and restored to them the privilege of working out their own salvation by their understandings and endeavours.... In [the] Scriptures all things needful for spiritual living and man's soul's health are mentioned and shewed. Consequently, faith and conscience,

---

[42] 'Memoir of John Disney', DWL mss., p. 35.

[43] 'Life of Jebb', p. 103.

[44] Blackburne anonymously attacked Samuel Johnson for his criticism of Milton's political principles in the *Lives of the Poets*. [Francis Blackburne], *Remarks on Johnson's Life of Milton* (1780).

[45] Francis Blackburne, *The Works Theological and Miscellaneous* (F. Blackburne jr. ed., 7 vols., Cambridge, 1805), I, p. iv.

[46] Blackburne, *Works*, I, p. lxxvii.

[47] Edmund Law was 'the only person who knew of *The Confessional* for some years, and actually suggested the title of it while the work was yet in embryo'. Blackburne, *Works*, I, p. lxxxviii.

having no dependence upon man's laws, are not compelled by man's authority.[48]

David Hartley had argued forcefully in his *Observations on Man* that the individual was duty bound to relentlessly pursue truth in all fields. Following the logic of this view Blackburne in effect declared as unchristian the practice of subscription to the Thirty-Nine Articles, even if a latitude of interpretation were allowed. The articles of the Anglican Church had been drawn up as statements of religious truth, he argued, and should be accepted or rejected as such – a latitude of interpretation was neither originally intended or possible. In arguing so Blackburne rejected the latitudinarian compromise whereby passive assent to the Thirty-Nine Articles was justified for practical reasons. The right and duty to espouse the truth as it appeared to one's conscience was more important, Blackburne argued, than the utility of requiring subscription to an orthodox doctrine.[49] Mainstream Whigs had long congratulated themselves on their toleration of Dissent. Blackburne, however, presented a powerful case for extending religious rights to allow Anglican clergymen to freely determine and preach their own sense of the doctrines contained in the Bible. This represented a broader, more positive conception of religious liberty which chimed with contemporary arguments for broader political representation and participation.

Archbishop Secker responded furiously to the *Confessional*, and sought out proof of the author. In the heated controversy that ensued, Blackburne's house became a centre for those favouring reform in Church and State (it was there that Joseph Priestley met Theophilus Lindsey in 1769). In the preface to the second edition, Blackburne claimed the popularity of the *Confessional* as proof 'that the love of RELIGIOUS LIBERTY is still warm in the hearts of a considerable number of the good people of *England*'. One of those people was John Jebb.[50]

GREEK NEW TESTAMENT LECTURES

The controversy occasioned by the *Confessional* no doubt encouraged Jebb's critical study of the Scriptures. Jebb's first significant contribution to the campaign against subscription was a course of lectures on the Greek New Testament, which he commenced in November 1768. As the heterodox flavour of these lectures became known throughout the University, the grumbling of conservatives became louder, and Jebb was 'branded with every name that the fiery spirit of *odium theologicum* could desire'.[51] One of the leaders of this condemnation was Thomas Rutherforth, the ageing Professor of Divinity (1756-71). Jebb's theological lectures were a direct challenge to this professor who had published works on moral philosophy and attacks upon Blackburne's *Confessional*, but gave no lectures on divinity. Infuriated by Jebb's lectures,

[48] Blackburne, *Confessional* (2nd ed., 1767), pp. 1-2.
[49] Fitzpatrick, 'Latitudinarianism at the Parting of the Ways', pp. 216-25.
[50] Blackburne, *Confessional*, p. i. For an overview of the controversy see John Disney, *A Short View of the Controversies Occasioned by The Confessional* (1773).
[51] 'Luther' [John Disney], *London Chronicle*, 19 February 1771.

Rutherforth responded by informing his ecclesiastical superiors of their nature while warning students against attending.[52] Eyebrows were raised throughout the University. A fellow of Peterhouse told a visitor Jebb promoted 'Socinianism and Fatalism' in his lectures, and 'laughs at the 39 articles in his room'.[53] According to William Cole, William Warburton informed Archbishop Cornwallis that lectures were being read at Cambridge in which 'the Arian Doctrine was taught and inculcated'. In response, Cole claimed, in the spring of 1770 Jebb wrote 'a most violent invective letter to the Bishop of Gloucester impeaching his Christianity and Humanity'. When no reply was made, Jebb wrote to the Archbishop, who responded with a letter of 'great Dignity, Moderation and Spirit', according to Cole, in which he 'blamed Mr Jebb's conduct'.[54] In Jebb's account, after Bishop Warburton had alleged he was 'endeavouring to overturn the established religion of this country', 'in the hope of softening the prejudices of some worthy men' he had sent an explanation and outline of his lectures 'to some persons of eminence in the Church'. But this had only made things worse, as 'accusations were everywhere multiplied'.[55]

In late 1770 Samuel Hallifax gave up the Arabic Professorship for the more prestigious chair of Civil Law (for which he had been designated successor). Yet Jebb had come to be seen as dangerous by too many members of the University and he was again passed over for the position in favour of a less controversial candidate.[56] He proceeded to publish *A Short Account of Theological Lectures now reading at Cambridge, to which is added a New Harmony of the Gospels* (1770), a tract that did nothing to allay orthodox concerns. Commenting on the second edition (1772), Cole noted that 'By the first paragraph expounding on *private judgement*, Reason, Civil and Religious Liberty one may guess at what he would be at'. Jebb's lectures had given 'great offence to those whose principles are steady to the Church of England and Orthodoxy', and 'it is said he explains away the Divinity of our Saviour ... and in other ways instils pernicious and dangerous Principles into his pupils, subversive to Religion and Government'.[57]

In addition to upsetting orthodox churchmen, Jebb succeeded in drawing some public attention. One writer urged the University not to impose any censure requested by the 'ungenerous, illiberal and interested' opponents of the 'worthy and ingenious Lecturer'.[58] Francis Blackburne reflected upon the

---

[52] 'Life of Jebb', p. 28; William Cole, BL Cole mss. 5873:52b.

[53] G.M. Ditchfield and Bryan Keith-Lucas eds., *A Kentish Parson: selections from the private papers of the Revd. Joseph Price, Vicar of Brabourne, 1767-86* (Kent County Council, 1991), p. 66.

[54] BL Cole mss. 5873:52b. Jebb later observed that Warburton had 'in a very public manner' accused 'a member of the Church of England of a departure from his subscriptions, but, though solemnly called upon, has not chosen to attempt a confirmation of his charge by the proper evidences'. 'Paulinus', *Whitehall Evening Post*, 21 January 1772, Jebb I, p. 174.

[55] *Short Account of Theological Lectures*, Jebb I, pp. 17, 7.

[56] 'Life of Jebb', p. 27.

[57] BL Cole mss. 5873:52.

[58] 'Hoadleianus', Winchester, 29 Sept. 1770, in Blackburne, *A Collection of Letters*, III, p. 242.

days when Cambridge was dominated by men 'of the most liberal sentiments' who encouraged learning and free inquiry. That these days were long past was attested by the opposition to 'this worthy Lecturer' by the 'Jesuitical clan' at Cambridge.[59] Blackburne claimed that the lecturer had 'submitted his plan to public judgement, to the no small mortification of his adversaries', and it revealed him as a man 'to whom much of the little credit' that Cambridge had left was owed. Lamenting the attempt to stifle Jebb's lectures by powerful men in the Church, Blackburne appealed to the popular political ferment surrounding Wilkes and America: 'Ye virtuous patriots, who have been so successful in laying open to your injured countrymen the iniquities of their *civil* oppressors (the principle fosterers of these men's ambition) have ye no drenches for these ecclesiastical cormorants?'[60] John Disney suggested that Jebb's predicament demonstrated how little the idea of religious liberty had progressed since the sixteenth century among those 'Protestant brethren' who still behaved like 'a conclave of Cardinals'. 'Thanks to heaven', he reflected, 'a different spirit prevails among the younger students'.[61]

Another correspondent observed that with the publication of Jebb's *Short Account* those who 'opposed him in the University by their *authority*, should oppose him in the face of the world by their *reason*', rather than simply whip up fear of his 'libertine' teaching. 'Last summer I met with a Lady who was under the deepest distress for a near relation of her's at Cambridge, because his Tutor was a follower of one Mr J-bb, who was a vile fellow, and taught such abominable doctrines that her relation, a man of consequence, was in danger.'[62] He called on the 'universal Dr Hallifax' to 'drop for the moment the weightier matters of the law, and take this opportunity of opposing the Lecturer like a *man*, [whom] he once opposed in the Affair of the Arabic Professorship like a *courtier*'.[63] In light of the strong reactions they provoked, we need to look closely at the method and theology espoused in Jebb's lectures.

In his *Short Account* Jebb tried to argue that he was not 'inculcating upon the minds of my pupils' a set of heterodox doctrine, but rather, promoting a method that would encourage study and facilitate private judgement. He refuted what he claimed were the two main accusations against him: denial of the Immaculate Conception and free will. Choosing his words carefully, he claimed that as the 'messiahship of Jesus' was proved by his miracles, belief in the Immaculate Conception 'follows of course'. In so arguing, Jebb sidestepped the real criticism: that he denied the full divinity of Christ. On the issue of free

---

59 'Cantabrigiensis', 4 Oct. 1770, in Blackburne, *A Collection of Letters*, III, pp. 244-45.

60 'Cantabrigiensis', Dec. 1770, in Blackburne, *A Collection of Letters*, III, p. 159.

61 'Luther', *London Chronicle*, 19 February 1771.

62 'P.P'. [J.F.] , 26 Feb. 1771, *London Chronicle*. This correspondent may have been John Firebrace, as John Disney inserted the initials J.F. next to the initials P.P. – see DWL mss. 87.6. Firebrace wrote elsewhere that had sixteenth-century Church reformers 'lived to see the improvement of scripture knowledge, upon the rational interpretations of *Locke, Clarke, Taylor, Law, Sykes, Benson, Dawson, [and] Jebb'*, they would not have drawn up the Thirty-nine Articles. [John Firebrace], *A Further Defence of the Present Scheme of Petitioning Parliament* (1771), p. 35.

63 'P.P'. [J.F.], 26 Feb. 1771, *London Chronicle*.

will, he admitted to being 'a little inclined to the system of Hartley and of Locke', but claimed the important point was that he had always believed that 'man is a moral agent, in the strictest sense'. At any rate, the lectures were designed to discourage philosophical and metaphysical speculation.[64] Jebb admitted that he had, after 'some years of incessant study ... deduced a system of faith and practice'. But he claimed that in his course of lectures he was not 'anxiously desirous' to impress this system upon the students. Any heterodox notions they arrived at were a result of the method, rather than direct instruction – the 'train of ideas arising in their minds' could lead to conclusions different to 'what the same Scriptures seemed to suggest in the time of our great reformers'. Such conclusions were the result of using the numerous learned commentaries on the Bible available in an enlightened age, and 'from a variety of other sources, which must crowd upon the mind of every candid thinking person'. Rather than adopting the 'groundless and odious supposition of my professedly inculcating a set of opinions', Jebb directed his critics to the effects of candid scientific study.[65]

Such a judiciously worded defence was designed to appeal to enlightened sensibilities, rather than silence orthodox alarm bells. While claiming that he was not 'inculcating' a set of doctrines, Jebb admitted that when examining texts used to prove 'certain doctrines', he stated what he thought to be the 'plain and natural meaning' of the passage. Pointing out to students that 'other worthy persons of the greatest name have been of different opinion from myself' can hardly have satisfied his critics.[66] Their concerns were justified. In his manuscript notes Jebb jotted: '"The most effectual way to overthrow error is to establish truth." A useful hint, and falls in with my idea of divinity lectures.'[67]

In the second edition of his *Short Account* (1772) Jebb compared his lectures to those of Edward Bentham, Professor of Divinity at Oxford.[68] Bentham's lectures discouraged 'that generous principle of free inquiry', and were designed to instil an acceptance of the orthodox interpretation. Jebb thought the comparison explained the opposition to his own lectures by 'the majority of the heads of houses, and almost every prelate who has the least connection' with Cambridge. The bishops opposed scientific study of the Bible. As the 'pontifical powers' had once feared that

> an inquiry into the operations of nature might shake down the philosophy of Moses, their lordships are alarmed, lest a mode of investigation, which succeeded so happily when the WORKS of God were the subject, might, if resolutely pursued

---

[64] *Short Account of Theological Lectures,* Jebb I, pp. 17-21.
[65] *Short Account of Theological Lectures,* Jebb I, pp. 25-6.
[66] *Short Account of Theological Lectures,* Jebb I, p. 35. Years later Jebb declared that in his lectures he always declared his own belief in the 'proper unity of God; and that He alone should be the proper object of religious worship'. J.J. to Dr William Chambers, 21 October 1775, 'Life of Jebb', p. 106.
[67] 'Theological Propositions', Jebb II, p. 159.
[68] Edward Bentham D.D., *Reflections upon the Study of Divinity* (Oxford, 1771).

> in the case of his WORD, prove fatal to that system of theological opinions, which, for certain reasons ... they now so strenuously uphold.[69]

A scientific approach to the Bible was necessary for a true conception of Christianity. Yet this kind of study was discouraged, Jebb claimed, because it undermined the doctrines on which the power and privilege of the ecclesiastical hierarchy were based.

Edmund Law did not play an active role in the *Confessional* controversy because he was a bishop with a large family whose future prospects he would not damage. Law's relative silence led conservatives to allege (with some justification) that Jebb was acting on his behalf.[70] Cole recorded that while preaching a controversial sermon on subscription in 1773, Jebb, 'looking up to the Heads laughed at the Bishop of Carlisle, who had his hand or cap before his face; this Mr Essex observed particularly who told me two days after, that he has frequently seen him do the same and the Bishop laugh [back?] at him; how ... in character [are?] both is easy to determine'.[71] Jebb boasted that 'many worthy characters' approved of his lectures. In response to rumours that he was acting on behalf of Law, he declared that he had commenced his lectures 'without the encouragement or suggestion of any person whatsoever'.[72] Yet it is clear that Law encouraged the studies from which the lectures resulted. At the start of the fourth volume of Jebb's interleaved New Testament he wrote the simple note: 'Newton – Locke – Law'. In 1767 Jebb had 'frequent communications with Dr Law', which John Disney considered 'an acknowledgement of the information he ever sought, and derived, from one so well informed in Scripture knowledge'. Jebb began his critical study of the Greek New Testament toward the end of that year.[73]

Echoing Edmund Law, Jebb directed those who claim that 'it is not likely that we should have a better knowledge of divine things' than in the past, to consider the advances in 'our works of elegance and taste'. In everything, 'orthodox taste' was 'giving way to nature in her loveliest simplicity, though improved by all the powers of art'. Likewise, we 'also see monkish superstition retiring before the powers of industry and common sense'.[74] Accordingly, he urged students of the Bible to 'make Newton our guide. Simplicity and magnificence in the works of God, the same to be searched for in the word'. He outlined four rules to guide his students throughout the course of the lectures:

1. Attend to evidence not imagination.

---

[69] *Short Account of Theological Lectures,* Jebb I, pp. 54-5.

[70] According to Warburton, Jebb was 'protected and encouraged' by Law. BL Cole mss. 5873:52b.

[71] BL Cole mss. 5873:53.

[72] *Short Account of Theological Lectures,* Jebb I, pp. 6, 54.

[73] 'Life of Jebb', p. 20. The first note in Jebb's interleaved Greek New Testament is dated 1767, and the second is 6 January 1768. Jebb completed his reading on June 7, 1768. His course of lectures commenced in November. DWL Jebb mss. I.

[74] DWL Jebb mss. IV.

2. Admit no opinion of mine unless you think it supported by proper evidence.
3. Hereafter reject any sentiment of mine if you perceive it false.
4. Keep your mind open to evidence.[75]

In a note written in June 1770 he observed how in the past many philosophers had accepted facts without rigorous examination, and so had invented hypotheses to solve them, which led to 'strange Doctrines' like the cycles and epicycles of Ptolemaic astronomy. Likewise, 'ill understood texts' were the bogus facts that gave rise to doctrines in religion such as the Trinity and Original Sin. 'The reasonableness of an Hypothesis does not prove it true', and empiricism should guide the study of both nature and the Scriptures. Only through 'experiment in philosophy', he argued, '[and] critical knowledge of the Scriptures ... [does] nature and Scripture stand evidently disclosed to our view'. 'Search the Scriptures', Jebb urged, 'search facts [and] use Newton's rule of philosophising'.[76]

Jebb's method was historical as well as critical. He acknowledged that many statements in the Bible had to be read with knowledge of their social, political and intellectual context. In this he was consciously following the influential work of Bishop Robert Lowth. An expert on Hebrew poetry, Lowth argued that the Scriptures must be studied as an expression of a former society, rather than as an outline of God's preferred form of government.[77] In this spirit, Jebb drew from Montesquieu the insight that 'we must not separate the Laws from the Circumstances in which they are made', as a guide to reading Scripture.[78] One should investigate the 'reigning ideas and controversies of the apostles' times, and by them interpret their words'. The New Testament was 'a history of discourses to particular persons, not a set of rules intended for all men indiscriminately'.[79]

Not only did the texts reflect the customs and concerns of the time, but they also reflected the ignorance and primitive language of the age. Jebb believed the evangelists had made a number of mistakes in their narration. Yet, while he thought Matthew was 'not a very judicious Historian according to our Ideas', he thought this was understandable because the evangelist wrote for his contemporary audience rather than later ages.[80] The Gospel writers at times

---

[75] DWL Jebb mss. VI.

[76] DWL Jebb mss. IV.

[77] Jebb placed at the start of his *Short Account* a large extract from Lowth urging study of the Scriptures and declaring that 'an opinion is not therefore false because it contradicts received notions: but, whether true or false, let it be submitted to a fair examination; truth must be the gainer by it, and appear with greater evidence'. *Short Account of Theological Lectures,* Jebb I, p. 4. See also B. Hepworth, *Robert Lowth* (Boston, 1978), chapter 1.

[78] The Epistles were important because so much orthodox doctrine derived from them. Locke had paid them particularly close attention, and observed that in Romans 13 Paul was silent regarding the right qualifications of the 'higher powers' that one must obey. John Locke, *A Paraphrase and Notes on the Epistles of St Paul* (Arthur W. Wainwright ed., Oxford, 1987 [1707]).

[79] 'As in I Cor 15:3', he added. 'Theological Propositions', Jebb II, p. 140.

[80] DWL Jebb mss. I; lecture 36, DWL Jebb mss. VI.

described things in 'general terms', and thus 'put their own words into the mouths of the speakers, to render it consistent', while Paul may have adopted the Jewish mode of interpreting scripture and arguing inconclusively.[81] The Bible was full of metaphorical statements: for example, that Jesus sits at the right hand of God and his enemies will be his footstool was a figurative expression.[82] On finishing the Greek New Testament, Jebb concluded that:

> The older a language is, the more corporeal it is, for all language derived itself from body prepositions denoting the relations of place, and many terms being purely corporeal at first therefore the figurative expressions would be more glaring. When they wanted to represent abstract or general ideas, particular names would be used instead of general names, as 'today' for 'the present time'.... Parables would stand for moral abstract truths, and justly for they raise the same affections. Everything, in short, would bc visible and tangible, rites and ceremonies would stand for doctrines and events, unity of existence for unity of design and opinion, local decent from Heaven stand for divine commission ... let no-one object that interpretation on such a plan is mystical or allegorical – it is literal though figurative. [83]

Behind primitive Biblical metaphor lay literal truth. To aid interpretation, one should study the language of 'barbarous nations' like the North American Indians, as 'they speak much in figure'. Jebb also thought it helpful to 'search the Koran for evidences and illustrations of scripture'.[84] Through this critical and comparative approach Jebb expected to uncover the true doctrine contained in the New Testament: 'As it appeared absurd to suppose, that the same passage could in fact admit of various senses, I was contented when I had found that one, which, from the consideration of its connection with the other parts of the discourse, appeared to be the meaning of the speaker, and, consequently, seemed to be that very sense, in which he would have wished to be understood.'[85]

Harmonising the Gospels was central to Jebb's method of reading the Bible. He instructed his students to draw four columns on a piece of paper – one for each Gospel. As they read the New Testament in Greek, they had to note the passages in each Gospel (if any) that dealt with each separate incident. Then, based only on the passages from Scripture that described an incident, the student had to write his own paraphrase. The student should confine himself to terms used in the Gospels and avoid adopting the language of scriptural commentators. This would lead the student to construct his own clear and concise account of the actions and teachings of Jesus. The aim was 'to imprint upon the mind such an idea of the actions and discourses of our redeemer, and of their most material concomitant circumstances, as may enable the student, from a consideration of

[81] 'Theological Propositions', Jebb II, pp. 144, 147.
[82] 'Theological Propositions', Jebb II, p. 138.
[83] DWL Jebb mss. I, p. 19.
[84] DWL Jebb mss. IV.
[85] *Short Account of Theological Lectures*, Jebb I, p. 23.

the particularities of time, place, and occasion, to form a just and accurate conception of all the Gospel doctrines'. Such accuracy could be achieved only if the student disregarded 'the manner of expression which he meets with in the Scripture, or in the commentators upon it'. The student must attempt to see through the figurative, rhetorical and generally distorted language of the texts, and construct his own paraphrase 'according to forms of expression conceived by himself'.[86]

The recently ordained Samuel Henley praised Jebb for entering in his prime upon endeavours which 'LOCKE and NEWTON, toward the close of life, regretted they had not earlier begun'. Where Francis Bacon had tried to 'strike off the shackles of the human mind' through 'the science of Nature', Jebb was attempting to do the same 'in the study of Revelation'.[87] Such praise was not entirely overblown. Theophilus Lindsey, founder of the Essex Street Unitarian church, declared in a private letter that 'of all persons I ever conversed with, [Jebb] has the most critical knowledge of the scriptures, and the best method of interpreting them'.[88] This was a considerable compliment when we consider that Lindsey stood at the centre of Rational Dissent and counted the likes of Richard Price and Joseph Priestley among his close friends. Priestley himself, however, was less enthusiastic about Jebb's very Baconian approach: 'If I were to lecture in divinity I would not take his method. It must be very tiresome to students and would keep them too long to one thing to the neglect of others. Besides, it is too timid a plan. Systems are the best for instruction, though they should be accompanied with particular instruction.' While he thought Jebb should have explicitly presented Unitarianism in his lectures, Priestley respected his knowledge of the Scriptures and included notes by Jebb in his own *Harmony of the Evangelists*.[89]

Jebb's method was eventually adopted by the 'Society for Promoting Knowledge of the Scriptures'. Established at the Essex Street Unitarian church in 1783 by the likes of Lindsey, Price and Andrew Kippis, Jebb wrote most of the Society's outline of intention.[90] Maintaining that 'the word of God ... like the book of nature, lies open to us all', the Society aimed to help remove 'the

---

[86] *Short Account of Theological Lectures,* Jebb I, p. 124.

[87] Samuel Henley, *The Distinct Claims of Government and Religion, considered in a sermon preached before the Honourable House of Burgesses, at Williamsburg in Virginia, March 1, 1772* (Cambridge, 1772), 'Dedication'.

[88] McLachlan, *Letters of Theophilus Lindsey*, p. 104.

[89] Joseph Priestley, *A Harmony of the Evangelists, in English, with Critical Dissertations ... Paraphrase and Notes* (1780); Joseph Priestley to Theophilus Lindsey, 27 January 1771 and 20 November 1777, Priestley, *Works,* I, pp. 130, 300.

[90] The original members of the Society were Theophilus Lindsey, John Disney, Andrew Kippis, Richard Price, Dr Chandler, the lawyer Michael Dodson, and the Rockingham Whig John Lee. The Society stagnated through a lack of original or 'ingenious' essays. Its 'plan was too circumscribed, and interfered too much with the larger, the more comprehensive, and more useful plan of the *Theological Repository,* at that time resumed by Dr Priestley'. In 1791 it was transmogrified into the more vigorous Unitarian Society. Belsham, *Memoirs of Lindsey*, pp. 131-32; Theophilus Lindsey to William Turner, 5 December 1785, DWL Lindsey-Turner correspondence.

cloud of human prejudices, which have so long obscured the heavenly light of truth' through an 'analytic' as opposed to the traditional 'synthetic' mode of inquiry. The Society would not accept essays 'written professedly in support of particular tenants or doctrines'. Contributors were to confine themselves to elucidating the rites, ceremonies, manners, or history of biblical times, or the language of the text. With a mind not 'warped in favour of any specific doctrine, or warmed with controversy', students of Scripture should sit down 'with the same calm and composed temper, with which we examine a passage in a Greek or Roman classic, whose genuine sense we are studious to explore'. The resulting correctly interpreted passages would, like 'a well-established experiment in philosophy', provide a sound empirical basis for the exercise of private judgement.[91]

SOCINIAN

We cannot know for certain the extent to which Jebb was disposed to Socinianism prior to his study of the Greek New Testament, but study of Hebrew, reading the Koran in Arabic and familiarity with Law's opinions suggest that Jebb was already far from orthodox. Indeed, the very act and manner of his study of the Greek New Testament suggest a mind wanting to explore, verify and willing to extend a heterodox tendency. His course of study had a profound effect: in June 1768 he finished 'the critical reading of all the Greek Testament (the revelations excepted for want of sufficient knowledge of history) … near 15 years after my admission to Dublin College, and upon the fairest review am persuaded of the truth of Christ's mission from the Almighty – and only lament that I had not performed this task 8 years ago and have only myself to blame that it was not so'.[92] In June 1760 Jebb had become a probationary fellow of Peterhouse and thus officially began his career in the Church. This and his ordination in 1762 does not preclude the possibility that he was already heterodox in his thinking. He chose Mark 8:38 as the basis of his ordination sermon: 'Whosoever, therefore, shall be ashamed of me and my words, in this adulterous and sinful generation, of him shall the son of Man be ashamed, when he cometh in the glory of his Father and with the holy angels.' This suggests that at this stage he was theologically an Arian, and shared widespread 'patriotic' concerns about moral and political corruption.

Whatever the nature of his prior theological opinions, his reading of the New Testament in Greek confirmed him as a Socinian – and it appears that had he been so in 1760 he may have pursued an alternative career. At the start of the first volume of his interleaved New Testament, Jebb noted:

> The idea which a person who reads the Scriptures in the English Bible or superficially in the original has of Christianity, differs as much from the notion he will have of it who studies the scriptures with critical exactness, as the sum

[91] *A Sketch of the Plan of the Society for Promoting the Knowledge of the Scriptures* (1783), Jebb II, pp. 239-53.
[92] DWL Jebb mss. I.

> of a long account consisting of pounds, shillings and pence, when the pounds are only reckoned, differs from the total sum when the shillings, pence and farthings are taken into the composition.[93]

Jebb evidently presented his lectures with the enthusiasm of one who had recently discovered truth. To understand the strong reactions they provoked, we need to consider the theology to which Jebb exposed his students.

One of the most important heretical doctrines held by Law, Blackburne and Jebb was that of 'mortalism' (known as the 'soul-sleeping system'). Exposure to debate over it during his undergraduate days may have set Jebb on the path to heterodoxy. This view considered the orthodox notion of the soul's existence in an intermediate immaterial state between death and the resurrection to be a Catholic corruption inspired by Greek philosophy.[94] This notion that the soul was insensible and 'slept' following death was popular among ultra-Protestants in the seventeenth century, and Blackburne found it implied in *Paradise Regained* when Christ utters: 'much of the soul they talk, but all awrie'.[95] Milton had championed 'the experimental knowledge of the Hebrews over the speculative knowledge of the Greeks', and there seemed to be no proof of an intermediate state for the soul in the Bible or at any time since. In many ways, mortalism represented 'a revolt by Protestant scripturalists against various strands of theological Platonism',[96] and it became a key issue in theological debate. Law defended mortalism in his doctoral examination in 1749 and published a tract 'concerning the use of the word SOUL in Holy Scripture; and the state of Death' in 1755.[97] Controversy over the issue raged during Jebb's undergraduate years, with Blackburne entering the debate on Law's side.[98]

In 1771 Professor Thomas Rutherforth (the main figure behind condemnation of his theological lectures) examined Jebb for a doctorate in divinity. The occasion provided Jebb with an opportunity to publicly challenge Rutherforth's theological opinions. To do so, he chose to argue the same thesis

---

[93] DWL Jebb mss. I.

[94] In his 32nd lecture Jebb discussed the nature of life after death. He noted the three Jewish sect's views on the soul and death: the Essenes believed in a separate state of the soul after death. The Pharasees believed in an *intermediate* state followed by a return to an *embodied state*. The Sadducees denied both. Jebb thought that Lucretious shared the Sadducee notion of the extinction of the soul upon death. However, 'the Christian if consistent in my Idea holds ... no intermediate state (Tim 1:10), which is one difference between the Pharasee and Christian'. DWL Jebb mss. VI.

[95] Milton, *Paradise Regained* (1673), iv, line 313. This text was the epigraph to Francis Blackburne, *A Short Historical View of the Controversy Concerning an Intermediate State and the Separate Existence of the Soul and the General Resurrection* (1765); Christopher Hill, *Milton and the English Revolution* (1977), chapter 25.

[96] B.W. Young, 'The "Soul-Sleeping System": politics and heresy in eighteenth-century England', *Journal of Ecclesiastical History*, 45 (1994), p. 74.

[97] Edmund Law, *Theory of Religion* (3rd ed., Cambridge, 1755), Appendix.

[98] Francis Blackburne, *No proof in the Scriptures for an intermediate state of happiness or misery between death and the resurrection* (1755). See also *The Autobiography of Joseph Priestley* (Jack Lindsay ed., Bath, 1970), p. 75.

on mortalism that had gained Law his doctorate. While, according to Disney, 'the disputation was conducted with ability and politeness upon both sides, and continued for a longer time than is generally employed in these exercises', Jebb's defence was declared unsuccessful. He responded with an attempt at public vindication through publication of his thesis.[99]

Jebb also gave an indication of his mortalism in the second edition of this *Short Account* when talking of the afterlife:

> The moral perfections of the soul, the virtues of the rational mind, touched by the rude hand of death, may perhaps, like the flower of the evening, close for a time their yet imperfect forms; but the gloomy night and darkness of the grave shall quickly pass, the morning of the resurrection shall arrive; they shall then expand their fragrant blossoms beneath the influence of brighter suns, and flourish in the possession of an eternal day.

At the resurrection we would rise 'from the bed of death'.[100] Mortalism touched the heart of Christian doctrine. It became a point of theological controversy that reflected deep philosophical differences, and the polarisation of political opinion.

Mortalism did not necessarily entail Socinianism. Francis Blackburne remained stoutly opposed to the latter position throughout his life, and thought the likes of Priestley, Lindsey and Jebb could hardly be considered Christians. Yet mortalism did lead many toward a heterodox view of Christ's person, and could even be a step toward making materialism palatable.[101] There seems to have been a substantial drift toward Socinianism among rational Christians from the late 1760s on, and in 1783 Edward Harwood could refer to the 'present triumphant Progress of *Socinianism*'.[102] Joseph Priestley was converted to the 'Socinian scheme' after reading Nathaniel Lardner's *Letter on the Logos* upon its appearance in 1768.[103] Jebb was familiar with Lardner's work, and the appearance of this book while he was immersed in study of the Scriptures can have had no small impact. According to Ronald Stromberg, Socinianism initially 'convinced few on scriptural grounds', and was effectively dismissed by Samuel Clarke. In the early decades of the century, interpreters were committed to rigid literalism, and found Socinianism 'too radical and too dubiously supported'.[104] The popularity of Socinianism in the later part of the century owed much to the

---

99 The question was: 'Status animarum in intervallo mortis atque resurrectionis agentium quicquam, sive sentientium ex sacris literis colligi nequit'. 'Life of Jebb', p. 29. For Jebb's *Thesis*, Jebb II, pp. 181-202.

100 *Short Account of Theological Lectures* (2nd ed., 1772), Jebb I, p. 51.

101 Hill, *Milton and the English Revolution*, pp. 317-33; While nobody was certain what Blackburne's view of Christ was, it is evident that he was at least not comfortable with the orthodox conception – he was probably an Arian.

102 Edward Harwood, *Of the Socinian Scheme* (2nd ed., 1783), p. 4.

103 Priestley, *Autobiography*, p. 93.

104 Samuel Clarke, *The Scripture-Doctrine of the Trinity* (1712); Stromberg, *Religious Liberalism*, pp. 41-2.

confident rationalism of the late Enlightenment and improving biblical hermeneutics.

Jebb considered Christ the last and greatest of a series of prophets.[105] He thought the doctrine of Christ's pre-existence to be both untenable and unnecessary.[106] Scripture showed Jesus to be a man, like David and John the Baptist, who had been chosen by God and invested with certain powers. John 11:22 revealed 'Jesus to be the son of God, declaring whatever he *asks* of God, God will grant him. [This is] a plain indication that He did not imagine that the title imported anything of equality, but only the Deity's affection.'[107] When Jesus talked of 'coming from God' he always used 'figurative language'; 'But he always appeals to his works ... [to] prove God *with him* not [that] he came *from* God'.[108] Praise was heaped upon Jesus because he was thought to be a new 'great king', not God.[109] That his Jewish opponents did not attack the doctrine of the Trinity suggested that Jesus was never identified in such a manner by himself or his immediate converts.[110]

Jebb also thought Christ's divine pre-existence philosophically unsound. One of several references to Lucretius is to a passage that seeks to demonstrate the union of mortal and immortal to be impossible.[111] Jebb thought it evident that Platonist theologians had created the Trinity through their own interpretation of the Gospels, and that the 'Holy Spirit' of the Scriptures was a figurative expression.[112] With regard to the Trinity and transubstantiation, he wrote: 'the evidence we have of the truth of the Gospels is not, cannot, be strong enough to support such violent departures from reason and common sense'.[113]

In what sense was Christ different from other mere mortals? Aside from his supernatural conception (a problematic doctrine eventually jettisoned by Priestley),[114] Christ had a greater degree of divine inspiration compared to

---

[105] Jebb referred to Jesus as 'the last great *Prophet*' who only taught more forcefully the doctrine of the Old Testament: love God and our neighbour. DWL Jebb Mss. IV.

[106] Jebb closed his lecture on the pre-existence of Christ with the observation that 'the question is therefore merely speculative ... [and] the example of Jesus [is] more forcible if he did not pre-exist'. Lecture 44, DWL Jebb mss. VI.

[107] 25 July 1772, DWL Jebb mss.

[108] DWL Jebb mss. VI, lecture 44.

[109] DWL Jebb mss. IV.

[110] DWL Jebb mss. III.

[111] Reference to Lucretius, *On the Nature of the Universe* (Harmondsworth, 1951), III 801; DWL Jebb mss. VI, lecture 44.

[112] '*That* by the intervention of which all things come to pass *is* God, *but*, by the intervention of the logos all things came to pass', thus 'the logos *is* God'. DWL Jebb mss. VI.

[113] DWL Jebb mss. IV.

[114] Joseph Priestley, *An History of Early Opinions concerning Jesus Christ, compiled from Original Writers* (Birmingham, 1786). In the words of McLachlan, 'in theological opinion Lindsey moved slowly, often reluctantly, forward under the influence of Priestley'. Rejection of the Immaculate Conception was one of the developments he found most difficult to accept. 'Fresh Light on the Life of Theophilus Lindsey, 1723-1808', in H. McLachlan, *Essays and Addresses* (Manchester, 1950), p. 53. When Priestley first talked of publishing his thoughts, Lindsey wrote: 'Still more will the outcry be increased against him, if it should

other prophets and evangelists. That Jesus could know 'of events beforehand' and predict 'the common occurrences of human life' in no way marked him out as the equal of God. Samuel had the same power, so 'the occasional knowledge of men's thought was communicated [by God, and thus was] not an inherent and a necessary power in our Lord'. Jebb offered a physical explanation for inspiration: it 'derived from the secret yet powerful influence of the wind, accompanied sometimes by an external symbol of the divine presence, as of a mighty rushing wind'.[115] Like miracles however, inspiration was only present in the world in Biblical times. Jebb concluded 'that the effusion of spirit ceased with the Apostles and that after the departure of the first converts from the world all inspiration ceased entirely and that the world is now governed by the ordinary providence of God'.[116] After listing texts where 'Jesus is compared to, or called by the names of various persons, substances, or mixed modes', Jebb noted that he was 'none of these in reality, all in figure'.[117] The simple 'matter of fact' was: 'God sent the Man Jesus, conceived in a supernatural manner, at the age of thirty to call men to repentance and to declare to them a future state. All the rest consists in allusions, applications of old scripture, prophecies, and Histories.'[118] Looking for a striking simile to explain Christ's status to his students, Jebb noted that 'Jesus appears to have been in his province as an *Agent* between the colonies and parent state.'[119] The resurrection remained as the only fundamental Christian revelation.[120] For Unitarians, Jesus was the greatest teacher of God's word who had shown the way to eternal life. Jebb was not troubled that the death of a human Jesus could not atone for human sinfulness,

---

appear that he has not proved his facts, and made good his accusation; which may be reasonably questioned in some instances. And not only myself, but Dr Jebb, and one other whom I have consulted, are persuaded that his chief argument fails him, when he would prove Christ's mistaken imperfect citation of the Old Testament similar to that of the rest of his countrymen, from Luke 24:27'. Lindsey later confessed that Jebb had not given the issue of the Immaculate Conception much consideration. Lindsey to Cappe, 2 December 1784 & 10 April 1787, Belsham, *Memoirs of Lindsey*, pp. 167, 175.

[115] See Acts 2:2, DWL Jebb mss. VI, lecture 45.

[116] DWL Jebb mss. VI, lecture 45.

[117] 'It is possible that the apostles might think that Jesus pre-existed when they remembered his strong impressions and when he talked of coming from Heaven. They mistook many other matters, why may not the notions of after ages arise from the highly figurative words of Jesus – from the attention paid by his hearers to those words, and from the metaphysical inquiring of after times'. DWL Jebb mss. VI, lecture 37.

[118] DWL Jebb mss. IV.

[119] Moses had likewise acted as an 'agent' of God. Jebb reminded his students that 'all similitudes are intended to illustrate', and it was the literal reading of these that had led to so much doctrinal confusion. Jebb Mss. VI.

[120] The narratives of the resurrection were 'not intended for evidence, but as a summary of things well known', the evidence being supplied first hand by those who ate and talked with Jesus. Jebb thought the resurrection was proved 'by considering Matthew's compendious account and his custom of attributing to many what was done by one'. Having Mary Magdalen see Jesus on her own was different to his usual way of relating things (having a group of men witness an event). This, Jebb thought, confirmed the truth of Matthew's account. Note written 26 September 1770, DWL Jebb mss. VI.

because he did not believe in original sin. There was no need for atonement, only for education.

Like most orthodox doctrine, Jebb sought to explain away atonement by uncovering its origins. 'Observe how Saint worship got in at the beginning of the fourth century', he wrote, 'and we shall see how the worship of Jesus got in at the beginning of the first'.[121] In the eighteenth century several writers developed the idea that the origin of sacrifice lay in primitive man's anthropomorphic notions of God.[122] Jebb likewise concluded that 'Rites are not parts, but helps to and symbols of Religion. Religion is the culture and right direction of the affections'. Sacrifice was 'an expression in symbols of those sentiments of the heart which now we express by words in prayer, and therefore had no value unless accompanied with such feelings of heart'.[123] The crucifixion of Jesus was, like the death of a soldier in battle, a necessary sacrifice for the greater good of the cause – but nothing more. There was no mystery, as Christ's death was easily explained 'from the history of what he attempted, and the circumstances of those times'.[124]

SCIENCE AND RELIGIOUS TRUTH

Jebb's criticism of orthodoxy must be viewed in the wider context of the Scientific Revolution and the Enlightenment – for him, the Reformation would only be complete when true Christianity stood firmly upon its scientific base, stripped of the encrustation of past superstition. In response to such attacks upon orthodoxy and episcopal authority, conservative Latitudinarians increasingly joined High Churchmen in criticising over-confidence in the powers of reason.

This is not to say that those of a conservative disposition did not embrace the Scientific Revolution. Most, like Samuel Johnson, were committed to the application of Newtonian methodology, but only when confined to natural philosophy.[125] Johnson emphatically denied the relevance of science to morality, and criticised John Milton for including natural philosophy in his school curriculum, as students should focus upon moral instruction that is best derived from 'poets, orators, and historians'. Beginning with his depiction of the 'mad astronomer' in *Rasselas* (1759), Johnson criticised the tendency to focus upon the achievements of science to the detriment of moral cultivation. 'The innovators whom I oppose are turning off attention from life to nature. They

---

[121] DWL Jebb mss. VI, 19 Nov 1772.

[122] *The Early Letters of Bishop Richard Hurd: 1739-1762* (Sarah Brewer ed., 1995), p. 154n; Arthur A. Sykes, *An Essay on the Nature, Design and Origin of Sacrifices* (1748); Joseph Priestley, *Institutes of Natural and Revealed Religion* (1774), esp. III, pp. 139-45.

[123] DWL Jebb mss. IV.

[124] 'Theological Propositions', Jebb II, p. 149.

[125] Richard G. Olson, 'Tory-High Church Opposition to Science and Scientism in the Eighteenth Century: the works of John Arbuthnot, Jonathan Swift, and Samuel Johnson', in J.G. Burke ed., *The Uses of Science in the Age of Newton* (Berkley, 1983), pp. 171-204; Stewart, 'Samuel Clarke, Newtonianism, and the factions of post-revolutionary England', pp. 53-72.

seem to think that we are placed here to watch the growth of plants, or the motion of the stars.'[126] Johnson also feared that an unrestrained and zealous faith in science may lead to proposals for radical political reform. In the words of Richard Olson, 'Johnson advocated no more than incremental change in material and political circumstances and no change whatsoever in religion'.[127] The fundamental difference between the likes of Jebb and Johnson was their attitude to religious truth: for conservatives, many distinctive Christian truths must, by their nature, remain forever shrouded in mystery. Yet for those committed to the ideal of a rational religion, all essential truths could be critically examined and better understood by the human mind.

Johnson reflects the general response of conservative Anglicans to the radical Enlightenment. Throughout the century the heterodox were accused of allowing reason and philosophy to capture their minds at the expense of the Scriptures. It was a criticism that they tirelessly denied and desperately tried to avoid. Samuel Clarke seems to have indicated why he made his Arian theology public in the form of a dense analysis of scripture when he wrote: 'the great objection against Men that think seriously and carefully about these things, is, that they are apt to adhere to their own *Reason* more than to *Scripture*: which is a most unjust Suggestion'.[128] Sixty years later Theophilus Lindsey resigned from the Church and established a Unitarian chapel based upon Clarke's revised doctrine and liturgy. His ecclesiastical superior, Dr Markham, the Bishop of Chester, chastised him for allowing 'carnal wisdom' to lead him away from orthodoxy. 'Philosophy will know everything', he wrote, 'and yet has discovered nothing; it is still a stranger to the essence of the meanest thing about us, and yet will know the essence of the Deity, and will say this and this is contrary to it. Our religion is supported by the fullest and clearest testimonies, and yet the whole is truly incomprehensible from the creation of man to his final resurrection.'[129] The reply from Lindsey was equally predictable: 'my faith is built not on a system of philosophy, but an impartial examination of the mind and will of God, as discovered in the Old and New Testament'.[130] As usual, the truth lay somewhere in the middle.

The Unitarians certainly did base their theology on intensive and critical reading of the Scriptures. But the defence of their reading of the Bible is reminiscent of the Baconian rhetoric of Robert Boyle and the early Royal Society for the Advancement of Science. Boyle argued that the Royal Society would discover and verify objective 'facts' through a carefully regulated collective process. Yet knowledge is never free from the attitudes and interests of its exponents. Boyle's program reflected his social and religious prejudices: a 'fact' was something assessed by a group of gentlemen guided by the 'right

---

[126] Samuel Johnson, 'Life of Milton', in *Poetry and Prose* (Mona Wilson ed., 1957), p. 822.
[127] Olson, 'Tory-High Church Opposition to Science', p. 199.
[128] Samuel Clarke to John Jackson, 23 October 1714, cited in Stewart 'Samuel Clark, Newtonianism and the Factions of Post-Revolutionary England', p. 58.
[129] Dr Markham, Bishop of Chester, to Theophilus Lindsey upon his resignation of the Vicarage of Catterick, 16 November 1773, Belsham, *Memoirs of Lindsey*, p. 385.
[130] *Memoirs of Lindsey*, p. 387.

reason' of a Christian.[131] We can reverse this insight for the rational Christians of the eighteenth century: they genuinely thought that they were conducting an impartial examination of God's word. Indeed, the Society for Promoting Knowledge of the Scriptures was an undertaking that in some ways mirrored the Royal Society. Yet aside from their social and political prejudices, the theology of rational Christians was influenced by their Baconian search for the 'facts' of revelation, and by their engagement with the philosophical context of the Enlightenment. In order to establish breathing space for science, Bacon had declared that religion and natural philosophy were separate and distinct types of knowledge. From the Cambridge Platonists onward, rational Christians denied the distinction, and by the late eighteenth century advanced rationalists were demanding that religion be treated like any other branch of science. Conservatives realised that behind contemporary heterodoxy lay the restless, unrestrained, and all-pervading critical attitude of the radical Enlightenment.

This is best illustrated by the three sermons Samuel Hallifax preached at Cambridge in response to the Feathers Tavern petition.[132] He condemned the 'airy pretensions to superior knowledge' or 'an overweening fondness for novelties, which seems to be an original frailty in some minds', and which meant that 'the teachers of false opinions have never failed of followers among the vicious or the vain'. John Disney identified such comments as personal abuse directed at Jebb (who attended the sermons).[133] In a clear rejection of his cousin's program of lectures, Hallifax observed that 'whenever the reapers of the word have given joyful expectations of a future harvest, the rank weeds of Heresy have secretly started up, and killed or stifled every cheerful hope of plenty'. In contrast to the 'modern innovators' within the Church (and in reference to Edmund Law), Hallifax asserted that the early Christians had 'studied the sacred oracles, not as containing a rule of Science, but a rule of Life: they were more busied in exploring the methods, by which the Evil of Sin could be done away, than in amusing speculations about its Origin; and little attentive to the Theory of Religion, their whole attention was directed to the Practice of it, by *Repentance toward God, and Faith toward our Lord Jesus Christ*'.[134]

To refute the 'favourite principle of these new gospelers, that the Redeemer was a *mere* Man', Hallifax pointed to the standard texts from the Gospel of John, and was content to pass over the arguments of the Socinians as 'they are such that every wise man must be ashamed of, and every Christian must abhor'. He concluded that the only thing left to complete the 'system of

---

[131] Lotte Mulligan, '"Reason", "Right Reason", and "Revelation" in mid-seventeenth-century England', in Brian Vickers ed., *Occult and Scientific Mentalities in the Renaissance* (1984), pp. 103-23; and 'Robert Boyle, "Right Reason", and the Meaning of Metaphor', *JHI,* 55 (1994), pp. 235-57.

[132] Samuel Hallifax, *Three Sermons preached before the University of Cambridge, Occasioned by an Attempt to Abolish Subscription to the XXXIX Articles of Religion* (Cambridge, 1772).

[133] 'Life of Jebb', p. 34.

[134] Hallifax, *Three Sermons*, pp. 3, 16.

Rational Christianity', would be interpreting 'the MIRACLES of Jesus as Allegories', as this was almost the only element of revelation that had 'yet escaped the polluted touch of modern Believers'.[135] The 'Theorists of our days', he declared, would not even allow Christianity to

> contain such difficulties as really belong to it: according to them, each circumstance in the *great Mystery of Godliness* is revealed in terms of the utmost perspicuity ... the veil, which was wont to hide the secrets of divine counsels from mortal eyes, is thrown aside, or at least made pervious to their understandings: they can force themselves into the very sanctuary of Truth, pervade her innermost recesses, and even seize her where she resides, in unclouded brightness, near the footstool of the Almighty.[136]

Much truth, particularly with respect to religion, was beyond the reach of rational scrutiny. Thus 'an article of religion is not *therefore* to be rejected, as unnecessary to salvation, because it is imperfectly understood by us'.[137]

Jonathan Clark uses these sermons to argue that conservative Latitudinarians began stressing the *truth* of orthodox doctrine in the face of the Feathers Tavern petition.[138] To an extent he is right, but we need to appreciate that in general their argument was a negative one, stressing the validity of orthodox doctrine in light of the limitations of reason. Jebb attended the sermons and claimed that Hallifax's language in defence of the Trinity was much stronger than what appeared in print.[139] Not surprisingly, High Churchmen found it easier to ridicule heterodox theologies and assert the truth of orthodoxy rather than explain Anglican doctrine. Good examples of this are the witty and abusive pamphlets of the 'high and dry' Tory, George Horne, whom Hallifax congratulated in 1782: 'I think your manner of treating the wretched attempts of modern infidels is much more likely to do good than a grave and formal answer would be. Your irony is admirable; and most happily blended with solid and serious argumentation, so as at once to entertain and instruct your readers'.[140] High Whigs and Tories like Hallifax and Horne became united in opposition to the confident rationalism that lay behind heterodox theology. According to the former, the petitioners were promoting a general contempt for 'religious obligations' that could be seen in

> a motley multitude of grotesque and uncouth appearances: now clad in the flimsy vest of French philosophy and critique;

[135] Hallifax, *Three Sermons*, pp. 35, 32-33, 48.
[136] Hallifax, *Three Sermons*, p. 36.
[137] Indeed, if this were the case, some of the 'most essential principles of Natural Religion' would also have to be set aside as incomprehensible. Hallifax, *Three Sermons*, p. viii.
[138] Clark, *English Society*, pp. 228-30.
[139] Apparently Hallifax declared that the Trinity 'were united though distinguished, distinguished though but one'. 'The expression was heard by hundreds', Jebb claimed, 'but, with many others of similar import, was not thought worthy of being retained in the printed copies'. *Short Account of Theological Lectures,* Jebb I, p. 171n.
[140] Samuel Hallifax, Bishop of Gloucester, to George Horne, 12 June 1784, cited in Nigel Aston, 'Horne and Heterodoxy', p. 908.

> now cloaked in the solemn garb of abstract speculation and enquiry; and now again, which is its usual form, in a disavowal of every moral principle, by an open and barefaced naturalism.[141]

In his *Short State of the Reasons for a late Resignation* (1775), Jebb argued that continuing worship of the Trinity was a great obstacle to the conversion of Muslims, Jews and unbelievers. A true 'manly piety' was only possible with a religion that could be rationally comprehended. He drew his familiar comparison with the progress of 'sound philosophy' based upon experiment, and declared that it was owing solely to a 'preposterous method of inquiry' that the Bible had come to be considered as contradictory, and containing 'the most fantastic doctrines'.[142] In response Edward Tew went through the standard orthodox dismissal of Socinianism, asserting that some truths are beyond rational comprehension. Toward the end he hit on the root of the conflict: 'Learn Wisdom, say you, from the *material* world. Let but the sources of religious Truth be explored in the same manner with the Laws of Nature; and the same success, the same just and easy explication, will follow.' While he agreed with Jebb's lament over the imperfect state of Scripture knowledge, he disagreed with his solution. Scientific method could not be applied to religion: 'No train of experiments whatever, [he writes] no critical patience or attention, could ever have suggested to our minds those sublimer doctrines of our Religion, which nevertheless we are bound implicitly to believe.'[143] This was the approach taken by conservatives. While thoroughly attached to Newtonianism as a bulwark of the Anglican establishment, they believed that an application of science to the mysteries of Christianity would threaten religious and political stability.[144]

Jebb's radicalism did not stem purely from his rejection of orthodox theology. Some who supported the Anglican establishment were more interested in its social and political utility than its intellectual credibility. Jebb's enthusiastic assault on orthodoxy and his political radicalism owed much to an intellectual confidence rooted in his combined religious and philosophical stance.

---

[141] Hallifax, *Three Sermons*, pp. 4-5

[142] Jebb II, pp. 206-18.

[143] Edward Tew, *Resignation No Proof, A Letter to Mr Jebb with occasional remarks on his Spirit of Protestantism* (Cambridge, 1776), pp. 56-57.

[144] F.C. Mather has written of the mathematician and bishop Samuel Horsley FRS, whose 'attachment to the Church was never free from self', that 'Devoted though he remained to Newton's mathematics, Horsley was never a consistent Newtonian. He drew back abruptly when science started to encroach on the freedom of God's dealings with the soul'. *High Church Prophet*, pp. 53-54. See also the collection of 'Sermons Preached at Lincoln's Inn 1765-1776', in *The Works of Bishop Richard Hurd* (1811), volume VI.

4

Religion and Moral Philosophy

According to Henri Laboucheix 'the philosophical culture of the reformers, with the exception of [Price,] Jebb or Priestley, was pretty scanty'.[1] When critics derided Jebb's pretence to having a 'superior system' and his mixing of philosophy with religion, they were referring to both his Socinianism and the accompanying determinist philosophy he derived from David Hartley. Orthodox theology rested upon a dualistic conception of the world as divided into matter and spirit. In this view, the physical was rationally comprehensible while much of the metaphysical could be said to be 'a mystery' and thus beyond rational criticism. It is not surprising that Jebb's confident rejection of orthodoxy was underpinned by a philosophy that rejected dualism.

A key aim of the Scientific Revolution was to reject the Aristotelian confusion of 'is' (truth) with 'ought' (good). But as John Gascoigne has pointed out, the desire to see a natural correspondence between the True and the Good lingered well into the eighteenth century. David Hartley's *Observations on Man* (1749) was a major attempt to demonstrate that the workings of nature corresponded perfectly with Christian revelation. Where Samuel Clarke had argued that the Newtonian universe demonstrated the existence of God, Hartley argued that the mechanism of the human mind revealed it to be a product of divine construction.[2] In doing so he inspired his adherents to adopt an unorthodox utilitarian Christianity. In 1793 Maximilien Robespierre declared that 'Man is good, as he comes from the hands of nature ... if he is corrupt, the responsibility lies with vicious social institutions'.[3] Jebb was neither a

---

[1] Henri Laboucheix, *Richard Price as Moral Philosopher and Political Theorist* (Studies on Voltaire and the Eighteenth Century, Oxford, 1982), p. 36.

[2] John Gascoigne, 'Science, Religion and the Foundations of Morality in Enlightenment Britain', *E&D*, 17 (1998), pp. 83-103.

[3] Cited in Norman Hampson, 'The Enlightenment in France', in Porter and Teich, *The*

Rousseauist nor a revolutionary, but he would have been inclined to agree with this statement, only adding that the hands of nature were attached to the God of Christian revelation.[4]

Hartley argued that the human mind was a dynamic process formed by sensory experience and the association of ideas. Individuals were part of a system designed by a just and benevolent God, in which humanity as a whole was slowly and inevitably progressing toward intellectual and moral perfection. This outlook fostered a distinctive approach to Christian piety that emphasised the importance of free enquiry and the candid expression of ideas.

The reputation the *Observations* attained owes much to the powerful effect it had upon a small but remarkably influential portion of the population, among whom we can number Joseph Priestley, Jeremy Bentham, James and John Stuart Mill and Samuel Taylor Coleridge.[5] Francis Blackburne said the *Observations* was a work 'to which ... Christianity is or will be more beholden, than to all the books besides of the last two centuries'.[6] Priestley wrote with respect to psychology: 'Something was done in this field of knowledge by Descartes, very much by Mr Locke, but most of all by Dr Hartley, who has thrown more useful light upon the theory of the human mind than Newton did upon the theory of the natural world'.[7] This was echoed by James Mill who thought the *Observations* the real 'master-production in the philosophy of mind'.[8]

It is clear that most of Hartley's eighteenth-century adherents were greatly impressed with his attempt to harness Christianity to a mechanistic psychology. In 1795 the Scottish clergyman James Wodrow complained that Paine's *Age of Reason* was 'one of the silliest and most childish books against revealed religion I have ever read'. In reply, his old Glasgow University student friend Samuel Kenrick recommended Hartley's 'defence of divine revelation'.

> Dr Hartley meets every objection ... sifts it with the cool penetration of a profound philosopher, and answers it with the meek spirit of a real Christian. How often I have wished that we had such a book in those youthful days of free inquiry in place of Deists. Nay even that our inquisitive instructors ... had seen it – how would they have rejoiced to meet so many congenial thoughts and such and honest and inquisitive mind.

Enlightenment in National Context, p. 49.

[4] Ann Jebb enthusiastically welcomed the French Revolution and blamed the religious and political establishment for provoking the violent actions of the people. *Two Penny-worth of Truth* (1792), pp. 11-12.

[5] The last named his son David Hartley Coleridge. On the influence of Hartley's work see R.K. Webb, 'Perspectives on David Hartley', *E&D*, 17 (1998), pp. 17-48.

[6] Francis Blackburne, *Works*, I, p. lxxviii. See also Francis Blackburne to Theophilus Lindsey, August 1770, DWL Blackburne correspondence.

[7] Joseph Priestley, *An Examination of Dr Reid's Inquiry into the Human Mind on the Principles of Common Sense, Dr Beattie's Essay on the Nature and Immutability of Truth, and Dr Oswald's Appeal to Common Sense in behalf of Religion* (1774), p. 26.

[8] John Stuart Mill, *Autobiography* (Jack Stillinger ed., Oxford, 1971 [1873]), p. 43.

Kenrick remembered that in 1749 he had been told about Hartley's book when in England, but only that he was 'an optimist'.[9] Such comments reveal how Hartley's influence was both confined and profound.

Again and again in the printed and manuscript sources, Hartley's influence on Jebb emerges – in direct references and in the general tone of his language. Joseph Priestley derived much satisfaction from a meeting with Jebb's father because he had been 'the intimate friend of Dr Hartley',[10] and Edmund Law corresponded with the author of the *Observations on Man*. Thus, through the combined influence of Law and his father it is highly conceivable that Hartley's book came into the hands of Jebb at a young age. His references to Hartley certainly pre-date the publication of Priestley's popular edition of the *Observations* in 1775.[11] When drawing up principles of conduct to follow as a doctor, Jebb repeatedly vowed to read Hartley: he urged himself to 'Employ the whole of every Sunday in sacred study, in reading Hartley', to 'read Hartley on ambition; and the proper and primary pursuits of man be diligently studied', and to act according to 'the three principles laid down by Dr Hartley, as the basis of right conduct, viz., piety, benevolence, and the moral sense'.[12] When Priestley dedicated his *Doctrine of Philosophical Necessity* to Jebb in 1777, he referred to 'our reverend master Dr Hartley' and hoped that as Jebb had 'followed the great Hartley in his application to theological, mathematical, and philosophical studies, and also in his profession of the theory and practice of medicine, you will still pursue his footsteps, in applying the elements of all these branches of science to the farther investigation of the phenomena of the human mind'.[13]

HARTLEY ON HUMAN NATURE

Hartley's work was an attempt to resolve the vigorous eighteenth-century debate over free will and determinism (or 'necessarianism'). The author of the *Observations on Man* has traditionally been seen as a rigid determinist for whom the mind is mechanically animated by sensory experience. In a major reassessment, however, Richard Allen has pointed out that Hartley did not see the mind as an independent entity which responds passively to stimuli, but rather as a 'dynamic construct, the totality of physiological and psychological processes' – a construct which develops and changes through interaction with its social and physical environments.[14] In doing so Hartley collapsed the traditional distinction between mind and body, allowed 'practical free will' within a necessarian framework, and held out the possibility of attaining moral and spiritual perfection in the temporal world. In what follows I will outline

[9] James Wodrow to Samuel Kenrick, 9 December 1795; Kenrick to Wodrow, 17 March 1796. DWL Wodrow-Kenrick correspondence.

[10] Joseph Priestley to Theophilus Lindsey, 20 April 1772, in Priestley, *Works*, I, p. 165.

[11] *A Short Account of Theological Lectures* (1770), Jebb I, p. 21.

[12] 'Life of Jebb', pp. 124-25, 136.

[13] Joseph Priestley, *The Doctrine of Philosophical Necessity Illustrated*, attached as an appendix to *Disquisitions Relating to Matter and Spirit* (2nd ed., 1777), pp. xv-vii.

[14] Richard C. Allen, *David Hartley on Human Nature* (New York, 1999), pp. 130-76.

Hartley's view of human nature and then discuss its practical implications as developed by Jebb and Priestley.

While admiring Alexander Pope as a 'moral poet', Hartley was concerned that the *Essay on Man* implied that 'the divine revelation of the Christian religion was superfluous, in a case where human philosophy was adequate'.[15] He saw the danger of Christianity being pushed aside by moral philosophers and sought to bring it back to rightful pre-eminence grounded on scientific demonstration. In doing so Hartley took up Newton's suggestion that the workings of the mind, like all subjects of natural philosophy, could be explained in simple material terms.[16]

Taking for granted that natural and revealed religion commanded the practice of virtue, Hartley decided early in his 'moral and Religious Enquiries' that 'the chief result of both Reason and Scripture ... is Universal Happiness in the most absolute sense ultimately'.[17] The doctrine of universal salvation was controversial, as many thought that it would encourage licentious behaviour and a disregard for morality. Hartley sought to demonstrate how the practice of virtue and the attainment of happiness were logically connected as a *necessary* consequence of the way God had designed human beings. In the words of one historian, Hartley was primarily a 'reconciler of competing philosophies: the philosophy of necessity and materialism, and that of Christian idealism'.[18] Accordingly, the *Observations* is set out in two parts: the first outlines the physical structure of the human 'frame', and how sense data is conveyed to the brain via vibrations along the nerves. Then Hartley shows how simple ideas produced in the brain by the senses are formed into complex ideas by a process of 'association'. This results in the various 'affections' or dispositions to which people are prone. In the second part Hartley discusses the moral implications of this view of human nature in relation to natural and revealed religion in a survey of the 'Duty and Expectations of Mankind'.[19]

Hartley thought that simple ideas were formed in the brain through vibrations in the medullary substance of the spinal marrow and the nervous system. By this means, sensory stimulation causes ideas in much the same way that the vibration of a string produces noise.[20] Where Lucretius made a distinction between *anima* and *animus* as separate and opposed substances, Jebb (following Hartley) claimed that they were both 'functions of our corporeal frame' which cease when the 'whole machine' dies, in the same way that sound stops 'when the wire is broken'. 'Lucretius supposes the motion of the fluid to

---

[15] David Hartley, *Observations on Man* (David Hartley jnr ed., 1791 [1749]), p. iv.

[16] Hartley, *Observations*, p. 6.

[17] David Hartley, 'The Correspondence of David Hartley and Rev John Lister', W.B. Trigg ed., *Transactions of the Hallifax Antiquarian Society* (1938), p. 234.

[18] Barbara Bowen Oberg, 'David Hartley and the Association of Ideas', *JHI,* 37 (1976), p. 442.

[19] On Hartley see Willey, *Eighteenth-Century Background*, chapter 8; Jack Fructman, 'Late Latitudinarianism: the case of David Hartley', *E&D,* 11 (1992), pp. 3-22; David Spadafora, *The Idea of Progress in the Eighteenth Century* (Princeton, 1990), ch. 4.

[20] Hartley, *Observations*, p. 298.

be from itself', Jebb continued, 'we, by impulse, and communicated vibrations from without'.[21]

The association of ideas, Hartley argued, resulted in the experience of 'affections' or dispositions which could be ranked in a cumulative hierarchy ascending from simple to more complex and refined: sensation, imagination, ambition, self-interest, sympathy, theopathy and the moral sense. The first four were the most common and basic affections, while the latter three characterised the development of a mature mind. All were interrelated and generated through a purely mechanical process:

1. *Simple ideas* are generated by sensory experience – this is the raw data that provides the basis for thought.

2. *Imaginative ideas* result from the perceived aesthetic quality of an object. As a scientific realist Hartley held a low opinion of imagination and thought it most vivid and useful during the infancy of both individuals and society. The Bible was characterised by figurative language, as were the beliefs of American Indians and other 'primitive' societies. Hartley thought that the mature individual (or society) should not indulge in the pleasures of the imagination, the evidence of which he saw to be the close connection between the 'polite arts' and all manner of vice. Yet while he criticised 'artificial beauty', he encouraged contemplation of nature, whereby the imagination could conjure up the vast complexity of God's creation.[22] Indeed, he argued that 'to the study of the word of God must be joined that of his works. They are in all things analogous to each other, and are perpetually comments upon each other.'[23]

3. *Ambition* is regulated by the praise or condemnation of others. Imagination plays an important part in fostering ambition and it can become a destructive passion if not harnessed and guided by development of the higher affections.

4. *Self-interest* is affected by the satisfaction or disappointment of our immediate desires and fears. This central affection (above which some never rise) Hartley divided into three categories: the most common is 'gross self-interest' under which is grouped the experience of sensation, imagination and ambition. The pursuit of a more 'refined self-interest' is encouraged by the happiness experienced through friendship and indulging in compassion, sympathy and religious thoughts. This in turn encouraged a 'rational self-interest' in which an 'abstract happiness' was affected by 'the hopes and fears relating to a future state'.[24] A sense of rational self-interest in turn forms the basis for the development of the higher affections.

5. The affections of *sympathy* (including compassion, mercy and sociability) are generated early in life through realising that your interests are connected to the fate of others, and that we can understand the pleasure or pain of a fellow creature. As one matures, the self-interested aspect of sympathy is

---

[21] 'Theological Propositions', Jebb II, p. 46.
[22] Willey, *Eighteenth-Century Background*, pp. 142-44.
[23] Hartley, *Observations*, p. 494.
[24] Hartley, *Observations*, pp. 272-275.

gradually replaced by a 'pure disinterested benevolence' according to which 'we must weep with those that weep, as well as rejoice with those that rejoice'.[25]

6. *Theopathy* is the happiness derived from cultivating a love of God. Even more so than benevolence and sympathy, the 'affections and actions enjoined by piety ... regulate, improve and perfect' the 'inferior classes of pleasure, viz. those of sensation, imagination, ambition and self-interest'. Pious reflection on God's goodness would strengthen one's ability to be virtuous, benevolent and spread the gospel. In thinking only of ourselves, Hartley observed, it is easy to become frustrated by a seemingly fruitless practice of benevolence, and begin to complain about the 'corruption and wickedness' of the world. But the pious individual who sees God 'as an inexhaustible fountain of love' will learn by His example to love both friends and enemies, 'and to labour, as an instrument under God, for the promotion of virtue and happiness'.[26]

7. While powerful, the feelings of piety are not as strong as those of the *moral sense*, which is affected by perception of 'moral beauty or deformity'. The moral sense is 'generated chiefly by piety, benevolence, and rational self-interest'. As a cluster of moral experience which judges new sensations and ideas through 'association', the moral sense provides the immediate guide to behaviour. According to Hartley, the moral sense: 'carries its own authority with it, inasmuch as it is the sum total of all of [the affections], and the ultimate result from them; and employs the force and authority of the whole nature of man against any particular part of it, that rebels against the determinations and commands of the conscience or moral judgement'.[27] As such it is effectively 'God's vicegerent, and the forerunner of the sentence which we may hereafter expect from him'.[28] While the Scottish philosophers were claiming that the moral sense was an innate human quality, Hartley argued that it was a mental process formed by experience and the association of ideas. As the moral sense is built up through the mechanical workings of the brain, 'the reiterated Impressions of those Associations will at last make Duty itself a Pleasure, and convert Sin into Pain'.[29]

Hartley believed he had shown how freedom could be exercised *within* a deterministic framework. He denied the existence of free will in the 'philosophical sense' that the mind has the 'power of beginning motion' and acting independently of circumstances, as it was inconsistent with God's infinite power and knowledge.[30] But he allowed free will 'under certain limitations' if defined in the 'popular and practical sense' whereby the mind is free to pursue that to which it is pre-disposed. This conception of free will entails no more than that 'voluntary and semi-voluntary powers of calling up ideas, of exciting and restraining affections, and of performing and suspending actions, arise from the

[25] Hartley, *Observations*, pp. 284, 474-78.
[26] Hartley, *Observations*, p. 490.
[27] Hartley, *Observations*, pp. 293-94.
[28] Hartley, *Observations*, p. 506.
[29] Cited in Willey, *Eighteenth-Century Background*, p. 146.
[30] Hartley, *Observations*, p. 348.

mechanism of our nature'.[31] Jim Dybikowski has described this version of necessarianism as *compatibalist*: 'to be free is not to be exempt from necessity, but to have the power to act as one pleases, unconstrained by *external impediment*'.[32]

Jebb clearly adopted Hartley's view of the mind. In a sermon he declared that 'we act in every instance upon an expectation of enjoyment.... This is the principle that guides the affections which direct the will'.[33] He wrote in his theological notes that 'the scripture-language and meaning confirms Hartley's doctrine of free-will'.[34] And while defending his theological lectures against the allegation of promoting 'fatalism', Jebb admitted to being 'a little inclined to the system of Hartley and of Locke', but assured his readers that he thought 'man is a moral agent in the strictest sense'.[35] Jebb's understanding of Hartley's concept of the will can be seen in his definition of three types of liberty: 'natural liberty' was a state of being free from physical defects and natural external restraints; 'political liberty' was freedom from the restraints of other men; 'moral liberty' however resulted when 'I have the will to act, and am not restrained by the prevalence of bad habits, which pervert that state of mind from being followed by actions or muscular notions. In this sense, every vicious man is really ... a slave'.[36] In effect, we are all slaves to circumstances and the morally corrupt are only acting in accordance with their cumulative experience. To exercise any degree of practical moral liberty, an individual had to be exposed to circumstances and education that would build up a strong moral sense. Thus, when encountering bad circumstances or tempted by self-indulgence, a well-developed moral sense would lead the individual to *rationally choose* the path of virtue.

Set within an optimistic metaphysical framework, Hartley's view of the mind placed great faith in the power of education. In justifying universal salvation, Hartley claimed that a merciful father would not condemn an errant son to eternal misery and that even the most hardened sinner was not beyond the reach of reform. 'For we are all alike in kind, and do not differ greatly in degree here. We have each of us passions of all sorts, and lie open to influences of all sorts; so as that persons A and B, in whatever different proportions their intellectual affections now exist, may, by a suitable set of impressions, become hereafter alike'.[37] Humans were only 'wicked' in the sense that they were limited, fallible creatures, who in an immature state pursue narrow self-interest. Jebb's student John Disney thought it would make as much sense to say it is sinful to have two hands as to say it is sinful to have human passions.[38] An

---

[31] Hartley, *Observations*, p. 297.

[32] Jim Dybikowski, 'Review of Peter N. Miller, *Joseph Priestley: political writings*', *E&D*, 15 (1996), pp. 117-27.

[33] Jebb II, pp. 57-8.

[34] 'Theological Propositions', Jebb II, p. 144.

[35] *A Short Account of Theological Lectures* (1770), Jebb I, p. 21.

[36] 'Theological Propositions', Jebb II, pp. 146-7.

[37] Hartley, *Observations*, p. 556.

[38] [John Disney], *Letter to the Rev Mr D--*, in *Tracts, printed and published by the Unitarian*

individual could be morally improved through exposure to the right influences and education. For Priestley, Hartley's account of the mind opened up the possibility of progress toward perfection, because through a systematic education 'children may be formed or moulded as we please'.[39]

From this notion of individual improvement it was easily assumed that a parallel increase in 'public happiness' would follow. Jebb believed that 'true enjoyment is only to be found in acts of social love',[40] and cultivating the moral sense was self-reinforcing as the pleasures derived from its exercise would stimulate one to greater benevolence and piety, and so on. Good circumstances would strengthen the higher affections and they in turn would lead one to seek and cultivate a good environment. Succumbing to the narrow 'gross self-interest' of sensation, imagination and ambition divorced from the higher affections was an ever-present danger, particularly if encouraged by a bad environment and circumstances – like a gang of thieves or a royal court.[41] You must avoid such circumstances and cultivate the moral sense: 'we *ought* never to be satisfied with ourselves, till we arrive at a perfect self-annihilation, and the pure love of God'.[42]

It was the duty of the rational Christian to help weaker souls to develop their moral sense and to promote, in every way possible, a physical and moral environment that would foster a virtuous society. Joseph Priestley devoted much of his time and energy to the theory and practice of education – and many of his most successful writings were designed to be used as teaching aids.[43] Jebb's efforts to improve the standard of education at Cambridge must be viewed in light of Hartley's claim that the educator was potentially 'the Instrument of Salvation, temporal and eternal, to Multitudes'.[44]

NECESSITY AND CHRISTIANITY

The scientist and Unitarian Joseph Priestley was the most prolific and influential of Hartley's followers. In part Priestley dedicated his *Doctrine of Philosophical Necessity* to Jebb in order to publicise the latter's resignation from the Anglican Church. Yet it is also evident that Jebb was one of the few people who sympathised with Priestley's philosophical stance.[45] While it is hard to gauge

---

Society for promoting Christian Knowledge and the Practice of Virtue (13 vols., 1791-1802), I, p. 98.

[39] Cited in Ruth Watts, ' Joseph Priestley and Education', *E&D*, 2 (1983), p. 87.

[40] Jebb II, p. 19.

[41] In the words of Brand Hollis, Jebb 'dreaded kings, from considering their education and the persons who frequent courts, where truth cannot enter'. Thomas Brand Hollis, 'A Character of Dr Jebb', in 'Life of Jebb', p. 233.

[42] Hartley cited in Fruchtman, 'Late Latitudinarianism', p. 14.

[43] This is a key theme of Robert E. Schofield, *The Enlightenment of Joseph Priestley: a study of his life and work from 1733-73* (University Park, Pennsylvania, 1998).

[44] Cited in, Spadafora, *Idea of Progress*, p. 162. Jebb observed that with knowledge comes the responsibility to act. Jebb II, p. 21.

[45] Jebb was greatly impressed by Priestley's controversial *History of the Corruptions of Christianity* (1782). Theophilus Lindsey to William Turner, 21 January 1783, DWL

how much, it is clear that Jebb and Priestley had some degree of personal acquaintance through their common friend Theophilus Lindsey. While spending winters in London with Lord Shelbourne in the late 1770s, Priestley regularly attended Lindsey's Essex Street Unitarian chapel, and there is at least one reference to his visiting Jebb at home.[46] In 1790 Priestley recalled: 'One day, I remember, I dined in company of an eminent Polish priest; the evening I spent with philosophers, determined unbelievers; the next morning I breakfasted with a most zealously orthodox clergyman, Mr Toplady; and the rest of that day I spent with Dr Jebb, Mr Lindsey, and some others, men in all respects *after my own heart*.'[47] And, it is worth noting, Priestley signed his dedication to Jebb: 'your affectionate friend, and fellow labourer'.[48]

The optimism of the Christian necessarians stemmed from their faith in Providence and the coming millennium. As Elie Halevy wrote, 'it must be borne in mind that [Hartley's] aim was to show in the mechanism of the laws of nature the justification of Christian optimism'.[49] Hartley avoided Hobbesian pessimism because he believed that a benevolent God could only have designed a system which naturally tends to generate human happiness. While happiness is not 'exactly proportioned to Virtue in the present life', Hartley believed that from the nature of things virtue was *in general* the safest and surest path to temporal happiness.[50] More important, the virtuous life would be rewarded at the day of judgement. 'Born again' Christians would escape 'the purifying lake of fire, whose smoke ascendeth up ... for ages and ages'. The price of eternal happiness for sinners was the 'tortures that are prepared for them ... in order to fit them for pure and spiritual happiness, to burn out the stains of sensuality and self-love'.[51] Orthodox Christianity relied upon fear of eternal damnation to enforce moral discipline. Starting with a theology of universal salvation, Hartley claimed that a natural 'sensual selfishness' could mechanically transform into altruism, 'a perfect self-annihilation, and the pure love of God'.[52]

Rational Christians were unsure as to whether the millennium would be inaugurated through gradual improvement or through a period of dramatic upheavals. As a result, their polemical writings often contained both calm philosophical reflections on the gradual progress of mankind, and passages that rang like an Old Testament prophet warning of impending doom. Either way, with an eye to the coming millennium their faith in progress was unshakeable,

---

Lindsey-Turner correspondence. It is also worth noting that Francis Blackburne wrote of Lindsey, Jebb and their fellow Essex Street Unitarians: 'These gentlemen are under the conduct of Dr Priestley, whose forte, as far as I can judge is not in the theological line'. Francis Blackburne to JW, 9 September 1783, DWL Letters of Lardner &c.

46 Theophilus Lindsey to William Tayleur, 24 April 1784, JRL Lindsey-Tayleur correspondence.

47 Priestley, *Works*, XIX p. 307; As Augustus Toplady died in 1778, this encounter must have taken place in the early or mid-1770s.

48 Priestley, *Doctrine of Philosophical Necessity*, p. xviii.

49 Elie Halevy, *The Growth of Philosophic Radicalism* (1928), p. 7.

50 Hartley, *Observations*, pp. 518-21.

51 Hartley, *Observations*, p. 565.

52 Hartley, *Observations*, p. 473.

and their challenge to existing authorities relentless.[53] As Fitzpatrick has observed, 'millennialism was by no means an eccentric import into Rational Dissenting religion. It was a consequence of their enlightened biblical studies and it was very much in the tradition which sought to integrate science and religion'.[54]

Hartley shared Edmund Law's view that human history was analogous to the growth of an individual through infancy and youth to maturity. When Lister asked him to explain this he replied that in the stage of infancy most people comprehended their world through 'Idolatry, Fiction and Fable'. During the world's youth 'supernatural communications' were confined to the Jews, and toward the end Jesus arrived to 'make the last and great Revelation'. Now, in the mature stage, mankind are left 'to compare all together [and] correct our own errors ... and Reason which without assistance could do absolutely nothing is now able on the footing of Revelation to discover and enforce true religion'. Hartley thought that the developments of 'the last two centuries seem to be presages and dawnings of the grand period of illumination'. Central to this process, he thought, was the spread of the 'doctrine of universal redemption and salvation'.[55]

Hartley believed that the dissolution of contemporary forms of political and religious government, the spread of Christianity to all nations, and the return of the Jews to Palestine would presage Christ's Second Coming. He thought it rash to predict when the millennium would begin. Nevertheless, in his conclusion Hartley implied that the last days had commenced, as 'the present circumstances of the world are extraordinary and critical, beyond what has yet happened'.[56] This was a powerful blend of moral critique, biblical prophecy and scientific confidence. As Jebb repeatedly read the *Observations on Man* for direction, he was no doubt inspired by the suggestion that 'we may perhaps say, that some glimmerings of the day begin already to shine in the hearts of all those who study and delight in the word and works of God'.[57] Joseph Priestley was certainly inspired. He wrote to their common friend Theophilus Lindsey in 1771: 'to me everything looks like that dismal catastrophe described, I may say predicted, by Dr Hartley in the conclusion of his Essay, and I shall be looking for the downfall of Church and State together. I am really expecting some very calamitous, but finally glorious, events.'[58] Nearly thirty years later, having witnessed two revolutions and the deaths of his wife and youngest son, he wrote to the same friend that 'it is nothing but a firm faith in Providence that is my

[53] Martin Fitzpatrick, 'Joseph Priestley and the Millennium', in R.G.A. Anderson and Christopher Lawrence eds., *Science, Medicine and Dissent: Joseph Priestley (1733-1804)* (1987), pp. 29-37; Fruchtman, 'Politics and the Apocalypse'; Clarke Garrett, *Respectable Folly: millenarians and the French Revolution in France and England* (1975), pp. 121-43; J.F.C. Harrison, *The Second Coming: popular millenarianism 1780-1850* (1979), pp. 3-10.

[54] Fitzpatrick, 'Heretical Religion and Radical Politics', p. 370.

[55] Hartley, 'Correspondence of Hartley and Lister', p. 259.

[56] Hartley, *Observations*, pp. 522-31, 523, 531, 574.

[57] Hartley, *Observations*, p. 530.

[58] Joseph Priestley to Theophilus Lindsey, August 1771, Priestley, *Works*, I (part 1), p. 146.

support at present; ... I read the introduction to the second volume of Hartley, and his conclusion, when I am most pressed'.[59] Hartley and his Unitarian followers believed in both general and particular providence, as indicated by Jebb's oft-repeated assurance that 'it is God's world, and I trust that he will order everything for the best.'[60] Yet determinism inevitably led to an emphasis on the general providential ordering of the universe – a belief that God *has* ordered everything for the best. As a result, according to Henri Laboucheix, Priestley's philosophical utilitarianism went further than Bentham's legal utilitarianism.[61]

In his edition of Hartley's *Observations*, Priestley casually suggested that the soul was corporeal. The resulting storm of allegations that he was no better than an atheist encouraged him to write the *Disquisitions relating to Matter and Spirit* (1777). As most people were staggered by the determinist implications of materialism, Priestley attached the *Doctrine of Philosophical Necessity* as an appendix in order to explain the mechanical nature of the human mind. In the 'Dedication' to Jebb, Priestley wrote an eloquent summary of their deterministic view of the world: 'Could we only, my friend, expand our minds fully to conceive, and act up to, the great principle asserted in this treatise, of the truth of which we are both of us convinced, nothing would be wanting for us to exert this, and every other effort of *true greatness of mind.*' 'We ourselves', he continued,

> complex as the structure of our minds, and our principles of action are, they are links in a great connected chain, parts of an immense whole, a very little of which we are as yet permitted to see, but from which we collect evidence enough, that the whole system (in which we are, at the same time, both *instruments* and *objects*) is under an unerring direction, and that the final result will be most glorious and happy. Whatever men may intend, or execute, all their designs, and all their actions, are subject to the secret influence and guidance of one who is necessarily the best judge of what will most promote his own excellent purposes. To him, and in his works, all seeming *discord* is real *harmony*, and all apparent *evil*, ultimate *good.*[62]

In this view all natural inequality and suffering could be accepted by focusing upon the providential unfolding of history. Thus, while suicide was not a civil crime, Jebb thought it a sin because it 'implies a want of trust in the goodness of providence, and indicates the greatest degree of self regard'. And he considered true religion as nothing more than a regulation of conduct 'suited to our state and circumstances in providence at any time'.[63] Reflecting upon the fate of those born in nations unexposed to the assistance of Christian revelation,

---

[59] Priestley, *Works*, I (part 2), p. 437.
[60] AJ to John Cartwright, February 1789, *Memoir of Ann Jebb*, p. 27.
[61] Laboucheix, *Richard Price*, p. 102.
[62] Priestley, *Doctrine of Necessity*, pp. vii-ix.
[63] 'Theological Propositions', Jebb II, pp. 139, 151.

Jebb preached: 'Let us be thankful for our better hopes; and leave the nations, which are involved in heathen ignorance, to the sure, though uncovenanted mercies of their God.'[64] Though facing many difficulties throughout his life, Priestley claimed that 'nothing has depressed my mind beyond a very short time'. This was owing to 'my firm belief of the doctrine of necessity, (and consequently that of everything being ordered for the best) has contributed to that degree of composure which I have enjoyed through life, so that I have always considered myself as one of the happiest of men'.[65] He counselled that the 'life of real piety and virtue' is attended by a 'perfect *serenity* and *cheerfulness'*.[66] As the following chapters will reveal, Jebb also took comfort from the doctrine of necessity during his frequent bouts of ill health and the frustration of his reform efforts.

The optimistic thrust of Hartley's necessarianism was strengthened by the materialist tendency of his disciples. While Hartley formulated a materialist understanding of the mind, he did not reject the immortality of the soul. Leaving the question open, he observed that it would not undermine the soul's immateriality if it could be proved that matter was 'endued with sensation'.[67] Priestley nevertheless decided that the notion of an immortal soul could be discarded, and was surprised that Hartley had not done so.[68] Citing the contempt with which the soul was treated in Holbach's *The System of Nature*, Priestley concluded that 'the state of things is now such that it appears to me to be absolutely necessary to abandon the notion of a soul, if we would retain Christianity at all. And, happily, the principles of it are as repugnant to that notion, as those of any modern philosophy'.[69]

The dedication of the *Doctrine of Philosophical Necessity* suggests that Jebb adopted Priestley's radical notion that matter was active rather than passive. Jebb also read Holbach, and while he makes no reference to Holbach's opinion of the soul, he agreed with his views on the Trinity and determinism. Like Priestley, Jebb felt that a Christianity purged of its irrational baggage would prove impervious to criticism by the likes of Holbach.

By the early 1770s Jebb had developed a physical explanation of the resurrection. He thought 'the materiality of man ie. extension of the conscious principle [is] a point sufficiently clear', and found evidence of this ('a medical incident properly attested') in an article placed in the *Public Ledger* by the 'Society for the recovery of Persons apparently drowned'. In copying out the extract he added some revealing comments of his own: 'Persons may by immersion in water have every corporal faculty (I would add mental) totally suspended, so that they may be to all appearance (I would say *actually*) dead for a considerable time. And yet it may be in the power of Art to recover them.'

---

64 Jebb II, p. 95.

65 Priestley, *Autobiography*, p. 123.

66 Priestley, *Doctrine of Necessity*, p. 165.

67 Hartley, *Observations*, p. 303.

68 Priestley, *Matter and Spirit*, p. 79.

69 Priestley, *Examination of Dr Reid*, p. 214; Alan Tapper, 'The Beginnings of Priestley's Materialism', *E&D*, 1 (1982), pp. 73-81.

This, Jebb thought, was 'a *real resurrection'*. He went on to reflect that 'the particles of those who are left alive may compose with different organisation the future body'. This led him to note that 'Chemistry shows great powers – no occasion for different matter – Christ perhaps now material – look around in nature, all material organisation and construction makes the difference between an oyster and a man, between a body in the womb and in life, so between a body in life and the next world.'[70]

Jebb was tending toward a materialist interpretation of Christianity in which the resurrection of Christ and his fellow human beings was a physical process. He was not alone in moving toward such a view: Edmund Law acknowledged the validity of a materialist conception of the soul in 1774, with a reference to Richard Watson's *Chemical Essays*.[71] In Jebb's case it is clear that he did not conceive of the soul as the traditional immaterial entity: 'The breath of God', he thought, 'added to flesh and blood makes men live' and at death 'the breath (ie. the soul) returns to God who gave it'. Rather than a spiritual substance, it was the 'added breath and heat' that made humans alive and conscious.[72] Samuel Taylor Coleridge later eloquently expressed such a view of the world:

> And what if all of animated nature
> Be but organic Harps diversely fram'd
> That tremble into thought, as o'er them sweeps
> Plastic and vast, one intellectual breeze
> At once the Soul of each, and God of all?[73]

In a series of letters, the genial Arian clergyman Henry Taylor (1711-85) pushed Ann Jebb for a clear explanation of this materialist reading of the soul. 'I laugh at the Theory' he confessed, 'because I can't conceive what they mean. I thought I would have got it out of you, as being one of the gang: but you won't squeak.... What you call the *breath of God* I suppose to be a *real Being*. What you suppose it to be, I cannot imagine.'[74] Taylor's perplexity is understandable, as irrespective of how the soul and matter are conceived, the problem remains as to how God (as a spiritual entity) can act upon the physical world.[75] Jebb's conception reflects the Newtonian view that passive matter is given life by God, and there is no direct evidence that he adopted Priestley's radical notion of active matter. Nevertheless, irrespective of his particular understanding of matter, Jebb's description of God's breath providing the 'heat' of life reveals a mind searching for a purely physical explanation of everything.

---

[70] DWL Jebb mss. VI, 47th lecture, note 1 April 1773.

[71] Edmund Law, 'Postscript', *Theory of Religion* (6th ed., 1774).

[72] See notes for the 47th and 48th lectures 'On promise of a Resurrection and the intermediate state of the dead', DWL Jebb mss. VI.

[73] Samuel Taylor Coleridge, cited in J.B. Beer, *Coleridge the Visionary* (New york, 1959), p. 95.

[74] Henry Taylor to Ann Jebb, [1773], CUL Taylor papers.

[75] A. T. Schwartz, 'Priestley's Materialism: the consistent connection', A.T. Schwartz and J.G. McEvoy eds., *Motion toward Perfection: the achievement of Joseph Priestley* (Boston, 1990), p. 119.

This lay behind Jebb's reading of Lucretius, a classical materialist whose philosophy could be contrasted to the platonic dualism that shaped orthodox Christian doctrine.

While we might say that Jebb adopted a materialism of sorts, the important point is that he saw any duality between the material and spiritual realms effectively dissolve.[76] In this vision, matter and spirit are conflated and the afterlife is populated by physical beings, including a human Christ. Such a view of the world was truly Unitarian, in that there is no substantial divide between matter and spirit, the temporal and eternal, God and man, or between the comprehensible and incomprehensible. As everything was material, everything had the potential to be understood, worked on and improved. This vision of a seamless creation indicates why Jebb and Priestley saw no conflict between reason and revelation, or between natural rights and utility. This confidence underpinned their focus on free inquiry and moral reform. In hindsight it is clear that Unitarian necessarians were, in the words of John Passmore, edging toward 'a theory of progress as "natural development", not as a mere consequence of the growth of knowledge, but as inherent in the very nature of the Universe'. At the same time, it is evident that they passed on the spirit of providential optimism to nineteenth-century utopians.[77]

FREE INQUIRY

Hartley convinced some Latitudinarians 'that moral authority resided in the individual's grasp of the world and in his ability to use his reason'.[78] In supporting the power of reason to uncover all important and practical truths, Hartley's system supported the argument for unrestrained free inquiry, undermined the practice of subscription and made the candid espousal of truth a central moral duty. In short, Hartley's *Observations* pricked the bubble of Latitudinarian complacency and encouraged a belief that all individuals should be able to *express* and *act* upon their ideas.

Traditional Dissent was fundamentalist and willing to believe anything that Scripture revealed to the individual 'seem it ever so incomprehensible to human Reason'.[79] As such, it lay open to the allegation that subjectively determined truth could lead to sectarianism and anarchy as witnessed in the English Civil War. Rational Dissenters, however, argued that it was not simply a matter of choosing between anarchy and established authority, because *reason* provided an authority to guide the individual. As Fitzpatrick has pointed out, they thought that the Bible 'was authoritative because it spoke the voice of divine reason'.[80] A rational God created humans with an ability to reason, and

---

[76] See Yannis Planngesis, *Matter and Spirit in Joseph Priestley's Philosophical Thought* (1991).

[77] John Passmore, *The Perfectibility of Man* (1970), p. 211.

[78] Fruchtman, 'Late Latitudinarianism', p. 22.

[79] Israel Mauduit, *'The Case of the Dissenting Ministers'. Addressed to the Lords Temporal and Lords Spiritual* (1772), p. 12; cited in Fitzpatrick, 'Toleration and Truth', p. 4.

[80] Fitzpatrick, 'Toleration and Truth', pp. 4-5.

provided two texts (Scripture and Nature) in which His will could be found and interpreted through the application of reason. Any irrational doctrine found in the Bible must stem *ipso facto* from either a mistaken interpretation, or from a willing distortion of the text out of political interest. There was no need for a powerful religious establishment to guard against and prosecute such misinterpretation of God's will (indeed, establishments tended to preserve and enforce misinterpretation). There would be no danger of sectarianism in an enlightened community, because wrong-headed notions of religion would be weeded out by the invisible hand of reason in a 'free-market' approach to religious opinion. An individual guided by reason could only do good; and the same went for a community of such individuals.

The *Observations on Man* appears to have helped propel some liberal Latitudinarians toward the ground upon which Rational Dissent stood. At the end of a discussion of religious doctrines, Hartley wrote: 'It is a great insult offered to the truths of religion, to suppose that they want the same kind of assistance as impostures, human projects, or worldly designs. Let every man be allowed to think, speak, and write, freely; and then the errors will combat one another, and leave the truth unhurt.'[81] God had ordered the world so that reason could (and should) seek out all those *important* truths that bore any relation to individual and social conduct.

Hartley opposed the imposition of any articles of faith because 'Men are to be influenced ... by rational methods only, not by compulsion'. While it was in the power of the magistrate to punish and restrict actions, opinions could not be so restrained. The irreligious can be made to 'appear to consent to anything, just as their interest leads them'. Hartley thought that this was the case with 'the great part of subscribers in all Christian communities. They have a mere nominal faith only'. More important, those who hold serious beliefs 'do proportional violence to these by performing a religious act out of a mere interested view'. Hartley thought even a subscription to the scriptures unnecessary. Diversity of opinion on speculative matters was inevitable, as evidenced by the failure of subscription to prevent the existing diversity within the Church. The answer was to abolish subscription and have preachers 'confine themselves to practical subjects'. 'If the scriptures cannot yet produce a true unity of opinion on account of our present ignorance ... how should articles do this?' No one had a right to make an article concerning an 'abstruse point' or 'metaphysical subtleties'. Rather, 'We are all brethren; there is no father, no master, amongst us; we are helpers of, not lords over, each other's faith. If we judge from other branches of learning, as natural philosophy, or physic, we shall there find, that the pure evidence of the things themselves is sufficient to overcome all opposition, after a due time'.[82]

Fitzpatrick has pointed out that in the hands of men like Jebb and Blackburne, Hartley's philosophy came to undermine the traditional Latitudinarian distinction between essential truths and 'things indifferent': 'Hartley allowed no room for the distinction between speculative and certain

---

[81] Hartley, *Observations*, p. 368.
[82] Hartley, *Observations*, pp. 513-15.

truths. In effect, he adapted the Christian humanist belief that 'ideally all man's faculties may be fused in the pursuit of that goodness which constitutes the highest truth', to the new spirit of the scientific revolution.'[83] Thus Jebb thought that where the exercise of reason is allowed free rein, 'true religion beams with unclouded luster on the mind'.[84] John Disney neatly summed up this confident belief in the unity of truth: 'The divine mind, seeing the whole compass of truth, and acting even to the extremest bounds of the universe, consequently sees and acts upon reasons unknown to us. But, as truth is *consistent*, that which is unknown to us cannot be *opposite* and *contradictory* to that which is known.'[85]

Hartley himself tried to play down the radical implications of his philosophy and sought to justify obedience to *forms* of worship imposed by civil authority. Impressed with Hartley's work, Blackburne also saw the implications for religious liberty: 'But he has joined *Necessity* and *Religion* together, – What of that? Ask the Church of England in her Articles'.[86] Following John Stuart Mill's fear of the tyranny of the majority, modern liberals see diversity of opinion as an end in itself, and believe that unanimity can be enforced only by an authoritarian regime. In the eighteenth century, however, there was a general desire for unanimity of thought – the main question being how to achieve it. Against authoritarian conformity, dissenters like Priestley, David Williams and Jebb argued that broad agreement on fundamental issues and principles would result from free thought.[87] This belief that free thought would ultimately produce harmony begged the question of how religion should be regulated.

It is instructive to compare Jebb's views on religious toleration with those of Joseph Priestley. As a Dissenter, Priestley argued that there must be a complete separation between Church and State because religious establishments inevitably tend to become authoritarian, control education and place restrictions upon the individual conscience. He claimed that the doctrine of necessity supported the idea of complete toleration: while the state was right to reward and punish behaviour, people should be free to have their knowledge shaped by the free exchange of ideas. Priestley argued that the government should concern itself only with actions rather than thoughts, and advocated unlimited religious pluralism, including toleration of atheism.[88]

In many respects Jebb embraced a similar commitment to religious liberty. While his writings contain phrases condemning 'Popery', he wanted full toleration extended to Catholics. As Colin Haydon has pointed out, the likes of Jebb and his mentor Edmund Law used the term as a synonym for 'ecclesiastical tyranny'.[89] Noting that the 'intolerant spirit ... more or less prevails in every

---

[83] Fitzpatrick, 'Latitudinarianism at the Parting of the Ways', p. 214, citing H.C. Baker, *The Wars of Truth* (Cambridge, Mass., 1952), p. 93. See also, Young, *Religion and Enlightenment*, pp. 43-44.
[84] Jebb III, p. 178.
[85] [John Disney], *Letter to the Rev Mr D--*, in Unitarian Society, *Tracts*, I, p. 93.
[86] Blackburne, *Works*, I, p. lxxxviii.
[87] Dybikowski, *On Burning Ground*, pp. 255-58.
[88] Priestley, *Political Writings*, pp. 59-60.
[89] Colin Haydon, *Anti-Catholicism in Eighteenth-Century England, c. 1714-80* (Manchester,

human establishment', Jebb often used the term 'papistic' in reference to the behaviour of the Anglican hierarchy.[90] Willing to grant toleration to all denominations (provided loyalty was sworn to the state), Jebb's enemy was authoritarian dogmatism. 'Our boasted Reformation', he complained, had done little more than change the 'spiritual head' of the Church. The continued imposition of the Thirty-Nine Articles 'as explanatory of the Scriptures, amounts to a solemn renunciation of the sufficiency of those Scriptures'. This, combined with 'a large portion of the intolerant spirit, the most odious concomitant of popish superstition', amounted to 'an authoritative renunciation of the Holy Scriptures themselves'.[91] As a result, the Church was spreading 'the contagion of corrupted doctrine, and unholy practice, through every rank and order of the state'.[92] Freedom of religious expression and practice (a right granted by 'the God of reason and the Gospel') was infringed and, in Jebb's eyes, 'the Reformation is so far from being completed that, in fact, with respect to a material part of it, it is but just begun'.[93]

Such sentiments could have come from the pen of a Dissenter. As an Anglican, however, Jebb was reluctant to give up the ideal of a national church charged with the responsibility of providing moral instruction. It has been noted that perceived liberalism with respect to theology has obscured the degree to which Latitudinarianism was the polite and rational face of religious dominance. In the last decades of the seventeenth century broad-churchmen championed a latitude of opinion *within* the pale of a comprehensive established church.[94] Jebb's vision of the religious constitution reveals how, in the wake of the *Observations on Man* and the *Confessional*, an advanced Latitudinarian endeavoured to combine his commitment to the utility of a national church with a broad conception of the right to religious liberty.

One of Jebb's first public contributions to the Feathers Tavern campaign was a letter praising Christopher Wyvill's *Thought's on our Articles of Religion, with respect to their supposed utility to the state* (July 1771). Jebb asserted that it was 'readily allowed that the power of the magistrate can only restrain the outward action'. Yet 'religion reaches to the heart, and regulates the springs which move the whole machine', and as such its true character was beyond the reach of the state to determine by either rewards or punishments. Jebb acknowledged that the 'unbounded liberty of conscience' that he advocated would find few supporters. So he conceded that if the government must promote religion to some extent, then it should confine itself to promoting only that which has a direct influence on human behaviour, such as 'the doctrine of an over-ruling providence, a future state, the happiness of the virtuous, [and] the

---

1993), p. 192.

[90] *Short Account of Theological Lectures*, Jebb I, p. 7.

[91] *Letters on the Subject of Subscription*, Jebb I, pp. 173, 161, 148.

[92] Jebb III, p. 164.

[93] *Letters on the Subject of Subscription*, Jebb I, p. 163.

[94] Richard Ashcraft, 'Latitudinarianism and Toleration: historical myth versus political history', in Richard Kroll et. al., *Philosophy, Science and Religion in England, 1640-1700* (Cambridge, 1992), pp. 151-77, at 155.

miseries which will hereafter prove the inevitable consequences of vice'. According to Jebb, only pure Christianity 'untainted by ... human error' espoused these simple doctrines; and only such a religion, with the primary aim of fostering 'social happiness', could claim the right to be an established religion.[95]

Jebb believed that extensive religious liberty could be accommodated within a national church and that its fundamentally Christian character would not be in doubt: 'The religion of the Gospel is the most useful to the community, and thus should be the religion of the state'.[96] Jebb's ecclesiology is most clearly stated in a controversial sermon he preached before Cambridge University on 27 December 1772. He began by outlining his understanding of a church as a voluntary society, which a member should be able to leave at any time without losing any 'privilege, dignity or emolument, to which he may be entitled as a subject of the civil power'. It cannot impose an orthodox doctrine because God provided the Scriptures for each individual to consult. Various churches can have different rights and ceremonies, which the individual may bend – 'his conscience must determine when the society becomes too corrupt, or contrary to what he thinks the truth.' After outlining his conception of a church, Jebb proceeded to the more controversial issue of how religion should be constituted within a nation. To begin with, he declared that 'All religious assemblies whatsoever, whether congregated in the name of Moses, the name of Jesus, or the name of Mahomet, have an equal claim to be protected by the state.' Jebb's view of the religious constitution was set within his Lockean conception of the state. Government was founded upon individuals giving up some of their civil liberty, and in effect delegating the power of civil reward and punishment to the state in the interests of protecting property, life and liberty. Yet the individual could never resign the right and duty to privately assess God's truth with 'my own eyes, and my own understanding'.[97]

Jebb thought that a public religion was still compatible with this broad conception of religious liberty. But as the formation of a public religion follows the 'social compact', it owes its form and existence entirely to the legislature and the 'ecclesiastical jurisdiction, as settled and defined by the state, should confine itself entirely to the regulation of the deportment of the established clergy'. The ecclesiastical hierarchy should not judge matters of faith, but only reward or punish the practical moral example set by clergymen. To support this utilitarian conception, Jebb claimed that those outside of the established church 'should not be obliged to pay for doctrines not useful to the state', and all religious societies had the same claim to 'security from interruption in our religious exercises'. Combined with such liberal toleration, the established 'form of public worship ... ought to rest upon the broadest basis'. For example, if there was a country with equal numbers of Jews, Muslims and Christians, then the publicly funded form of worship should 'be framed in such a manner as to comprehend them all'. In a revealing footnote, he explained:

---

[95] 'A Whig' [JJ], *London Chronicle*, 6 July 1771, Jebb III, pp. 1-4.
[96] 'A Whig' [JJ], *London Chronicle*, 6 July 1771, Jebb III, p. 4.
[97] 'A yoke upon the necks', Jebb II, pp. 114-15, 118-20.

> The idea is not so impracticable, as may at first be thought. Jews, Christians and Mahometans, &c. united under the same government, and the same laws, receive national blessings: why should they not unite in returning national praise, and national thanksgiving? Securing to them, however, the right of separate congregations, if they are desirous of making their acknowledgements of *any other than national concerns*. [my emphasis]

The picture Jebb paints is of a national church with rituals and moral instruction designed to serve social and political needs of the state, with a plurality of *forms* of worshipping God determined by individual congregations and ministers. The 'power of revising and correcting such an establishment, according to the improving judgement of the nation, should not be foreclosed by sanguinary and oppressive law'. In a predominantly Christian country the national religion should be based upon a belief in the New Testament, but should not formulate a doctrine and liturgy 'obviously exclusive of particular sects, professing obedience to the same common master'. What is more, an unlimited toleration should be allowed, and 'each particular religion' should receive a 'proportional part of the public fund appropriated to the religious service of the nation'. And those who pay tax and yet dissent from the established church should not be excluded from 'places of secular dignity and trust', provided they obey the bounds of civil and criminal law.[98] Jebb's vision was of a religious constitution in which a national church is sanctioned by a majority in the legislature, but those who dissent are still be able to hold public office *and* draw on the public treasury for support of their own dissenting churches.

Jebb wanted religious pluralism both within and without an established church. But where should the boundaries of that church be drawn? When talking of the religious constitution Jebb tends to confine himself to the varieties of monotheism, which aids his emphasis upon the common ground shared by different religions. But would a polytheistic church be able to claim funding from the government? Probably, as Jebb considered orthodox Christianity itself to be a form of polytheism. Yet in the end, Jebb does not pay much attention to the difficulties of a constitution in which a plurality of religions is tolerated and even funded by the state. This is because, like Priestley, he believed that mature and candid individuals would inevitably converge on an agreed, rational understanding of religion. It could not be otherwise, because free from the distorting influence of falsehood supported by political authority, the human mind would, through the association of ideas, necessarily arrive at a true understanding of natural and revealed religion.

As rational Christians jettisoned theological doctrines they placed an increasing emphasis on the practice of candour. Priestley even went so far as to suggest that candour might be more valuable than the 'right decision in any controversy'. The important thing was that all parties to a debate display a 'truly

---

[98] 'A yoke upon the necks', Jebb II, pp. 120-22.

Christian temper' and 'love of truth'.[99] Despite its complex and at times confusing semantics, Alan Saunders claims to have discerned a change in the way Rational Dissenters used 'candour': from 'meaning impartial as between persons, [it] came eventually to mean being impartial as between ideas'. According to Saunders, the result was a vacuous Rational Dissent 'largely without positive content', which reached its apotheosis in the 1790s in welcoming the French Revolution and Paine's *Rights of Man.* Confronted with the 'vengeful, murderous forces of Jacobinism' the exponents of candour appeared 'either deluded or deluding'. This partly explains how Rational Dissent was, if not intellectually defeated, then at least shouted down by a loyalist reaction supported by the government.[100] But such an assessment is too harsh and dismissive. The likes of Jebb and Priestley were not naïve and hollow people 'who distract your attention with polite conversation while somebody else is trying to pick your pocket'.[101] Had they been so, they would have stayed at home by the fire with a glass of port, and not written controversial pamphlets and books, or harangued meetings, or formed committees and associations, or worked for political, religious and humanitarian reform. Their position was akin to Voltaire's supposed famous declaration that 'I may hate your opinions, but would die defending your right to express them'.

It is true that, like virtue, candour featured prominently in eighteenth-century cant, but the sincerity with which Rational Dissenters used the term should not be underestimated. A commitment to the candid expression of ideas did not lead to an undiscriminating and intellectually permissive stance, because their intellectual method was backed up by a practical 'sense of religion' equal in substance to the most devout manifestation of orthodox Christianity.

'A SENSE OF RELIGION'

Jebb claimed that the Anglican Church should be reformed because 'it does not tend to generate, to inculcate, and to cultivate the sense of religion in the minds of men'.[102] The reformers argued for free inquiry so that they could cultivate 'a sense of religion' that would translate into practice. As Hartley had written, anyone could put his hand to an empty and insincere religious confession, but candour and free inquiry were essential for the cultivation of a benevolent, pious and moral disposition. To be an instrument of the will of God and help fulfil the designs of providence, one had to live with an honest sense of religion. In the words of Ann Jebb: 'that faith which doth not produce good works we are tempted to disregard: a precept may enter in at the ear, but it is a good example

[99] Cited in Fitzpatrick, 'Toleration and Truth', p. 27.

[100] Alan Saunders, 'The State as Highwayman: from candour to rights', in Haakonssen, *Enlightenment and Religion*, p. 249.

[101] Saunders, 'The State as Highwayman: from candour to rights', p. 271.

[102] *Letters on the Subject of Subscription* (1772), Jebb I, p. 169; At the close of his memoirs, Priestley expressed satisfaction that his children enjoyed good health, 'good dispositions, and as much as could be expected at their age, a sense of religion'. Priestley, *Autobiography*, p. 127.

which maketh it reach the heart. The clergy therefore should be doers of the word, not preachers only'.[103]

Jebb's 'rational religion, with mutual love and charity its fairest fruits', was in many respects closer to deism than to orthodox Christianity.[104] In this guise, Christianity loses its mystical and sacrificial aspects, and is reduced to an ethical code. In Jebb's words, 'pure Morality ... [is] the great point aimed at in both the Jewish and Christian dispensations'.[105] But to say that Christianity was *reduced* to a mere moral code implies that Jebb's view was less 'religious' than other versions of Christianity. This is an assumption that has traditionally permeated the writings of commentators on eighteenth-century thought. A dry, minimalist rational Christianity has been contrasted with sacramentalism, Evangelical Christianity and romanticism. This assumption lay behind E.P. Thompson's dismissal of the cold, polite religion of Rational Dissent as having little appeal to the lower classes.[106] In a perceptive study, however, Robert Webb has pointed to the neglected phenomenon of enlightened rational piety, of which he sees Jebb as an exemplar.[107] In her immensely popular *Practical Piety; or, The Influence of the Religion of the Heart on the Conduct of Life* (1811), the Evangelical Hannah More declared that Christianity was not a religion of 'forms, and modes, and decencies', but rather a transformation of the heart, an 'inward devotedness' in the service of God. As religion was designed to govern 'the movements of the rational machine', piety must lead to action. As Webb notes, it is suggestive that More did not criticise religious rationalists for a lack of piety.[108]

Despite their theological, philosophical and political differences, More's words could have flowed from the pen of Jebb, whose emphasis upon the practice of piety grew in proportion to the theological baggage he discarded. Jebb reminded his students at Cambridge that 'I have always earnestly exhorted you to consider religion as a science, which has for its proper object the culture of the human heart'.[109] From rational apprehension of the benevolent God of nature, 'arise those pious affections of gratitude and love, and upright conduct' that are our duty. 'This is true religion, the religion of the heart'.[110] While Christianity was supported by evidence that commanded rational assent, Jebb could also assert that the Gospel 'chiefly aims at our conversion, by the milder powers of persuasion, and a generous appeal to the uncorrupted feelings of the uncorrupted heart'.[111]

---

[103] 'Priscilla' [AJ], 'To Rev Dr Randolph', *London Chronicle*, 26 December 1771.

[104] Jebb I, p. 171. Paul Hazard did not blink at calling Priestley 'a deist ... of the "enlightened Christianity" school'. *European Thought in the Eighteenth Century* (Harmondsworth, 1965 [1946]), p. 137.

[105] DWL Jebb mss. IV.

[106] Thompson, *The Making of the English Working Class*, p. 31.

[107] R.K. Webb, 'Rational Piety', in Haakonssen, *Enlightenment and Religion*, p. 296.

[108] Cited in Webb, 'Rational Piety', pp. 290-91.

[109] *The Excellency of the Spirit of Benevolence, a sermon preached before the University of Cambridge on Monday, December 28, 1772* (1773), Jebb II, pp. 5-6.

[110] Jebb II, p. 34.

[111] Jebb II, p. 11.

Jebb was far from wanting a religion purged of emotion, and thought the stoic repression of all desires absurd, unnatural and unreasonable.[112] Rather, he espoused a 'Christian stoicism' in which one sought happiness through the imitation of Jesus, suffering the immediate and short-term frustration of one's benevolent efforts knowing that future 'happiness' was accruing on God's balance sheet of reward and punishment. While their method and doctrine differed, Jebb's heart was no less warm than John Wesley's.[113] Jebb's close friend Theophilus Lindsey claimed true Christians were distinguished by their fraternal love rather than commitment to any specific doctrines.[114] As Knud Haakonssen has neatly put it, 'for the Rational Dissenters who rejected original sin, self-betterment and piety were no longer a compensatory mission but a fulfilment of God's promise for the future'.[115]

Nowhere is the influence of Hartley better illustrated than in Jebb's sermon on the 'Spirit of Benevolence'. He declared that 'the principle of unlimited benevolence' was 'the great characteristic of the religion of the Gospel'. Our love of pleasure, power and praise, he suggested, 'are in a manner congenial with the human mind: they appear necessary movements in our frame'. These affections were entirely natural, and their highest state of satisfaction was found in promoting the happiness of others. Jebb pointed to the pleasure derived from making one's children happy, and to the kind of 'filial love' commonly expressed by the citizens of Sparta and Rome (though the latter was 'an almost antiquated passion'). While 'every social and disinterested affection is gradually formed in the heart, by a kind of mechanical process', this process was augmented by the hopes and fears derived from revealed religion. At length, the heart comes to consider 'every increase in the happiness of others, as an addition of happiness to itself'. It follows from this that those blessed with the advantages of birth and education should work for the common good, as 'he that increaseth knowledge, increaseth sorrow, if he toileth only for himself'. 'Let not then the light of science shine inward only on thy self', Jebb urged, 'let it radiate thy neighbour's footsteps with it's friendly beam: let it light him on his

---

112 Jebb II, pp. 30-31.

113 Jebb told the Methodists that he often defended them 'on account of your zeal for what you think the real doctrines of revelation.... But that you should oppose the scheme of abolishing a subscription to any human Articles whatsoever, I own, amazes me'. *General Evening Post*, 3 September 1772. DWL Disney mss. 87:II:118. Likewise, Hannah More respected Jebb's practise of piety: 'Being one day in a large company, who all inveighed against Lindsey, and Jebb, and other Socinians who had deserted the Church, because they could not subscribe to the Articles, I happened to say that I thought sincerity such a golden virtue, that I had a feeling bordering on respect for such as had apostatized upon principle: for when a man gave such an unequivocal proof of his being in earnest, as to renounce a lucrative profession, rather than violate his conscience, I must think him sincere, and of course respectable'. Hannah More to Horace Walpole, *The Yale Edition of Horace Walpole's Correspondence* (W.S. Lewis ed., 48 vols., New Haven, Conn., 1937-83), XXXI, pp. 328-29.

114 Theophilus Lindsey, *The Catechist* (1781), p. xi.

115 Knud Haakonssen, 'Enlightened Dissent: an introduction', in *Enlightenment and Religion*, p. 10.

dark and dangerous way through the wilderness of life'. The pious heart should 'overflow with the milk of human kindness', and openly rejoice with the happy, while crying with the distressed.[116]

The deist David Williams wrote that Jebb 'harassed his friends with reveries'.[117] But Jebb was only reflecting in a strong light the eighteenth-century revolution in sensibility that gathered momentum in the 1760s and 1770s.[118] Norman Fiering has traced the development of what he calls the notion of 'irresistible compassion', illustrated by Thomas Jefferson's declaration that 'nature hath implanted in our breasts a love of others, a sense of duty to them, a moral instinct, in short, which prompts us irresistibly to feel and to succour their distresses'. According to Fiering, during the Enlightenment 'the trust in certain qualities of human emotion was unbounded, as impressive certainly as the more often noted trust in rational faculties'. This increasingly widespread doctrine reflected the optimism of the Enlightenment and contributed to the humanitarianism that lay behind modern political radicalism.[119] Belief in a natural disposition toward virtue and benevolence was a common feature of Enlightenment thought.

There are similarities between the emotional style of Jebb's 'reveries' of rational piety and Rousseau's religion of nature. While there is no evidence that Jebb read Rousseau, the latter's important influence upon the English reading public in the 1760s is well attested. While most looked upon Rousseau as an eccentric French oddity, his writings, along with those of Lawrence Sterne, fostered a general interest in 'natural sentiment'.[120] Jebb evidently read Sterne, and he became acquainted with Thomas Day, an eccentric Rousseauist.[121] Although the direct influence of such writers on Jebb was probably minimal, his espousal of a rational piety must be set in the general context of the rise of sentiment. Jebb blended aspects of both Christianity and Enlightenment humanism into an exalted view of God's providence.

While he did not believe in original sin, he did think that poor education or bad circumstances could lead one into the pursuit of narrow self-interest. It was this that caused most of the trouble and suffering in the world, and thus one of Jebb's most-often-used dictums was that 'this world is a good world, and those who say otherwise should mend themselves'.[122] Providence had designed the world with 'evils' in order to remind humans of their mortality,

---

[116] *Spirit of Benevolence,* Jebb II, pp. 1-26.

[117] Cited in Dybikowski, *On Burning Ground,* p. 44n.

[118] The writings of Laurence Sterne both contributed too, and illustrate the development of 'sentiment' in the 1760s and 1770s in Britain: *Tristram Shandy* (1760-67) and *A Sentimental Journey* (1768).

[119] Norman S. Fiering, 'Irresistible Compassion: an aspect of eighteenth-century sympathy and humanitarianism', *JHI,* 37 (1976), p. 195.

[120] Edward Duffy, *Rousseau in England: the context of Shelley's critique of the Enlightenment* (Los Angeles, 1979), pp. 1-30.

[121] Jebb started one of his 'Every Man his Own Priest' letters with a quote from Lawrence Sterne: 'An ounce of a man's own sense, is worth a ton of other peoples.' 24 October 1772, Jebb III, p. 196.

[122] John Disney, *Memoirs of Thomas Brand Hollis* (1808), p. 43.

and thus prompt them to focus on the prospect of eternal happiness in the afterlife. Such an optimistic attitude only appears naïve, and even cruel, when one ceases to be convinced of the existence of an afterlife. Jebb experienced his fair share of illness in an age in which a minor ailment could quickly become life threatening. He always looked upon these bouts, which culminated in his death at the age of fifty, as a spur to greater application in fulfilling his duties to God and man.

In *On the Nature of the Universe,* Lucretius (to whom Jebb refers several times in his lecture notes) attacked the way men have worshipped and feared their gods. He portrayed 'true piety not as the traditional rigmarole of Roman ritual but as an almost mystical quietude in nature'.[123] In this spirit Jebb thought that true religion should dispel fear and encourage trust in God and the ultimately benign nature of his providence. 'Religious awe weakens the mind', he declared. One should only fear giving offence to God, 'but be bold and intrepid in every other matter relating to religion'.[124]

Substitute 'God' for 'Nature', and Jebb was in essential agreement with the view expressed in Holbach's *The System of Nature.*[125] The atheist Holbach argued that traditional religions reflect a primitive personification of nature, and had caused much harm by preaching fear and superstition. 'Nature' dictated that humans were neither innately good nor evil, but that virtue should be cultivated under rational laws to promote social happiness.[126] Jebb could agree with the anti-religious thrust of Holbach's work because he thought the philosophes were merely reacting to an irrational and despotic Catholicism. He, on the other hand, as an English rational Christian, knew that true religion was 'intelligible to every sensible being': 'Every virtuous man is its priest; errors and vices are its victims; the universe its altar; and God the only divinity it adores. Morality is the sum and substance of this religion. When we are rational, we are pious; when we are useful, we are virtuous; when we are benevolent, we are righteous and just.'[127] Access to the simple revealed word of God contained in the Gospels only made one better equipped to practice rational piety. But if anyone should live in this manner, 'we pronounce him to be actuated by a "principle of piety and benevolence", or, in other words, we attribute to him justly, whatever be his mode of faith, or outward worship, the honourable appellation of the "religious man"'.[128]

In accordance with these views, Jebb thought that the liturgy of the Church should be revised. Though it would be impossible to devise a liturgy that would reflect the sentiments of all people, Jebb believed 'an affecting and unexceptional form of public worship' could be agreed upon.[129] Toward the end

---

[123] Wilfred Cantwell Smith, *The Meaning and End of Religion* (New York, 1963), p. 22.
[124] 'Theological Propositions', Jebb II, p. 139.
[125] 'Theological Propositions', Jebb II, p. 168.
[126] William Wicker, 'Helvetius and Holbach', in F.J.C. Hearnshaw, *Social and Political Ideas of Some Great French Thinkers of the Age of Reason* (1930), pp. 195-214.
[127] 'God no respecter of persons', Jebb II, p. 105.
[128] Jebb III, p. 198.
[129] Jebb III, p. 45; Jebb I, p. 141n.

of 1772, David Williams asked Jebb to join him as minister at his Margaret Street chapel. In *The Philosopher* (1771) Williams had advocated universal toleration, the abolition of articles of religion and creation of an ecumenical Unitarian liturgy. Jebb replied that both he and Edmund Law had read the *Philosopher* with approval, and confessed that 'it has long been my persuasion that a real Reformation in the Liturgy must be effected by the spirited efforts of a few individuals'. As such, he welcomed the Margaret Street venture, as a rational liturgy 'held out to the observation of mankind in the capital city will do more than ten thousand times ten thousand *Candid Disquisition's* on the subject'. Nevertheless, he declined to join Williams as a minister at the chapel as he was committed to reforming the national church from within.[130]

Jebb gives an insight into the optimism and faith in Providence that underpinned such views when he outlined how he thought it was possible to avoid scepticism 'after painful reflection, upon important subjects':

> Attend to the duties of life, respecting of parents, loving of friends; and seek the situation which is most agreeable to nature, (a country life, if not with children, yet with pupils), and the convictions which nature warrants, will then arise in their proper course ... Take the season of temperance, benevolence, and health, and the secondary affections will then point at truth; and nature, rightly conceived of, will lead to nature's God.[131]

This echoes the Latitudinarian belief that faith enabled the Christian to exercise a superior form of 'right reason'. Jebb defined 'right reason' as the 'the analogy of faith, and sound criticism'.[132] Hartley constantly insisted upon the rational advantages of the believer, which in turn strengthens faith and dispels scepticism.[133] In efforts to draw out and manifest the potential good in nature and society, Jebb saw himself as engaged in the practical, every-day worship of God. This attitude lay behind his criticism of the prevailing doctrine, liturgy and structure of the established Church. Thus Jebb defined a Protestant as one whose 'chief characteristic is a mild, forbearing, tolerating spirit, which rises to zeal, when the sacred rights of humanity are invaded, under a pretence to orthodoxy'.[134]

Piety and benevolence were ultimately motivated by the contemplation of eternal happiness. Like Hartley, Jebb did not believe in eternal punishment, as it would serve no purpose, and go against the nature of a benevolent God. Indeed, he noted that 'Intolerants, and persons who maintain eternal punishment and atonement, are more unfit for society than atheists'.[135] He even thought it possible that animals would enjoy eternal life as they 'differ from us in degree

---

[130] JJ to David Williams, 26 October 1772, in Martin Fitzpatrick and James Dybikowski, 'David Williams, John Jebb and Liturgical Reform', *E&D*, 9 (1990), pp. 106-13.
[131] 'Theological Propositions', Jebb II, p. 166-67.
[132] *Short Account of Theological Lectures*, Jebb I, p. 145.
[133] Hartley, *Observations*, p. 511.
[134] 'Definitions' [JJ], 3 March 1774, Jebb III, p. 256.
[135] 'Theological Propositions', Jebb II, p. 145.

rather than kind'.[136] The afterlife was best considered as a place in which we 'will be happy or miserable by natural consequence as we behave here'.[137] As outlined above, Hartley thought that all would eventually be granted eternal life and happiness, though 'the wicked' would first have to be cast into a 'purging fire' where they would suffer 'according to their demerits' and thus be cleansed and prepared for an eternal life of pure happiness.[138] If the path to eternal life was not in some way like this, Jebb thought, what use would there be 'in the improvement of our faculties, or by acting in support of religious liberty, and taking pains in the scriptures. But if we live again every improvement will remain'.[139] The more rational and pious one lived on earth, the more one would appreciate and enjoy eternal life.[140]

Jebb was attracted to Richard Price's argument that friends will know one-another in the afterlife, and claimed that 'I do not know any consideration half so animating ... it is sufficient to convert a person'.[141] In like manner, Priestley wrote in his final years: 'I think more of my departed friends, Mrs Rayner, Dr Price, Dr Jebb, and others who have been my chief friends and benefactors, ... forming conjectures (wild ones no doubt) concerning our meeting and future employment hearafter'.[142] Upon his deathbed he reflected that all friends would be reunited after 'different degrees of discipline, suited to our different tempers', in a life of eternal happiness that would 'afford us ample field for the exertion of our faculties'.[143] There would be no idle lounging in angelic clouds in this Unitarian vision of the afterlife, but rather a heaven in which friendship and industrious employment could proceed uninhibited.

Hartley thought that corruption was so rife among the governing class of Britain that there was a real danger that 'an independent populace may get the upper hand and overset the state'. As a mainstream Whig, Hartley thought that resistance should be an act of last resort. He recommended that individuals continue to fulfil their obligations while promoting moral and institutional reform. In this manner, in the days preceding the Second Coming the torment 'brought upon us by our excess of wickedness' may be 'delayed, or alleviated, by reformations public and private'.[144] On the other hand, Hartley warned 'that the worldly-mindedness, and neglect of duty in the clergy, must hasten our ruin', especially by the 'superior clergy' who were 'in general, ambitious, and eager in the pursuit of riches; flatterers of the great, and subservient to party interest'. On the last two pages of the *Observations* he urged the clergy to adopt the 'zeal, and

---

[136] Jebb II, p. 39; Hartley, *Observations*, p. 563.
[137] 'Theological Propositions', Jebb II, p. 152; DWL Jebb mss. VI, 30 December 1774.
[138] Hartley, *Observations*, p. 561.
[139] 'Theological Propositions', Jebb II, p. 161.
[140] Jebb II, p. 25.
[141] 'Theological Propositions', Jebb II, pp. 151-52. See Richard Price, *Four Dissertations* (1769), no. III; see also Theophilus Lindsey to William Turner, 1 September 1783, DWL Lindsey-Turner correspondence.
[142] Joseph Priestley to Theophilus Lindsey, 15 April 1803, Belsham, *Memoirs of Lindsey*, p. 417.
[143] Priestley, *Autobiography*, p. 138.
[144] Hartley, *Observations*, p. 565.

concern for lost souls' of the Methodists without their sectarian peculiarities, for the world will only be converted by those 'who are of a truly catholic spirit'.

It would not be too much to say that the *Observations on Man* served Jebb as a manifesto for reform. 'Let those worthy clergymen', Hartley concluded, 'who lament the degeneracy of their own order, inform the public what is practicable and fitting to be done in these things. I can only deliver general remarks, such as occur to a bystander'.[145] Hartley was an Augustan and conservative by temperament, yet the thrust of his thought had radical potential when adopted by a younger generation surrounded by political and intellectual dispute. In the ears of some, at least, his general remarks rang loud.

[145] Hartley, *Observations*, pp. 570-72.

5

A Second Reformation

Jebb's religious and philosophical views mark him out as a representative of the radical late Enlightenment in Britain. He supported Francis Blackburne's neo-puritan demand that the Anglican clergy be given the right to freely exercise their private judgement. Yet Jebb also argued for greater religious liberty on utilitarian grounds, claiming that unrestrained free inquiry was necessary to ensure progress and religious stability in a changing world. For Jebb, extensive religious liberty was both a natural right and a practical necessity. His dogged efforts to act upon these convictions saw him become a leader in the campaign against subscription, with one Cambridge conservative describing him as a 'most turbulent, busy Spirit'.[1]

THE FEATHERS TAVERN PETITION

In 1767 Francis Blackburne first suggested that those clergy who shared his feelings of 'political dissent' should petition parliament to remove subscription.[2] With Theophilus Lindsey in the chair, twenty-four supporters of the *Confessional* gathered at the Feathers Tavern in the Strand on 17 July 1771 to discuss and agree on the proposed petition.[3] The participants left with a determination to circulate the petition throughout the country and gather signatures. In November Jebb's 'Circular Letter' publicly outlined the case for the petition. It asserted that liberty of conscience was the defining right of all Protestants, including Anglican priests; claimed that subscription obstructs progress toward a better understanding and comprehension of the true content of

[1] William Cole, BL Cole mss. 5378:53.
[2] Belsham, *Memoirs of Lindsey*, p. 35.
[3] Blackburne, *Works*, VII, p. 3-4.

the Gospels; and that an oath of allegiance to the state and the Scriptures was sufficient. It was evident that the bishops had no intention of acting to alter the situation, and, irrespective of their social status, it was the duty of 'Protestants and Englishmen' to petition for their rights.[4] In the months following the first meeting, members of the Feathers Tavern association busied themselves with gathering signatures for the petition.

While the reform-minded clergy were organising to meet at the Feathers Tavern in July 1771, Jebb's friend Robert Tyrwhitt made the first practical move against subscription at Cambridge. It was obligatory for all recipients of degrees to subscribe to three articles in the sixth and thirtieth canons of the Church of England, along with the Oath of Supremacy. This requirement had been introduced in 1616 at the command of James I in an effort to counter the influence of Puritanism in the University, and had remained in effect except during the Civil War and Protectorate. A correspondent to the *London Chronicle* thought it a ridiculous requirement that 'the generous youth, who has been permitted to bring Locke and Newton to the bar of reason, and occasionally to differ from and even correct them, must be bound by the narrow views of a paltry canonist'.[5] Tyrwhitt presented a proposal to remove subscription to the University's governing Caput, and it was rejected unanimously.[6] Samuel Hallifax, a member of the Caput, argued that subscription was required by a statute law, and thus it was beyond the ability of the University to modify or repeal. While this was true, the unfavourable disposition of the Caput toward the proposed reform was apparent and grounded in a fear that it would open the University to Dissenters.[7] Tyrwhitt was a politic choice to introduce the reform, as he was, in Robert Plumptre's words, 'a serious, studious man of exemplary character and far from any interested, factious or enthusiastic disposition'.[8] He put forward a second proposal that sought exemption for only those taking BA degrees, which was also rejected.[9]

Writing as 'Paulinus', Jebb addressed four letters to the undergraduates, urging them to take subscription seriously and suggesting that they examine the substance and coherence of the Articles. This should not be done by looking into 'those ingenious expositors, who will torture your imagination with a thousand interpretations'. Rather, they should pursue a course of study 'similar to what you are now pursuing in philosophical subjects', and in doing so try to reconcile

[4] *'Circular Letter' of the Feathers Tavern Petition* (November 1771), Jebb III, pp. 12-23.

[5] [Anon.], *London Chronicle*, 8 June 1771.

[6] The Caput was composed of Vice-Chancellor Sumner, Smith, Hallifax, Coligan, Farmer and Bates. [anon.], *Whitehall Evening Post*, 25 June 1771. One correspondent referred to this Caput as 'Agents of the Antichrist', and hoped that the next Caput would let Tyrwhitt's grace go before the University Senate. 'Luther', *London Chronicle*, 8 August 1771.

[7] 'Atticus', *London Chronicle*, 9 January 1772.

[8] Cited in Winstanley, *Unreformed Cambridge*, p. 305.

[9] Michael Tyson observed that the grace regarding subscription for degrees 'which made such a noise last Term, is again sent to the V.C., with alterations by Jebb'. Michael Tyson to Richard Gough, 21 November 1771, cited in Nichols, *Literary Anecdotes of the Eighteenth Century,* VIII, p. 572.

the doctrine of Athanasius with the 'unsystematic language of the New Testament; and his intolerant spirit with the mild and meek demeanour of your saviour'. After outlining the contents of the articles and pointing out some contradictions, Jebb urged the students to subscribe if, after study and careful consideration, they perceive them to be in accord with the contents of 'that sacred book, which holds forth a religion, reasonable, important and true'.[10]

Charles Crawford, a rowdy fellow commoner of Queens' College, organised a student petition to the Vice-Chancellor requesting that they be relieved of subscription. When presented on December 31 the petition was ignored. Crawford called on the Vice-Chancellor and requested action, as 'all mankind, with one voice, cry out against the imposition we speak of as absurd and illegal, which an arbitrary Stuart, in the wantonness of his power, had pleased to establish in the University'.[11] Not surprisingly, he was flatly informed that nothing could be done. While Jebb kept his distance from this agitation, it is worth noting that the petition was centred on Queens' College, where a number of those involved would have been under Jebb's tuition. M.L. Clarke is not unjustified in observing that 'the ingenious attitude of Crawford and the skilful phrasing of the petition were probably inspired by Jebb'.[12]

Following the defeat of the Feathers Tavern petition, Sir William Meredith MP decided to introduce a bill for relief of the laity in the universities, as many speakers who had opposed abolition of subscription for the clergy had suggested that the laity were a different case. After consultation with lawyers, the university authorities 'discovered' that they did have the power to remove subscription for BAs. In order to counter the threat of parliamentary intervention, the Vice-Chancellor formed a committee to consider the appropriate action. By June 1772 it had resolved to replace explicit subscription to the Articles with the oath: 'I declare that I am, bona fide, a member of the Church of England as established' – which was just another way to ensure subscription. This continued insistence on a test incensed the reformers. Jebb argued that 'as degrees are the testimonies and rewards of literary merit' they should 'lie open to every son of science, without distinction of party, sect or nation'. Even if he conceded the 'illiberal idea' that the universities should

---

[10] 'Paulinus' [JJ], 'An Address to the Gentlemen of the University of Cambridge, who intend proposing themselves, the ensuing January, as candidates for the degree of Bachelor of Arts', *Whitehall Evening Post*, 23, 30 November and 5, 12 December 1771, Jebb I, pp. 182-222, at 183, 185, 215-16. Jebb also addressed a public letter to the new Vice-Chancellor, Dr James Brown, master of Pembroke Hall, reminding him that 'the public' was astonished by the refusal to allow Tyrwhitt's motion to go before the Senate. He asked Brown, as the head of the new Caput, to allow the motion to pass – if not, then he should encourage lectures explaining the contents of the Articles in each of the colleges. 'A Member of the Senate' [JJ], *London Chronicle*, 30 November 1771, Jebb III, pp. 23-25. Jebb also criticised W.S. Powell for republishing his 1757 sermon in which he assured everyone that subscription only implied a 'general belief' in the articles. W.S. Powell, *A Defence of Subscription* (Cambridge, January 1772 [1757]); 'Camillius' [JJ], *London Chronicle*, 25 January 1772, Jebb III, pp. 50-52.

[11] Cited in *Letters on Subscription* (1772), Jebb I, p. 210.

[12] Clarke, *Paley*, p. 19.

remain institutions propagating 'one particular set of doctrines', there could be no cause for concern that the Dissenters would take over, because college fellowships would remain the province of members of the established Church.[13] Arguments such as this, however, were to no avail. Many of the dons seem to have been of Dr Johnson's mind, who declared 'that our Universities were founded to bring up members of the Church of England, and we must not supply our enemies with arms from our arsenal'.[14] Religious tests for non-clerical degrees remained in place until the late nineteenth century.

While the Feathers Tavern campaign is well known and treated by historians, most studies have relied upon the pamphlet literature. The newspapers, however, were of equal if not more importance in the cultivation of public opinion. Through studies of petitions to Parliament we know that the proportion of the population interested in politics was much greater than the number officially included in the political nation through the franchise.[15] In the smoke-filled coffee-houses newspapers were read and their contents enthusiastically discussed. A culture had developed in which a Swiss visitor could claim that 'workmen habitually begin the day by going to coffee-rooms in order to read the latest news'. Similarly, when an Irish clergyman visited London in 1775 he was struck by an example of 'English freedom' in a coffee-house when 'a whitesmith in his apron and with some of his saws under his arm, came in, sat down and called for his glass of punch and the paper, both of which he used with as much ease as a Lord'.[16] According to one observer, Cambridge scholars were 'so greedy after news ... that they neglect all for it ... which is a vast loss of time ... for who can apply to a subject with his head full of the din of a coffee-house?'[17]

Letters to the papers were designed to be read quickly and stimulate conversation through a potent mix of coffee and forceful opinion. With an eye to sales, newspaper proprietors were keen to stoke the fires of controversy. Before the development of the 'editorial', the eighteenth-century newspaper conveyed opinion in three ways: essays printed as letters to the press, short paragraphs and occasional extracts from correspondence. The first was the most important, and the leading letter was usually given a prominent title on the front page.[18] Several times John and Ann Jebb contributed the leading letter to the *London Chronicle* and the *Whitehall Evening Post*. A reading of the newspapers during the Feathers Tavern controversy reveals how heated the debate could become. It also reminds us that the Anglican Church existed in an increasingly plural and commercial society. Letters on religion sit between the lottery results, shipping

---

[13] *Letter to Sir William Meredith*, 31 August 1772, Jebb I, pp. 260-61.

[14] Samuel Johnson quoted by James Boswell, 21 March 1772, cited in Searby, *A History of the University of Cambridge: volume III*, p. 409.

[15] John A. Phillips: 'Popular Politics in Unreformed England', *Journal of Modern History* 52 (1980), pp. 599-625; and *Electoral Behaviour in Unreformed England: plumpers, splitters and straights* (Princeton, N.J., 1982).

[16] Cited in Porter, *Enlightenment*, p. 36.

[17] Cited in Knight, *University Rebel*, p. 29.

[18] Verner Crane, *Benjamin Franklin's Letters to the Press 1758-75* (1950), p. xxiii.

news, society gossip, political correspondence and the latest cure for everything from headache to venereal disease.[19]

Not surprisingly, the most vocal and enthusiastic opponents of the petitioners in the press were those High Church clergy like William Jones and George Horne who had no second thoughts when it came to asserting the *truth* of orthodox doctrine. Jones likened the petitioners to a swarm of rats who were trying to eat away the foundations of the house in which they sheltered.[20] The petitioners constantly tried to say that doctrine was not relevant to the debate – they only wanted the freedom to express their opinions. Lindsey thought allegations that the petitioners held dangerous and heterodox opinions were 'nothing but Episcopal cant ... Our petition has nothing to do with particular doctrines'.[21] When told that theology was irrelevant to the question, George Horne (writing as 'Clericus') replied that 'orthodoxy and heterodoxy are but other terms for right and wrong, applied to the doctrines of religion'. He disliked the tone of intellectual superiority affected by the petitioners and resented that 'Anti-Clericus' 'advises me to read upon the subject "if I dare"; as though every reforming pamphlet were a cannon; and, like a monkey, I should have my head blown off by peeping into it'. For Horne the matter was simple: orthodox doctrine was true and there was no need for reform.[22] Most reformers thought their opponents resorted to such polemical abuse and ridicule because orthodox doctrine could not stand up to critical scrutiny.[23]

Jebb weighed into the debate over the petition with several eloquent contributions. Seeking to generate momentum for the petition, he asserted that it would be 'criminal' for any clergyman on either side of the debate 'not to take an animated part', and concluded in a triumphant tone that: 'A British parliament shall decide upon the justice of our claims ... The time is approaching, when the ... ghost of the *Alliance* shall shrink into itself; [and] the heroes of a second reformation will arise'.[24]

In refutation of the 'Circular Letter', 'No Bigot' advanced a negative conception of liberty, claiming that private judgement was in no way infringed because nobody was forced to become a member of the Anglican Church. Jebb replied:

---

[19] See, for example, the front page of *The London Chronicle*, 12 January 1772, where an advertisement for a Yorkshire association to support the clerical petition is sandwiched between an advertisement for cough medicine and a cure for venereal disease which could be taken 'without confinement, hindrance of business, or amusement'.

[20] [W. Jones], 'Fable of the Rats', *General Evening Post*, 5 December 1771.

[21] Theophilus Lindsey to William Turner, 12 April 1772, DWL. Mss., 12.44.5.

[22] 'Clericus' [George Horne], *General Evening Post*, 19 September 1771. Horne was one of the most prominent Tory High Churchmen of the period; see Aston, 'Horne and Heterodoxy', pp. 895-919.

[23] 'A Layman', *London Chronicle*, 2 January 1772; [Anon.], *London Chronicle*, 11 January 1772.

[24] 'Laelius' [JJ], *London Chronicle*, 16 November 1771, Jebb III, pp. 8-12. Bishop William Warburton's *Alliance between Church and State* (1736) was an influential statement of conservative Latitudinarian ecclesiastical theory.

> The man that forces me by fear of death, or duress of imprisonment, to resign my liberty of action; and he who endeavours to engage me in the support of his unworthy purposes, by taking every unfair advantage, which my youth or ignorance supplies him with, or holding forth the splendid offers of riches, pomp and power in order to seduce me; exercises an equally unjustifiable dominion over my will, equally obstructs the exercise of private judgement.

The champions of Church authority only wanted to 'prolong the existence of superstition and fanaticism, in the midst of an enlightened and improved people'.[25]

Jebb's main contribution to the debate was in the form of four letters to a member of Parliament. The key problem, he thought, was that an authoritarian ecclesiastical hierarchy would not allow diverse opinions to be expressed within the Church of England. Jebb sought to sketch how this situation had evolved: in the second and third centuries the Christian church drew persecution upon itself owing to the 'ambitious claims and practices of its prelates'. Nevertheless, they were ultimately successful, and the conversion of the Roman Empire to Christianity could be described as a victory of church over state. The claims of the clergy continued to increase until the civil rights of men were 'annihilated or absorbed in an all-devouring power and patrimony of the church'. A clerical despotism combined with an 'absurd and senseless superstition ... soon entombed in one gloomy grave whatever was valuable of the arts, the learning, and the religion of mankind'. The advent of powerful popes only changed the government of the church from aristocratic to monarchical, and at the Reformation England simply replaced pope with monarch. Bishop Warburton's alliance between Church and State was only an attempt to justify and preserve a High Church in practice. In principle the Church has no real authority over Englishmen, 'like other corporations, [it] has no authority to enact or impose anything which affects the liberty of the subject'. But the bishops have great power and cannot be expected to alter a system in which they possess enormous privileges. Yet without allowing preachers to express their own interpretation of the Scriptures, the Church would increasingly appear absurd in an enlightened age. It is plain, Jebb contended, that a man could be 'a good Christian, a good master, a good husband, a good citizen, and a good friend' without believing the Articles.[26]

Ann Jebb also took up her pen in an attempt to rouse the majority of clergymen from their 'lethargic ignorance'.[27] She proceeded to address three public letters to Dr Thomas Randolph in reply to his defence of faith over works. He had, she thought, confirmed the general suspicion that men destitute

---

[25] 'Collatinus' [JJ], *London Packet*, 3 and 8 January 1772, Jebb III, pp. 30-50, at 33, 49.

[26] 'Paulinus' [JJ], *Whitehall Evening Post*, 28, 31 December 1771 and 14, 21 January 1772, Jebb I, pp. 137-181, at 150, 147, 159-60, 162, 168-70. These letters were gathered together and printed as a pamphlet at the end of January.

[27] 'Priscilla' [AJ], *London Chronicle*, 9 November 1771.

of virtue may rise in the Church provided they were seen to be orthodox.[28] Ann turned the traditional justification for orthodoxy around and argued that it was the cause of division and retarded the study of Scripture. She asked Randolph how he could be content to concede that the Church had lost many learned men as a result of the subscription requirement:

> At a time when vice not only stalks fearless through the streets at midnight, but rides triumphant even at noon day; when the places of public resort are filled with people who scoff at religion, and make a mock of sin; and when the Scriptures by many are disregarded as a worn out tale, can anyone at such a time venture to say that we have not wanted the assistance of every sincere, learned, and worthy man in the kingdom!

The Articles were 'high walls' that concealed 'the greatest beauties of the structure', and their removal would see the conversion of many to true Christianity.[29]

Ann observed that a problem for the orthodox had always been that those branded heretics have generally been among the most pious and virtuous of clergymen, and proceeded to ridicule Randolph's means of determining the sense of the Articles 'from the plain, usual and literal signification of the words'. But how could this be done when he had already asserted that many of the Articles had been purposely worded in general terms so as to encompass the theological diversity present in the sixteenth-century Church? 'It might not be easy to find out the *general* doctrine, or how far persons might differ in explaining particulars, before they deserved to be called *unsound in the faith*'. Randolph had pointed to the 17th Article concerning predestination as one that could be subscribed to in a general sense. But, Ann claimed, non-Calvinists could no more sincerely subscribe to this article than Unitarians could give assent to the later part of the 1st Article outlining the Trinity. In light of such vagueness and contradiction, she claimed, it was best to remove subscription to any doctrine.[30]

Theophilus Lindsey is said to have covered two thousand miles on horseback in his canvass of the north of England.[31] Yet despite such efforts, no more than two hundred clergy of generally low status, and fifty lawyers and physicians put their names to the petition. Many joined with William Paley in his famous declaration that he 'could not afford to keep a conscience'. Such cautious and pragmatic well-wishers were thought to have done the cause great harm.[32] Jebb addressed a public letter to a clergyman who had turned down his

---

28 'Priscilla' [AJ], 'To Rev Dr Randolph', *London Chronicle*, 26 December 1771; Thomas Randolph, *Reasonableness of Requiring Subscription to Articles of Religion from Persons to be Admitted to Holy Orders* (Oxford, December 1771); W.R. Ward, *Georgian Oxford* (Oxford, 1958), p. 246.

29 'Priscilla' [AJ], 'To Rev Dr Randolph', *London Chronicle*, 4 January 1772.

30 'Priscilla' [AJ], 'To Rev Dr Randolph', *London Chronicle*, 18 January 1772.

31 Belsham, *Memoirs of Lindsey*, p. 35.

32 'Priscilla' [AJ], *London Chronicle*, 9 November 1771.

request to sign the petition: 'you read the petition with attention. I saw the movements of your inmost soul ... You confirmed by the inflexions of your voice, the truth and importance of the matter contained in the petition'. But 'the danger of forfeiting the favour of an earthly patron, by bearing testimony to the truth' meant that no signature was forthcoming. This was to be lamented, as 'by the better temper of the times, that celebrated engine of Church despotism, if unaided by the secular power' would be rendered powerless. It was for this reason that the petitioners were appealing to the 'suffrages of every friend to public virtue'.[33]

Such pleading was of little avail. The 'Whig Dr Johnson', Samuel Parr, thought that the petition 'grasped at too much at once'.[34] And in a particularly damaging move, Richard Watson writing as 'A Christian Whig' distributed *A Letter to the Members of the House of Commons* (January 1772) prior to the presentation of the petition. While favourable to the aims of the petition, he thought that it should properly be presented to the bishops rather than the Parliament.[35] Jebb criticised the action of 'A Christian Whig' and observed that 'the injudicious friends of the petition' were wrong to suggest that a modification or reduction of the number of articles would be sufficient. The petitioners wanted to see the right to impose subscription to *any* articles removed, and they would never 'quit their Protestant ground'.[36]

In the face of hostility from High Churchmen and Methodists, and disapproval by the King, Sir William Meredith presented the petition to the Commons on 6 February 1772. This precipitated what a historian has referred to as 'one of the most eloquent debates in the whole century'.[37] Sir Roger Newdigate, the member for Oxford, rose and denounced the petitioners, declaring that 'prudence will confine them within certain bounds and prevent the nation from being overwhelmed with a deluge of impiety and blasphemy. If you remove this institution I cannot see how the state can for a moment subsist'. Newdigate argued that the coronation oath and the Act of Union with Scotland meant that any alteration to the Anglican Church would violate the constitution. Hans Stanley warned of a revival of the 'commotions raised by Sacheverell' if Parliament acted on the petition, and Charles Jenkinson concluded: 'Stir not the plague from the pit in which it is buried! If you once kindle the flame of theological dispute, you know not where it may end'. Lord George Germain replied that such fears were absurd in so 'enlightened an age'. 'What think you of Clarke and Hoadly, of Locke and Newton?' he asked; their writings reveal that, if alive, they would support the petition. Thomas Pitt, Dunning, and Sawbridge followed in pronouncing as indefensible subscription to 'strikingly

---

[33] 'Laelius' [JJ], 'To the Reverend —', *London Chronicle*, 28 December 1771, Jebb III, pp. 26-9.
[34] Clarke, *Paley*, p. 20.
[35] Richard Watson, *Miscellaneous Tracts: on religious, political and agricultural subjects* (2 vols., 1815), II, p. 4.
[36] *Letters on Subscription* (1772), Jebb I, pp. 217-22.
[37] Ward, *Georgian Oxford*, p. 247. See also Ditchfield, 'The Subscription Issue', pp. 45-80.

absurd' articles. Yet the vote did not depend upon such partisans, but rather the mainstream members of both the government and the opposition who were in favour of maintaining the *status quo*. Lord North agreed that it was best not to 'wake that many-headed hydra, religious controversy'. After asserting Parliament's right to act upon the petition, Edmund Burke argued that it should be ignored because it was concerned with 'abstract principles'.[38]

Such was the sense of the House that proceeded to reject the Feathers Tavern petition 217 votes to 71. Nevertheless, it was far from a resounding victory. W.R. Ward has observed that in the absence of anyone in the Commons willing to 'claim the virtue of truth for the articles, the only defensive arguments were those of expediency'.[39] Writing after witnessing the vote, Lindsey reflected that seventy-one was a respectable minority, though he was disappointed that Burke spoke against the petition and seemed to be expressing Rockingham's sentiments.[40]

PRUDENCE AND UTILITY

The reformers had drawn predictable condemnation from High Churchmen such as George Horne and William Jones. But to understand the defeat of the Feathers Tavern petition, we need to appreciate the way the *Confessional* brought Whig clergymen into open conflict. We can see this reflected in the political and religious alignments at Cambridge: while Peterhouse has long been recognised as a centre for those seeking 'further reformation' within the Church, St John's College, under the mastership of William Powell, acted as a bastion of conservative Whig ideology. To understand this division, we need to see the regulation of religion in the wider context of debate over how to best serve the common good.[41]

To some extent debate was polarised between two concepts of liberty: conservatives stressed the negative liberty of Englishmen in being free *from* oppression and able to pursue private interests and opinions unmolested by the state. Reformers, on the other hand, were advocating a more positive view of liberty which entailed the right to participate in the religious and political culture of the state regardless of one's particular opinions, provided an oath of loyalty were sworn. In response to 'Wilkes and Liberty', the American Revolution and the campaigns for religious reform, High Churchmen and conservative Latitudinarians found themselves closing ranks.

Latitudinarians agreed that an established Church was justified on the grounds of political and social utility. In the debate over subscription they were split over the character and the constitution of that Church. Conservatives

---

[38] Richard Burgess Barlow, *Citizenship and Conscience: a study in the theory and practice of religious toleration in England during the eighteenth century* (Philadelphia, 1962), pp. 150-56; *The Annual Register* (1772), pp. 86-90.

[39] Ward, *Georgian Oxford*, p. 248.

[40] T. Lindsey to W. Turner, 7 and 28 February 1772, DWL Lindsey-Turner correspondence.

[41] Peter N. Miller, *Defining the Common Good* (Cambridge, 1994).

defended the Articles as a defining 'bond of union' that distinguished the Anglican Church from other denominations. On the other hand, Jebb and the petitioners rejected the utility of subscription, arguing that it actually undermined the effectiveness of the Church as an institution charged with providing moral instruction to the nation. As explained in the previous chapter, Jebb thought that free inquiry and the candid exchange of ideas was the only way to ensure social progress, spread Christianity and obtain a uniform religious practice. During the Feathers Tavern controversy the senior prelates tended to remain aloof from the fray, content to allow their subalterns to carry the fight to the petitioners. We can see how debate over the utility of subscription was played out through the way John and Ann Jebb engaged with some of the conservative Whig champions.

The traditional practice of Latitudinarian polemicists was to stress the expediency of subscription and pass over the truth of orthodox doctrine. They claimed that an established Church, combined with toleration of Dissent, was a fundamental support of those English liberties praised by Voltaire. The classic statement of Court Whig ecclesiology was William Warburton, Bishop of Gloucester's, *Alliance between Church and State* (1736), which had been attacked by High Churchmen for defending the established Church through its civil utility rather than divine sanction. Nevertheless, Warburton had managed to put forward a realistic defence of the established Church as subordinate to the state, but also owed a duty of protection. Bishop of Gloucester from 1760 until his death in 1779 (when he was succeeded by Samuel Hallifax), Warburton stood as the patriarch of the conservative Whig clergymen who went into battle against reform. In the words of Leslie Stephen, 'Warburton led the life of a terrier in a rat-pit, worrying all theological vermin'.[42] A more recent and sympathetic assessment has depicted him as 'a polemic divine' who 'dictated much of the intellectual agenda at mid-century'.[43]

As indicated in the previous chapters, conservatives argued that the scope of reason to uncover truth was limited. Following Warburton, William Samuel Powell explicitly stated: 'No body ever asks concerning a petition or a rule, whether it be true; but whether it be decent, proper, reasonable, useful'.[44] According to this prudential view, anarchy would reign without an orthodoxy supported by authority. Jebb condemned the 'Heads of the Gloucesterian Alliance' for their efforts to 'throw an Odium' upon the petition.[45] Likewise, Francis Blackburne recognised that Warburton's argument had become the mainstream defence of the established Church, and accused them of 'dropping indeed the point of *right* to establish them as tests of truth, but insisting largely on their *utility*'.[46]

In 1769, a year after becoming Professor of Arabic, Jebb's cousin Samuel Hallifax preached a 30th of January sermon before the House of

---

[42] Stephen, *English Thought*, p. 293.
[43] Young, *Religion and Enlightenment*, pp. 13, 167-212
[44] Powell, *Defence of Subscription*, cited in Miller, *Common Good*, p. 309.
[45] 'Collatinus' [JJ], *St James's Chronicle*, 26 November 1772.
[46] Blackburne, *Confessional* (1767), p. 51.

Commons (to commemorate the martyrdom of Charles I). He eulogised George III and the political establishment upon which British civil and religious liberty rested. Dismissing the rhetoric of reform, he warned that the danger to liberty, 'if there be any, is from ourselves; lest our love of liberty degenerate into licentiousness, and our private vices and party quarrels defeat [the King's] endeavours, and counteract his designs for the public welfare ... the reformation, for which some amongst us are so clamorous, may, on enquiry be found to be only wanting in themselves'.[47]

Hallifax delivered three sermons before the University of Cambridge in January 1772, and in Jonathan Clark's words, his tone was 'urgent and agitated'.[48] His sermons were rushed into print at the request of the Vice-Chancellor and the heads of colleges as expressing the official stance of the University with respect to the Feathers Tavern petition. Hallifax cited Warburton on the virtues of an arrangement whereby an orthodox established Church tolerated orthodox Dissent. Yet as noted in chapter 3, he was appalled at the resurgence of heterodox thinking, which involved 'a disavowal of every moral principle, by an open and barefaced naturalism'. In response to this challenge, he parted from traditional Latitudinarian convention and asserted the *truth* of orthodox doctrine, claiming that if the Trinity and the Atonement were rejected the 'very *being* of the National Church' would be undermined.[49] According to Lindsey, Hallifax observed the parliamentary debate on the petition and 'seemed disappointed that his violent nonsense had produced so little effect on the House'.[50] Writing after the defeat of the petition, Ann Jebb criticised the aggressive tone of Hallifax's sermons, and claimed that she was confused as to his conception of the Trinity, the existence of which he supported with texts quoted out of context.[51]

In light of the arguments put forward by the majority of MPs during the vote on the Feathers Tavern petition, Thomas Balguy, archdeacon of Winchester, sought to defend subscription independent of the truth of orthodox doctrine. In 1769 Balguy had preached a sermon in which he restated Warburton's argument in favour of an established religious authority. According to Blackburne, 'Warburton's system was Hobbism trimmed and decorated with various distinctions and subterfuges', and Balguy was the only one 'fully appraised of the latent meaning of his master Warburton, to whose "little senate" he was said to have belonged'.[52] Among others, Joseph Priestley attacked Balguy for implicitly justifying all established religions.[53]

---

[47] Samuel Hallifax, *A Sermon Preached before the Honourable House of Commons ... on Monday, January 30, 1769* (Cambridge, 1769), pp. 13-14.
[48] Clark, *English Society*, p. 228.
[49] Hallifax, *Three Sermons*, pp. 3-4, 23.
[50] Belsham, *Memoirs of Lindsey*, p. 44.
[51] 'Priscilla' [AJ], *London Chronicle*, 24 March 1772.
[52] Blackburne, *Works*, I, p. xxxv.
[53] Thomas Balguy, *A Sermon Preached at Lambeth Palace* (1969); Joseph Priestley, *Political Writings* (Peter Miller ed., Cambridge, 1993), pp. 73-4, 102-03.

Following the failure of the Feathers Tavern petition Balguy published *A Charge Delivered to the Clergy of the Archdeaconry of Winchester in the Year 1772*. He claimed that removal of subscription would lead to the abolition rather than the reform of the national church, while conceding that 'neither the truth, nor the importance, of the Articles of the Church of *England* is in any way concerned in the present debate'. The issue was whether any '*human formulary*' could be imposed as a religious test by a Protestant church. From this he proceeded to argue that 'the opinions of the People are, and must be, founded more on Authority than Reason'. Most ideas and beliefs are derived from parents, teachers, and governors. He denied that the 'bulk of mankind' had the time, inclination, or ability to engage in rational study, and thus must be content 'with that religion which chance has thrown in their way; because they *can* do no better'. The press should be open for the airing of different opinions, but the pulpit should be kept free from controversy. Religion was most effectively spread by adopting a '*uniform appearance*' he argued, and allowing the preaching of different theological opinions within the national church would only 'introduce doubt and perplexity into the minds of the people'. What would the people make of differing views of the person of Christ being preached from the same pulpit? 'Would you have them think for themselves? Would you have them hear and decide the controversies of the learned? .... There are *more* men capable ... of understanding Newton's Philosophy, than of forming any judgement at all concerning the abstruser questions of Metaphysics and Theology'.

Balguy openly admitted that his argument could be used to defend both Catholicism and pagan religions, and declared that 'false religion' was preferable to having no established religion at all. As the notion of having contrary religions supported by the state was absurd, he argued that the real issue raised by the Feathers Tavern petition was: 'are we to have *any* Establishment or *none*?' Those who realised that the state could only support one kind of religion must be hoping that 'after a short conflict of parties ... their *own* System' would emerge as the new orthodoxy. Locke and Warburton had demonstrated that the 'Magistrate has no concern in the Truth or Falsehood of the doctrines he establishes: but undoubtedly', Balguy went on, 'he is concerned to establish such doctrines, as will promote the peace and safety and happiness of his Subjects'.

Balguy turned to consider the criticisms levelled by the petitioners that subscription was unjust, inexpedient and unnecessary. In the first case, the exercise of private judgement was widely tolerated, while the state had a right to appoint those it thought qualified to be 'Publick Teachers'. Second, subscription did not limit the ability of the clergy to defend Christianity by binding them to *'the doctrines of dark and ignorant ages'*, evidenced by the fact that the best apologists for Christianity were members of the Church of England. Aside from this, the nature of orthodox doctrine was not relevant to the issue, as the state had the right to support whatever form of religion it thought proper. Balguy admitted that imposing an orthodox creed meant that those whose opinions had changed would be forced to resign from the profession to which they had devoted their life. This was 'truly a case of compassion: but it is a case that admits no remedy. Would the objector themselves pay any regard to this plea, if urged in favour of a professed *Roman Catholic*? .... Accidental inconveniences will ever arise from all general rules; yet rules must be made, and must be observed'. Third, the claim that the oaths of supremacy and allegiance made subscription to the Thirty-Nine Articles unnecessary only shifted the problem, as some will regard any oaths as an unjust imposition. The oath of supremacy was a religious test that imposed upon individual consciences, without ensuring religious uniformity or restraining 'the Teachers of hurtful doctrines'. A subscription to the Scriptures was consistent with 'every imaginable absurdity and mischief'. As the established religion must have some defining articles, Balguy concluded that the petitioners must declare what form of religion they would have the state endorse, and what forms would be excluded.[54]

Ann Jebb thought Balguy was wise in not resting his case upon the truth of the Articles, but suggested that he had misunderstood the nature of the petition. The question was not whether the government endorse all ministers of religion, but rather, whether the government should support all Protestant ministers who 'promise to teach [Christianity] as they shall find it in the Scriptures, and to conform to the established Liturgy, and ecclesiastical government of the Church of England'. As to Balguy's claim that the 'bulk of mankind' could not reason on religious matters, Ann replied that Jesus had preached a plain and rational Christianity designed to be comprehended by uneducated people.[55] How could Balguy encourage learned men to discuss theology and pursue religious improvement if doing so could lead to heterodoxy and undermine their career? Rather than preserving harmony, the obscure nature of the Articles was the main reason that the pulpit had become the site of religious controversy. Where was Balguy's boasted uniformity in a church that encompassed Calvinists, Methodists, Arians, Socinians and crypto-Catholics?[56] In contrast, Ann argued, 'altho' freedom of enquiry through the folly of some, and the prejudices and passions of others, may for a time be productive of discordant opinions and dissensions amongst men; yet, that is the only way by which we can ever hope to arrive at perfect knowledge of those sacred truths revealed in the gospel, and therefore, that it must in the end, lead to the blessings and unity of peace'. Balguy's rhetoric was designed to kindle fear among his readers. If the law cannot protect property and the oath of allegiance maintain the security of the state, 'in vain should we fly for security to the bare subscription of the hand'. Indeed, Ann concluded, 'a state is more frequently overturned by the obstinacy of its governors, than endangered by their patient attention to ... the civil or religious grievances of a naturally brave and loyal people'.[57]

---

[54] Thomas Balguy, *A Charge Delivered to the Clergy of the Archdeaconry of Winchester in the Year 1772* (1772), p. 4-9, 16, 19-23.
[55] 'Priscilla' [AJ], *London Chronicle*, 19 December 1772.
[56] 'Priscilla' [AJ], *London Chronicle*, 26 December 1772; 'Priscilla' [AJ], *London Chronicle*, 12 January 1773.
[57] 'Priscilla' [AJ], *London Chronicle*, 23 January 1773.

Henry Taylor was impressed by Ann Jebb's letters, and pasted them into the front of his copy of the *Charge*. He thought Balguy 'has no ground but what belongs to the Jesuits to stand upon ... [and it] gives way under him; nothing but an Irish bog-trotter can travel upon it'. Taylor was particularly incensed that Hoadly had been quoted as supporting subscription without acknowledging other opinions that would show him as favourable to the petition.[58] Ann's letters seem to have been quite effective, with William Paley declaring that 'the Lord hath sold *Sisera* into the hands of a woman!'[59] Her letters were said to have irritated Hallifax so much that he called upon Wilkie, the publisher of the *London Chronicle*, and demanded that he print no more letters by 'Priscilla', because 'it was only Jebb's wife'.[60] For whatever reason, no more letters appear in the *Chronicle* after 26 January 1773, except for two more replies to Balguy in early 1774. In a letter to Ann, Henry Taylor railed against the printers of the *Chronicle* as 'illiberal Rag-stainers'. 'I pity you more because I have met with the same Fate. These Dunghill Cocks are no judges what Jewels they spurn. Their ignorance and nothing else can excuse them'.[61]

A year later (prior to the second submission of the petition) the front page of the *Chronicle* was filled with Ann's fifth letter to Balguy. In this she directly addressed Balguy's prudential argument: 'The Magistrate, in consequence of his power derived from the people, hath a right to restrain the liberty of his subjects, so far as may be found necessary for the good of the whole. But it seems to be public utility alone, that can give sanction to any act which restrains the liberty of the subject.' By excluding many talented clergymen from the Anglican Church the Articles worked against the welfare of society. Balguy supported his argument with appeals to past religious conflict. In reply, Ann claimed that both religious conflict and subscription were the product of a 'dark and ignorant age', and in the more enlightened 'present times' subscription was obviously unjust, inexpedient and unnecessary.[62] In her final letter, Ann criticised Balguy's claim that a subscription to the Scriptures was consistent with every imaginable absurdity. While some parts of Scripture may prove difficult for the uneducated, the central doctrines 'which are necessary to salvation may be said, in this our day, to be plain and easy' for any careful reader to discover. The gleaning of absurd doctrines from the Bible was not the fault of the text itself, but rather the ignorance of past times. In an environment in which free inquiry is encouraged, simple religious truth will triumph over absurd and wrong-headed notions. This is what Balguy should be promoting, she concluded, rather than arguing that people should subscribe as true 'abstruse metaphysical articles', which he confesses few can hope to understand.[63]

In August 1772 Jebb published a *Letter to Sir William Meredith* in which he sought to answer the 'darling argument' of the opponents of the

---

[58] Henry Taylor to Ann Jebb, [February?] 1773, CUL Taylor papers.
[59] 'William Paley' in *DNB*.
[60] Meadley, *Memoir of Ann Jebb*, p. 12.
[61] Henry Taylor to AJ, [?] 1773, CUL Taylor papers.
[62] 'Priscilla' [AJ], *London Chronicle*, 22 January 1774.
[63] 'Priscilla' [AJ], *London Chronicle*, 26 March 1774.

petition, that the Church must have 'some test expressive of the sense in which we understand the scriptures'. He was directly responding to *An Apology for the present Church of England as by Law established* (December, 1771), by Josiah Tucker (1713-99), Dean of Gloucester.[64] Rather than treat the Church as 'the creature and servant of the state', for the sake of argument Jebb accepted the Warburtonian view that it was an independent body allied to the state. To analyse the issue, he drew an analogy with a philosophical society set up to 'diffuse the light of science'. The aim of such a society, he argued, should not be confused with its 'bond of union' or its rules of conduct. The bond of union was the oath every member swore to perform their duties and promote the 'laudable end of their association'. The rules of conduct were to be suggested by individuals, and decided upon by the society as a whole. It is here that the members could differ over the means by which their collective task is best pursued. If the Parliament, or the King 'by his own mere notion', should grant the body a charter owing to its public utility, then they have the right to a say in how the association is governed. If, however, the members of the society should allow the state to influence their conduct in such a manner as to undermine their overall aim, then they would be breaking their bond of union. This, Jebb thought, was the state of the Anglican Church. The Church was designed to spread knowledge of the gospel and promote piety. The clergy must be 'honest, sincere and zealous', encourage study of Scripture, provide instruction and act as an example of virtue and piety. The controversy over subscription was really a debate over what rules of conduct would encourage clergymen to fulfil these duties.

Subscription, according to Jebb, encouraged clergymen to be insincere (and even lie) in order to preserve their livelihood. Even if he could agree with Tucker that an orthodox doctrine was necessary to the definition and preservation of the Church, Jebb argued that the Articles should be rejected because 'a bond of union, which is to serve six millions of people, should be plain and simple' rather than 'complicated and mysterious'. As the Church of England was not the only Christian church, and no church could claim authority in matters of faith, Jebb suggested that some system should be devised in which several churches, with their separate rites and ceremonies, 'may be formed into one collective whole'.[65]

In the face of such arguments, conservative Whigs hardened in their defence of orthodoxy. By 1775, with the American colonies in open rebellion, Balguy's declarations were becoming more strident: 'The benefits of society cannot be obtained, unless each person submit his private opinion to public authority. ... In all ordinary cases, it is the duty of a churchman, as well as of a citizen, to submit quietly to *the powers that be*: not to indulge himself in a fruitless, perhaps hurtful inquiry, how they *might* have been more wisely

[64] George Shelton, *Dean Tucker and Eighteenth-Century Economic and Political Thought* (1981). Jebb thought Tucker should 'be ashamed of a Cause unworthy of his Abilities; unworthy of a Spirit of Freedom, the Exertion of which did him so much Honour in his earlier years'. 'Collatinus' [JJ], *St James's Chronicle*, 26 November 1772.
[65] *Letter to Sir William Meredith* (August 1772), Jebb I, pp. 227-61.

constituted'. Balguy drew an analogy with the law, and argued that as individuals submit themselves to a law imposed by the Parliament, they should support the religion chosen by the Parliament, while retaining the right to passive dissent.[66]

The debate over subscription helped define the emerging split between conservative and reform-minded Latitudinarians. The former increasingly relied on Warburton's utilitarian defence of the Church. As Langford has observed, 'most of the non-resistance theory rehearsed in 1775 and 1776 smacks rather of Hobbes filtered through Blackstone and Johnson rather than Filmer revived'.[67] Both sides believed that liberty was an essential component to any definition of the common good, but they differed in their concept of liberty and how it could be secured. The use of prudential arguments by conservative Whigs fed the perception of a Tory resurgence. Theophilus Lindsey observed that the principles Balguy expressed in his 1775 *Charge* were those of 'James and Charles I', but 'I am told [he] actually deprecated those very articles he now extols in some of his first charges to his Archdeaconry before the turn of the times'.[68] When the Bishop of Lincoln declared that the Dissenters were not oppressed, that the dissatisfied clergy should resign, and supported government policy in respect to America, Lindsey wrote: 'I do not wonder at this turn in this man – who was formerly a high Whig'. The Bishop was now connected to his neighbour Lord Sandwich, and was expressing the very sentiments that 'the King is equally stiff in'.[69] Jebb read the political landscape in the same way. Following his resignation from the Church, Jebb wrote that 'I am not offended with the Tories, they act according to their nature; the prostitute Whigs offend me more, and the slumbering Whigs most of all'.[70]

Nowhere is the influence of David Hartley's *Observations* more strikingly illustrated than in two sermons Jebb preached at Cambridge University on 27 and 28 December 1772. They are also an early indicator of the political dimension of Jebb's reform interests. Both sermons are shot through with Hartlean language, and he even cites the *Observations* to support his assertion that a morally compromised clergy will contribute to the 'increasing dissipation, and profligacy of manners, in all ranks of people'.[71] Jebb opened by claiming that orthodoxy had been established upon the 'ruins of right reason'. Allowing clergy to preach the 'native purity' of the gospel was necessary to encourage 'public virtue' and ensure 'the lasting establishment of those constitutional privileges, which, as Englishmen, it is our duty to revere'. He set

---

[66] Thomas Balguy, *A Sermon Preached in Lambeth Chapel, on the consecration of the Right Reverend Richard Hurd and the Right Reverend John More* (1775), pp. 4,5,15.
[67] Langford, 'English Clergy and the American Revolution', in Hellmuth, *Transformation of Political Culture*, pp. 284-5.
[68] Theophilus Lindsey to William Turner, 2 February 1775, DWL Lindsey-Turner correspondence.
[69] Theophilus Lindsey to William Turner, 6 October 1774, DWL Lindsey-Turner correspondence.
[70] 'Life of Jebb', p. 109.
[71] 'A yoke upon the necks', Jebb II, pp. 107-33, at 128.

forth his vision (as discussed in chapter 4) of a religious constitution with unlimited toleration and a narrowly utilitarian national church in which the hierarchy could only dispense reward and punishment according the moral behaviour of clergymen. Such a system, Jebb maintained, would prove 'a permanent foundation for the real glory of the state' by encouraging 'public virtue, public honour, and a vital religion founded upon the scriptures and embraced with fervour'. Subscription, he concluded, required clergymen to submit their 'better judgement, to an authority, not less despotic than the antichristian power of Rome'.[72]

John Disney felt justified in reprinting this sermon because the argument was more condensed and forcefully stated than in Jebb's newspaper letters, and on account of the 'conversation' it caused at Cambridge. William Cole referred to it as the 'infamous Sermon he preached at St Mary's'.[73] Having provoked much 'conversation', Jebb followed with his sermon on 'The Excellency of the Spirit of Benevolence'. Yet he did not back away from controversy, and proceeded to make explicit the connection between rational piety and 'that sacred ardour which glows in the patriots breast'. He assured his listeners that the true Christian, whether from

> a sense of high dessert he treads the path of public virtue … [or] dissolves in tears at the prospect of the impending desolation of his country, yet, assisted by the power of faith, he directs his view to those improved forms of civil polity which future ages shall disclose in happier climes; and, enraptured with the glorious prospect, enjoys a source of satisfaction, which the sceptred king may envy – which the selfish cannot feel.[74]

In this sermon we can see the way Jebb's rational piety helped foster an early belief in the need for parliamentary reform. Indeed, he reprinted this sermon in 1780 and 1782 in an effort to encourage the people of England, Ireland and America to 'curb the violence of passion, without impairing the vigour of our virtuous efforts for that which we think right'.[75]

DEFEAT OF THE PETITION

Ann Jebb praised those who signed the petition and were 'deaf to the advice of worldly minded friends – deaf to what the world weakly calls prudence'.[76] One petitioner lamented the opposition to reform by 'political men, who are governed by what they call prudential maxims'.[77] A 'thinking layman' thought subscription of no demonstrated 'utility' to the constitution, and that the petitioners had been opposed by nothing but 'the most futile, contemptible

---

[72] 'A yoke upon the necks', Jebb II, pp. 110, 130, 134.
[73] 'A yoke upon the necks', Jebb II, p. 108n; BL Cole mss. 5873:53.
[74] Jebb II, p. 23.
[75] 'Life of Jebb', p. 44.
[76] 'Priscilla' [AJ], *London Chronicle*, 9 November 1771.
[77] 'P.Q.S'., *London Evening Post*, 2 January 1772.

sophistry'.[78] Jebb's frustration with the opposition is evident in a handful of letters not included in his *Works*. 'Here then, ye Balguys, ye Rotherans, ye Ridleys, ye Tuckers, the words of [John] Jortin', he thundered: 'The Scriptures, say the Protestants, are the only Rule of Faith in Matters pertaining to Revealed Religion, and they say well: there is no other *Christianity* than this, no other *Test* of Doctrine than this, no other *Centre of Union* than this. Whatsoever is not *clearly* delivered there may be *true,* but it cannot be *important.*'[79] There were broadly three options facing the petitioners following the initial rejection in February 1772: leave reform in the hands of the bishops, resubmit the petition, or resign from the Church.

By the end of 1772 Lindsey was complaining that not only were 'the whole bench of bishops' against them, but that a 'dissident party' among the petitioners wanted to compromise in order to 'get what reformation they can'.[80] Some of what the Duke of Grafton referred to as 'the more cautious' petitioners broke away from the main movement. In late 1772 Frances Wollaston, Beilby Porteous and Dr Yorke (who became Bishop of Ely) sought to prevent a split within the Church by privately asking Archbiship Cornwallis to persuade the bench of bishops to review the liturgy and articles. Cornwallis replied on 11 February 1773 that 'nothing can in prudence be done in the matter'.[81]

Most of the petitioners rejected this approach from the start, and were angry that the bishops had been approached. They clung to their demand for greater religious liberty. Jebb wrote: 'I view our late application; not in the light of a petition for relief to a few individuals, who cannot bring the articles of our church to square with their own private interpretations of scripture; but, as an attempt to restore the genuine splendour of the gospel, by vindicating the right of every individual in these kingdoms, to interpret scripture for himself.'[82] Subscription to any doctrine, no matter how revised, was a restriction of their Protestant rights. But more importantly, for Jebb, it impeded the discovery of truth.

The petitioners were genuinely annoyed that some of their opponents on the episcopal bench were lax in their own private religious opinions. Ann Jebb lamented that the petitioners were 'condemned to hear the scoffs of the Stalled Infidels, and the unrelenting frowns of Mitred Prelates'.[83] Foremost among these was Archbishop Frederick Cornwallis (1768-83), who had studied

---

[78] 'An Old Bystander', *Middlesex Journal*, 9 November 1771.

[79] 'Collatinus' [JJ], *St James's Chronicle*, 26 November 1772; John Jortin, *Remarks on Ecclesiastical History* (1751-54), p. 85; see also, 'An Englishman' [JJ], *General Evening Post*, 30 June 1772.

[80] McLachlan, *Letters of Lindsey*, p. 48.

[81] Francis Wollaston, *An Address to the Clergy of the Church of England in particular, and to all Christians in general* (1772); R. Hodgson, *The Life of Beilby Porteus, late Bishop of London* (5th ed., 1811), pp. 39-41.

[82] JJ, 18 July 1772, in a letter to (in Disney's words) 'a greatly esteemed character', explaining why he would not support a mere revision of the Articles. 'Life of Jebb', p. 39.

[83] 'No Petitioner but a friend to the Petition' [AJ], 'To the Archbishops and Bishops of the Church of England', *Whitehall Evening Post*, 14 April 1772.

under Edmund Law at Cambridge, and was an ambitious and worldly aristocrat in clerical robes.[84] Jebb publicly chastised him for defending what he must know are absurd articles owing to the education he had received.[85]

Ever persistent, John and Ann Jebb were at the forefront of efforts to have the petition resubmitted to Parliament, despite clear indications that it would be rejected. During the debate on the clerical petition, Lord North had suggested that a petition by the Dissenting ministers might be acceptable to the House. A petition was quickly put together and presented to the Parliament, with the Dissenting ministers anxious to distinguish between their circumstances, and those of the Anglican clergy. Despite heated opposition from Methodists and some orthodox Dissenters, the petition successfully passed through the Commons, but was rejected by the Lords. Priestley observed that their success in the House did not bode well for a resubmission of the clerical petition, because almost all the speakers stressed the difference between the two.[86]

The Jebbs continued to work at keeping the issue of subscription in the realm of public debate. On 28 March 1773 Jebb preached another controversial sermon at Cambridge, from the text 'Let your light so shine before men, that they may see your good works, and glorify your Father, which is in heaven' (Matthew 5:16). It was during this sermon that Cole claimed Jebb looked up and 'laughed' at his mentor Edmund Law. Again, the influence of Hartley's view of religion and psychology is evident throughout. The gospel could only be spread, Jebb declared, by 'an experimental display of its reforming powers upon themselves'. But the British were in no state to do this because of 'the present state of our national manners and religious polity'. Jebb accused the orthodox of failing to defend the theology of the articles, and resting their argument upon 'political convenience'. He concluded that the 'religion of Jesus' could not be carried to other countries until it was established in Britain itself.[87] Once again, William Cole gives us an insight into how Jebb's sermon was received by the orthodox:

> he told them last Sunday, that by Prophecy and Revelation the Christian truth was to be propagated in *every country in the world*, but that the Honour of doing so was not to be expected by *this nation*, who enslaved *Peoples Consciences* by *Articles* and *Subscriptions*; and that Religion ought to be free to every sect of Christians, and even to *Pagans* and *Mahametans* who were to be tolerated; to every one in short, *but to the Antichristian Church of Rome*.[88]

---

[84] Alfred W. Rowden, *The Primates of the Four Georges* (1916), pp. 311-12.
[85] 'Cornelus' [JJ], 'To the most Rev. the Archbishop of Canterbury', *London Evening Post*, 25 August 1772, Jebb III, pp. 83-90.
[86] Kippis, *Vindication of the Protestant Dissenting Ministers*, pp. 9, 12; Priestley, *Works*, I, p. 164.
[87] 'Let your light so shine', Jebb II, pp. 51-67, at 53; and Jebb III, pp. 233-41, at 235, 240-41.
[88] William Cole, BL Cole mss. 5873:52.

Amongst her other letters, Ann Jebb wrote to the *Whitehall Evening Post* in the guise of a congregation of farmers. Their parson had just died, which they did not really regret as he was 'a kind of methody man' who 'talked of Hell and Damnation, and articles, and a Light within us'. They had asked their landlord to grant the living to a neighbouring curate whom they had heard preach 'some good plain doctrine'. But they were puzzled that he declined, saying that he had '*thirty-nine* reasons for refusing' the offer. When they offered the curate more money, he explained that he could not subscribe to the articles. After pondering the curate's predicament, the farmers decided to examine the articles and the prayer book, 'and though we laboured harder than if we had been at the plough, we could scarce understand any of them'. 'We don't see anything they are fit for', they concluded, 'except to keep honest men out of the ministry; our friend the Curate out of a good Living, and deprive us of a good Parson'. To ease their developing concerns about attending communion, the curate lent them *The Rational Christian's Assistant to the worthy receiving of the Lord's Supper*. 'The gentleman who wrote it tells us it is an abridgement of Bp Hoadly; but that does not matter'. Though unable to 'write a clever petition' to Parliament, they would talk to their MP about their concerns, and support any scheme to remove religious impositions.[89]

The petition was resubmitted to Parliament on 5 May 1774 and, after a four-hour debate in which most MPs restated their positions, it was dismissed without a vote. This fact, combined with the minuscule number of resignations from the Church which followed, has led historians to conclude that the Anglican desire for reform was not very widespread, despite the rhetoric of the petitioners.[90] Most politicians and clergy seem to have been content to maintain the status quo and avoid any innovation during a period of growing conflict with the American colonies. Richard Farmer, a staunch opponent of Jebb's reform activities at Cambridge, articulated the nub of conservative concerns on 18 February 1773: 'Suppose the Remedy should prove worse than the disease – it would at least make one *Schism* more – We should have the *old Liturgists*, and they joined by the *Methodists*, would make a formidable figure. Those, who are able to find Difficulties in the old Form, are able likewise to explain them: and these bear a very small proportion to the Bulk of Mankind.' The reformers carried on, Farmer thought, 'as if Religion was intended for Nothing else but to be mended'.[91] This attitude prevailed among the political and ecclesiastical hierarchy, and by mid-1773 it was clear that the petitioners would have to live with the Articles or resign.

---

[89] 'The Farmers of …' [AJ], *Whitehall Evening Post*, 14, 18, and 23 December 1773, and 20 January 1774; John Disney published an abridged edition of Benjamin Hoadly's *Rational Christian's Assistant to the Worthy Receiving of the Lord's Supper* (1774).
[90] Sykes, *Church and State*, p. 38.
[91] Cited in Ditchfield, 'The Subscription Issue', p. 51.

A UNITARIAN CHURCH

Living with orthodoxy posed real difficulties for the petitioners, especially for those whose self-definition was increasingly bound up with the ideal of a candid disposition. Conservatives relentlessly urged the simple solution: leave the Church. But to give up a secure income in the only profession for which one was qualified was no easy solution – especially in light of family obligations. So most Anglicans who rejected the Trinity and original sin soldiered on in their country parishes, attempting to preach in a manner that did not entail compromising their beliefs at the least, or outright dishonesty at worst.

While Jebb indicated his Unitarian beliefs in his lectures, he was plagued by an 'uneasiness' in reading the church service, and eventually resigned in 1775 because 'to officiate in a liturgy which is formed upon the Athanasian system, struck me as a singular impropriety of conduct; and as an inconsistency of behaviour not to be defended'.[92] During the Feathers Tavern campaign, John Disney was permitted to omit the Nicene Creed and the entire liturgy from his services by a liberal-minded congregation and ecclesiastical superiors who turned a blind eye. When the petition ultimately failed, he resumed the established service and returned to study of the Scriptures in the hope of reconciling himself to orthodoxy.[93]

Unease over his position in the Church had driven Theophilus Lindsey to become the 'Principal Conductor' of the Feathers Tavern petition (during which time he struck up a close friendship with Jebb).[94] In the months following defeat of the petition, Lindsey's dissatisfaction increased as it became evident that the bishops were almost entirely opposed to the repeal of subscription. A public letter by Jebb (under the pen-name 'Laelius') moved Lindsey to write: 'I cannot say that I have been, for many years, a day free from uneasiness' at the thought that the spread of 'irreligion and infidelity' were encouraged by the moral inconsistencies of the established clergy.[95] While he continued to support the efforts to resubmit the petition, he thought the prospect of success extremely slim, if not hopeless. In a series of letters under the pen name of 'A Mortal Man' he lamented the authoritarian spirit of orthodox clergymen, pointing to the attacks upon the 'reverend and learned John Wesley' by Calvinist Methodists.[96]

Lindsey was always a disaffected Anglican, waiting in the wings and hoping for a reform of the doctrine and liturgy of the established Church. But as the years ticked by, and High-Church rhetoric increasingly poured forth from the cathedrals, it became clear that, at least in Lindsey's lifetime, attention must be directed to building the Unitarian faith outside the Anglican fold. With friends such as Benjamin Franklin and Joseph Priestley providing moral support, he decided to establish a Unitarian chapel in London. This was far from being an easy step. It meant leaving behind friends and financial security in Yorkshire, to

---

[92] 'Life of Jebb', pp. 106-07.

[93] DWL 'Memoir of Disney', pp. 25, 38.

[94] Ditchfield, 'The Subscription Issue', p. 51.

[95] 'Laelius' [JJ], *London Chronicle*, 27 February 1773, Jebb III, pp. 138-42; Belsham, *Memoirs of Lindsey*, p. 51.

[96] 'A Mortal Man' [T. Lindsey], *London Chronicle*, 11 June 1772.

establish an illegal church in London. His resignation was also criticised by his father-in-law, Francis Blackburne, who felt that he had 'lost his right arm', and chastised Lindsey for undermining the cause of reform within the Anglican Church.[97] Despite initial fears and difficulties, Lindsey opened the Essex Street Unitarian chapel on 17 April 1774. While the clergyman Augustus Toplady thought Lindsey an indifferent preacher who avoided controversial political issues, the church was well patronised by people of high social, political and intellectual status.[98]

Not for the last time, Lindsey asked Jebb to join him as co-minister of the new Unitarian church, but the latter declined.[99] There is no record of when the two first met, but most likely it was at or around the time of the first meeting at the Feathers Tavern in July 1771.[100] Along with William Turner, Jebb acted as a confidential friend and adviser to Lindsey as he set about establishing his chapel. Jebb revised Lindsey's *Apology on Resigning* and subsequent publications, provided advice on Biblical texts, helped him modify his liturgy, and regularly attended Essex Street when in London.[101]

Jebb first suggested to a few friends that he might resign from the Church in August 1773.[102] Having just received confirmation that Lindsey was resigning, Jebb made a public display of his defiance of the ecclesiastical hierarchy.[103] It would seem that he hoped to provoke a dramatic instance of clerical persecution. Fortunately, we have two accounts of the event: one by Jebb and the other by William Cole as the incident was related to him by a witness.[104] Dr Goodall, the Archdeacon of Suffolk, advised Jebb that he would visit his church at Flixton on 25 September, and say prayers for the surrounding parishes that were outside his diocese. According to Jebb, 'I appointed myself preacher, and gave a discourse upon subscription' (the same sermon he had preached at Cambridge the previous March).

---

[97] Blackburne to Lindsey, [1773?], DWL Blackburne correspondence.

[98] John Seed, 'Gentlemen Dissenters: the social and political meanings of Rational Dissent in the 1770s and 1780s', *Historical Journal*, 28 (1985), pp. 299-325.

[99] Lindsey to Jebb, 1 January 1774, Belsham, *Memoirs of Lindsey*, p. 68.

[100] The first mention of correspondence between them has Lindsey informing Jebb of his intention to carry the petition around the north of England. Belsham, *Memoirs of Lindsey*, p. 35.

[101] Belsham, *Memoirs of Lindsey*, pp. 57n, 103; 'Life of Jebb', pp. 83-5.

[102] 'Life of Jebb', p. 52.

[103] Lindsey had sent the manuscript of his *Apology* to Turner in June 1773. On 17 September he related that he had informed Blackburne of his intention to resign. He also wrote to Jebb 'about the same time', and according to Belsham this letter 'crossed upon the road' with one from Jebb indicating that *he* would resign at sometime in the future. As Disney tells us that Jebb first indicated his intentions to some friends in August 1773, this suggests that the Jebb-Lindsey letters crossed upon the road in early September. If so, then this means that Jebb knew of Lindsey's resignation prior to confronting Archdeacon Goodall. Belsham, *Memoirs of Lindsey*, p. 56.

[104] Dr Gooch was the Vice-Chancellor that Jebb first approached with his academic reform proposals.

> The Archdeacon was greatly enraged, although a Wollastonian; and publicly rebuked me before the clergy at the public house where we met: much altercation ensued, yet, I trust, I kept my temper. I told him that I had a right to preach every day in the week, if I thought proper: he was at liberty to retire, if he disliked my doctrine; he talked of authority, complaining to the diocean, &c. but, I resolutely told him, I should have used the same language to the bishop, had I met with equal provocation. At last he thought it best to hold his tongue, and be quiet. Much more was said, but this was the substance. For some days I expected a summons to Norwich, but have heard no more of it. I acted thus, with a view to call the attention of the Norwich clergy to our cause, and have in part succeeded.[105]

Jebb's superiors were wise not to respond to his taunt, but William Cole reveals the degree to which he tried to provoke them. According to the account he had been given, Jebb appeared in the church with his curate 'and neither in Gown, Cassock or even Band ... being the first time Dr Gooch ever saw the like'. By appointing himself as preacher rather than the Archdeacon, Jebb demonstrated contempt for the ecclesiastical hierarchy. He also cast aside the priestly robes that marked the clergy out as a privileged religious cast. Jebb proceeded to preach 'a very good sermon ... for about twenty minutes, and concluded with an invective against the Liturgy, Articles, and Clergy'. Goodall had not met Jebb before, and afterwards congratulated him on the first half of the sermon, but expressed the desire that he had 'left off where it was proper'. Upon this, 'Jebb flew in a Passion, and told him that he would preach at Flixton what he thought proper, that he disclaimed his jurisdiction and that he did not make use of him as a gentleman'. Goodall declared that his 'discourse was improper' and suggested he 'lay aside a gown he seemed so ashamed of'. When Jebb declared that he would resign if the Archdeacon also did likewise, Goodall replied that he was content with the Church and its articles. The altercation continued when they retired to dine and Goodall asked the other clergy if he had been rude to Jebb. When one affirmed that he had been well mannered, Jebb declared that 'the company were ready to say all that the Archdeacon would have them say'. Goodall threatened to inform his superior, and 'Jebb set the Bishop at defiance [as] he knew the man, and had talked to him on the occasion, and told the Archdeacon that he would never wait on him again'. The meeting ended after Gooch accused Jebb of being 'too warm', and in response Jebb 'fell foul on him'.[106]

With his friend Lindsey having resigned from the Church, Jebb was evidently eager to take a stand for his principles and cause. Uneasy about performing the liturgy while openly professing Unitarianism in his lectures, Jebb observed in October 1775 that 'for two years past, I have declined all discharge

---

[105] 'Life of Jebb', p. 54. He preached the sermon that he had delivered earlier in the year at Cambridge: 'Let your light so shine before men that they may see your good works'.
[106] William Cole, BL Cole mss. 5873:53.

of duty'. This would mean that in the autumn of 1773 he stopped reading the service – just after the confrontation at Flixton.[107] It was clearly an important occasion for Jebb, and there is probably little exaggeration or injustice in Cole's account. We know from other occasions that Jebb's idea of 'keeping his temper' did not preclude forcefully and bluntly speaking his mind. That he expected to be summoned to Norwich to justify his actions is revealing. Lindsey had voluntarily resigned and John Disney was able to continue within the Church for many years using a revised liturgy. The problem was that apart from the prosecution of Edward Evanson in the late 1770s for openly preaching Unitarian doctrine, there was little or no *active* oppression of the heterodox within the Church.[108] Clergymen who had scruples regarding Anglican orthodoxy were left in their quiet country parishes to ponder the moral dilemma of receiving payment for preaching falsehood.

Before resigning, Lindsey's mind was occupied with the idea of composing a list of 'Unitarian martyrs', to which he thought quite a few names were about to be added. However, while heterodox Anglicans felt weighed down by their consciences and had no prospect for promotion within an orthodox Anglican Church, there was no great instance of unjust persecution. Even Lindsey's Unitarian Chapel was left alone and actually patronised by people of wealth and power, though he was technically in breach of the law prohibiting anti-trinitarian preaching. Under a relatively enlightened Church and State, 'oppression by neglect' would seem to sum up the extent to which heterodox Anglicans suffered at the hands of ecclesiastical authority. Jebb certainly had the rhetorical skill to turn any prosecution of his actions into valuable publicity for the cause of reform – but it was not to be.

Conservatives constantly warned that any modification of the religious constitution would fuel social and political unrest. 'T. Lovechange' scoffed at Jebb 'making everyone his own priest', as 'Whitefield has got the start on you, and there are amongst the Methodists [many] Cobblers, Taylors, Shoe-makers, Weavers, and Drummers, who have become priests not only to themselves, but to others more simple than themselves'. He warned that Jebb's principles would lead to the same troubles as 'in Oliver's time, when men fought with the scriptures, and with the sword'.[109] Another referred to the petitioners as an 'enthusiastical set of Puritans'.[110]

The reformers were often willing to make the connection between their cause and a perceived need for political reform. One correspondent accused George Horne of promoting the prosecution of Edward Evanson for preaching Unitarian doctrine, and declared that every act that limited religious liberty was 'a repeal of the *Magna Charta* of Christians, and consequently null and void'.[111] Edmund Law thought that the practice of imposing an orthodox measure of faith was the cause of both infidelity and the increasing tendency to 'thoroughly sift

---

[107] 'Life of Jebb', p. 106.
[108] Ditchfield, 'Ecclesiastical Policy Under Lord North', p. 233.
[109] 'T. Lovechange', *Whitehall Evening Post*, 12 March 1774.
[110] [Anon.], *St James's Chronicle*, 13 January 1774.
[111] L.L.B., *Whitehall Evening Post*, 11 January 1774.

our Constitution'. This was to be expected, in light of the 'increase of general knowledge, and no less general taste for liberty' among a growing proportion of the population. The clergy of the established Church laboured in a 'confused state of things' from a lack 'of those timely revivals, and gradual reformations, which might enable it to keep pace with each improvement in every branch of science round us'.[112]

John Disney anonymously and publicly urged Jebb to continue his letters to the newspapers: 'This century has not produced a time when there was a greater need of a clear and methodical prosecution of the idea you have taken up, than the present moment: a moment when the Hierarchy are actively serving the interests of Bigotry, Superstition and Intolerance.' He urged Jebb to take up his pen again, so that 'through the means of a paper of extensive circulation, the laymen of Great Britain may know their rights, and be roused to assert them. Associations among *them* must be formed in every county in the kingdom, for the better establishment of Christianity'.[113]

In a society where religion and politics were intertwined, the political implications of the common people 'associating' to discuss and reform Christianity were obvious. Under the pseudonym 'An Englishman', Jebb wrote (echoing Priestley) that 'every person who is acquainted with the first principles of government' knows that 'the legislature of this kingdom, consisting of King, Lords, and Commons, is accountable for their trust to the general body of the nation'. As a result, 'the people have a right of remonstrating to their deputies, when their interests, either civil or religious, are affected by an absurd, unjust, or an oppressive law'.[114]

---

[112] Edmund Law, *Considerations on ... Subscription* (1774), pp. 51-2.
[113] 'A Country Gentleman' [J. Disney], *Whitehall Evening Post*, 27 February 1773.
[114] 'An Englishman' [JJ], *General Evening Post*, 30 June 1772; Joseph Priestley, *Essay on the First Principles of Government* (1768).

6

A Storm in Cambridge Teacups

As Malcom Muggeridge has observed, 'to the liberal mind, education provides the universal panacea'.[1] It is not surprising that Jebb turned his energies to educational reform when it became clear that Parliament would not address the grievances of the petitioning clergy. The best way to obtain reform was to change the minds of Britain's governing class. Reform of education provided to future clergymen and politicians by Cambridge University would be an important step toward this end. Jebb's attempts to reform education at the University, however, were strenuously opposed by those who objected both to his religious and political views, and also to any diminution of the power of the colleges. Jebb promoted these reforms at a time when he was supporting his friend Theophilus Lindsey in establishing a Unitarian church in London. Whenever he visited London Jebb attended the Essex Street church, which was supported by many socially and intellectually eminent people, such as the politician Sir George Savile, the Duke of Grafton (Chancellor of Cambridge), and two noted exponents of education reform, Joseph Priestley and Benjamin Franklin.[2] The experience of associating with such company in London must have fuelled his dogged pursuit of reform at the University. The development of determined opposition to his proposals for education reform further illustrates an increasing polarisation between conservative and liberal Whigs at Cambridge.

---

[1] Malcom Muggeridge, 'The Great Liberal Death Wish', in Russell Kirk ed., *The Portable Conservative Reader* (Harmondsworth, 1982), p. 621.

[2] Gascoigne, 'Latitudinarianism, Rational Dissent and Radicalism', p. 230; Joseph Priestley, *An Essay on a Course of Liberal Education for Civil and Active Life* (1765); Watts, ' Joseph Priestley and Education', pp. 83-100.

THOUGHTS ON EDUCATION

As a university examiner in the early 1760s, Richard Watson reflected upon 'defects in the University education, especially with respect to noblemen and fellow commoners ... and strongly insisted on the propriety of obliging them to keep exercises in the schools'. In 1766 he recommended 'annual examinations, in prescribed books, of all orders in the University', stressed the need for more time devoted to examination, more academic supervision, and examination for honours in subjects other than mathematics – in particular ethics and metaphysics.[3] Working with Watson as an examination moderator, Jebb shared his desire for such reforms. In November 1772 William Cooke (1711-97) became Vice-Chancellor of the University and made a speech in which he stressed the importance of academic education. Jebb sent Cooke his 'long projected' ideas on educational reform, noting that, as some influential members of the University were 'prejudiced against me', such reform would have a better chance of success if introduced by the Vice-Chancellor. Four days later Jebb discussed the proposals with Cooke, and left with the impression that he was favourably disposed towards them. However, no action was forthcoming over the next four months, and during a couple of subsequent visits Cooke was guarded and expressed himself 'in general terms'.[4] In response, Jebb published his *Remarks upon the Present Mode of Education in the University of Cambridge* (6 April 1772), and distributed copies to the heads of colleges.

To the modern reader Jebb's proposals seem sensible and moderate, but he was proposing to alter an institution with roots firmly planted in the Middle Ages, and in which vested interests abounded. In particular, his reforms would have enhanced the role of the University in shaping the curriculum, and consequently have undermined the autonomy of the colleges to some extent (though how much was the subject of hot debate). Cambridge was also a leading seminary of the Church. In an age of innovative political and religious ideas, any proposal to alter the structure of university education, no matter how innocuous, was bound to draw opposition from conservatives.[5] Nevertheless, Jebb was keen to increase the 'public utility' of Cambridge through reform proposals rooted in his Hartlean view of the human mind. To enable Cambridge to help combat the

---

[3] R. Watson, *Anecdotes*, pp. 46-7.

[4] 'A Narrative of Academical Proceedings Relative to a Proposal for the Establishment of Annual Examinations in the University of Cambridge' (20 December 1773), attached to the *Remarks upon the Present Mode of Education in the University of Cambridge: to which is added a proposal for its improvement* (Cambridge, 4th ed., January 1774), Jebb II, pp. 315-16.

[5] In 1750 the Duke of Newcastle had encouraged efforts to improve standards of behaviour at Cambridge. Regulations were introduced that sought to curb extravagant behaviour, drunkenness, and 'keeping evil company, breaking windows, making and fermenting riots and disturbances'. Understandably, these regulations were not popular with the students and their rebellious behaviour was encouraged by High Church pamphlets attacking the Chancellor's interference in university matters. Wordsworth, *Social Life at the English Universities*, pp. 67-68.

'present alarming crisis in national manners',[6] Jebb sought to achieve two broad aims: to improve the study habits of the entire student body, and to broaden the curriculum.

As noted in chapter 1, life in the universities reflected the wider social patterns of eighteenth-century England.[7] At the top of the heap were the noblemen and fellow commoners, who enjoyed numerous privileges and nominal examination. Naturally, young noblemen were much sought after because they brought wealth and the prospect of future patronage to colleges and their fellows. But some fellow commoners also caused considerable disruption among the undergraduates by encouraging riotous behaviour and contempt for the dons. Jebb observed that the fellow commoner, often residing in college for only a year or two, is left to 'aim at distinguishing himself in every fashionable mode of dissipation'. This was an 'evil the more to be lamented, as the superiority of fortune in that order of our students, would render their literary attainments more extensively beneficial to their country'. As things stood, Jebb believed that 'a licentious and infidel spirit, diffusing itself from the metropolis as its centre, at length hath penetrated these retirements; and hath produced appearances, peculiarly unbecoming a place, set apart for the purposes of learning and religious education'.[8] As noted in chapter 2, Jebb joined in widespread criticism of the British elite for indulging in fashionable luxury. In support of his education reforms, Jebb cited John Brown's influential *Estimate of the Manners of the Times* (1757), which emphasised the importance of education to the safety of the state and argued that it should inculcate habits of rational self-regulation.[9]

In contrast to the generally easy and indulgent life-style of the wealthy young gentry and aristocrats, students from less affluent and even poor backgrounds often found themselves in the awkward position of having to succeed academically, but needing to mix socially with those who offered the prospect of future patronage. With assessment postponed until the end of three years of residence, there was plenty of opportunity and encouragement for students to neglect their academic studies – especially under the spendthrift influence of fellow commoners. As a result, many awoke from idleness in their final year and 'broke their brain' preparing for examination. William Paley thought the system (with competition for honours in the final year) unhealthy,

[6] *Remarks upon ... Education*, Jebb II, p. 262.

[7] Lawson, *Social History of Education*, pp. 109-18; George C. Brauer, *The Education of a Gentleman: theories of gentlemanly education in England, 1660-1775* (New York, 1959), pp. 52-67; Sheldon Rothblat, 'The Student Subculture and the Examination System in Early Nineteenth-Century Oxbridge', in Lawrence Stone ed., *The University in Society* (1974), I, pp. 247-303.

[8] *Remarks upon ... Education*, Jebb II, pp. 268, 262.

[9] *Remarks upon ... Education*, Jebb II, p. 372. Jebb clearly agreed with much in Brown's analysis: the importance of a broad rational education based on a Lockean epistemology and praise for Sparta and its public education system 'suited to the Genius of the State'. That which he disagreed with, such as Brown's denigration of women, he could put down to Brown's reputation as a peculiar, even mentally unbalanced character who eventually slit his own throat in 1766.

because 'the stimulus is too strong: two or three heads are cracked by it every year.... Why, some of them go mad; others are reduced to such a state of debility, both of mind and body that they are unfit for anything during the rest of their lives'.[10] In 1781 Edmund Law similarly observed that many young men often sacrificed their 'whole stock of strength and spirits' in trying to get high honours, and ended up 'hardly good for anything else'.[11] Jebb also observed that the tendency to cram in the final year involved 'an obstinate course of labours which enfeeble the central powers of the student, ... [and] have not infrequently been known to be destructive of his health'.[12] Even if we allow for some exaggeration in such observations, it is clear that many students pushed themselves in their final year in an effort to avoid falling back into the obscurity and marginal existence that was the fate of many 'common people'.

Jebb's proposals to reform the study habits of all undergraduate students reflect the view of psychology and religion he derived from Locke and Hartley.[13] A moderator five times and a tutor for more than fifteen years, Jebb felt his 'knowledge of our form of literary discipline, and ... acquaintance with the movements of the youthful mind' made him well placed to advocate reform. He argued that traditional forms of 'severe discipline' were not suited to producing 'a decent and regular deportment' in an enlightened age. He believed that the contemporary laxity among students stemmed from 'the denial of indulgence to a virtuous affection of the soul, formerly cultivated with the most assiduous care ... as a passion, productive of the most salutary consequences to the public welfare'.[14] Rather than trying to stifle natural youthful passions, educators should harness them to literary and intellectual pursuits. 'I am inclined to prefer that mode of reformation', Jebb wrote, 'which gently leads the minds of youth from the pursuit of each inferior gratification, by proposing to their view such objects as are truly deserving of their attention; which ... rouses to the practice of every manly virtue, by the animating prospect of reward'. He argued that in the period of youth, 'the spirit of EMULATION is found in greatest force; it constitutes a motive, more generous than the selfish, sensual passions, which, according to the usual course of nature, prevail in earlier life; but less exalted than the fervent love of human kind, which is intended by the author of our being to be the incentive in maturer age'. This echoes Hartley's necessarian view of the mind as developing, as a result of experience and organic growth, through the stages of infancy and youth to maturity. According to Jebb:

> It has frequently been observed that the affections of the human mind rise by a necessary progress, in beautiful succession, each being introductory to affections of a nobler kind; that each has a limited time of acting ... and that if, in particular, the season, when the emulative affections most

---

[10] Cited in Clarke, *Paley*, p. 25.

[11] Edmund Law, 'Preface' to King's *On the Origin of Evil*, pp. xx-xi.

[12] *Remarks upon ... Education*, Jebb II, p. 266.

[13] John Locke, *Some Thoughts Concerning Education* (John W. and Jean S. Yolton eds., 1989).

[14] *Remarks upon ... Education*, Jebb II, pp. 261, 263.

> prevail, should be neglected, it will be in vain that we afterwards endeavour to impress the mind with the ardour of improvement, or to stamp it with the image of each sterling virtue.[15]

The age at which young men attend university was crucial in determining their lifelong development. If their ambitious affections were not directed toward literary pursuits and the cultivation of morality and religion at this age, they would be condemned to a morally enfeebled life – slaves to narrow self-interest.

Jebb was full of praise for those offering lectures in both the colleges and the University, in particular the recently appointed Professor of Modern History, John Symonds. Yet he believed that the University should support such efforts to promote learning by instituting a greater prospect of academic honour, and corresponding threat of disgrace. The carrot-and-stick mechanism central to Jebb's hedonistic moral philosophy lay behind his argument that the University should 'endeavour to confirm habits of application' learned at school by a 'more extensive exercise of the emulative affections', through having students compete for examination honours and prizes. Jebb proposed that the noblemen and fellow commoners should be examined annually, and other undergraduates examined in their second year. Aimed squarely at disciplining the fellow commoners, this proposal was not without appeal or support within the University. The Chancellor, the Duke of Grafton (to whom Jebb had dedicated his *Remarks upon ... Education*), made it clear that he wanted something done about the riotous lifestyle of the more wealthy students. Jebb suggested that the incoming first-year students of 1773/74 could be examined in May 1774, and speculated that the 'native candour, and ingenious manners' of those students already at the University would see them 'cheerfully' submit to be examined under the new programme.[16]

As noted in chapter 1, by the mid-eighteenth century the teaching of Newtonian natural philosophy dominated the curriculum at Cambridge. Both college and private tutors undertook most teaching, and students tended to become well versed in established mathematical knowledge without being exposed to any original research. The focus on inculcating orthodox Newtonianism also restricted time spent on other subjects.[17] While Jebb had excelled at mathematics, his religious and political interests led him to argue that moral and political instruction should receive more official encouragement. Jebb thought the emphasis upon Newtonian mathematics was no 'less reprehensible' than the failure to examine the fellow commoners. A 'moderate attention' to such studies provided a good training in rational thought, expanding and elevating the mind. But study of mathematics and 'nature's operations, should not entirely engross the youthful mind', since 'inquiry into metaphysical and moral truth' was necessary to prepare students for their future public and private lives. Mathematics and natural philosophy, 'however excellent in many respects, certainly has not a reasonable claim to the distinguished privileges, which it

---

[15] *Remarks upon ... Education*, Jebb II, pp. 264-65.
[16] *Remarks upon ... Education*, Jebb II, p. 274, 267, 281.
[17] Gascoigne, *Cambridge*, ch. 6; Wordsworth, *Scholae*, pp. 65-128.

enjoys at present in this seat of literature', as it does not prepare students 'for a general commerce with the world'.[18] The student must turn to the classics 'if he wishes to excel in just sentiment, and expressive diction'. Yet the University, aside from a few small prizes, did not reward such study. Likewise, the study of history was 'not sufficiently encouraged', and elocution 'utterly neglected'.[19] In short, each of these branches of 'useful literature' was 'defrauded of its proper portion of praise'. In this respect the curriculum at Cambridge compared poorly with the leading Dissenting academies, where students were given a comprehensive education in both science and humanistic studies. Jebb believed the student left Cambridge ill-prepared for public life: 'his acquisitions appear unimportant in the eyes of his fellow-citizens; and he, therefore, either resigns himself to despondency, or seeks for happiness in the gratifications of a dissipated life'.[20]

Jebb argued that the quality of education would improve if the University were to conduct annual examinations of all students. Under the mastership of William Powell St John's College held regular half yearly examinations to improve the academic ability of its students, no doubt with an eye to their claiming honours in the Senate House examinations. While applauding this example, Jebb argued that such examinations could not be introduced in the smaller colleges. He briefly sketched his proposed reforms at the end of his *Remarks*: annual examinations could be held in the Senate House; the subject matter should encompass 'the law of nature and of nations, chronology, history, classics, mathematics, metaphysics, and philosophy natural and moral'; no student would be allowed to 'plead his order, as an exemption from attending' the examinations; at the start of each academic year the University should nominate particular classical authors and portions of history as the subject of examination, and establish awards for each subject and year level; limitations should be set on the particular portions of mathematics and natural philosophy to be examined, so students could focus their studies and not have all of their time consumed in studying these subjects; to encourage students to excel in 'Latin or English composition', they should be awarded 'books of the most elegant editions' with 'inscriptions suitable to the occasion' and the engraved arms of the University; in the final examination for the BA, students should be tested on their knowledge of the Scriptures.[21] Jebb lamented that the custom of providing theological lectures in the colleges had waned. He thought that a BA student should be 'tolerably well versed' in the original Greek text of the four Gospels and Hugo Grotius's writings in favour of Christianity and religious toleration. However, those intending to enter the Church should ideally

---

[18] *Remarks upon ... Education*, Jebb II, pp. 269-70.

[19] According to G.M. Trevelyan, 'No lecture was delivered by any Regius Professor of Modern History at Cambridge between 1725 and 1773; "the third and most scandalous" of the holders of that Chair dies in 1768 from a fall while riding home drunk from his Vicarage'. *English Social History* (1944), p. 366.

[20] *Remarks upon ... Education*, Jebb II, pp. 271-73.

[21] *Remarks upon ... Education*, Jebb II, pp. 275-79.

be encouraged to stay on at the University and undertake some post-graduate study in theology.[22]

Jebb's proposals had the capacity to attract substantial support as a means of promoting greater discipline. Yet such reforms could also be seen as a threat to college autonomy, an affront to the aristocracy and a Trojan horse for new and unorthodox curricula. Such fears were fuelled by the fact that Jebb's proposals clearly stemmed from his religious, philosophical and political concerns. Openly involved in the Feathers Tavern petition, Jebb claimed the right to propose academic reform because he possessed 'a voice in the legislature of our little republic'. Admitting that the proposals were far from perfect, he argued that a 'reformation of the most material errors in our practice, may prepare the way for more desirable improvements'. He offered his proposals because 'it is incumbent upon every citizen to contribute whatever may lie in his power to the advancement of the public welfare'. Finally, implying intellectual deficiencies on the part of the existing clergy, Jebb suggested the reforms would induce senior members of the University 'to devote themselves, with increasing application, to such parts of literature, as may be eminently beneficial to them in their profession as divines'.[23]

Supporters consciously linked education and religious reform: Henry Taylor thought the continuing support for orthodox theology 'arises from a neglect in our University Education' and in particular the 'slovenly way of using words'.[24] Writing of the Feathers Tavern petition, Ann Jebb claimed that while 'religious superstition' had helped guide moral behaviour in the past, with the decline of superstition 'in this enlightened age' a continuing increase in immoral behaviour would be inevitable if 'true Religion be not planted in its place'.[25] Likewise in his *Letter to Sir William Meredith* (1772), Jebb declared that 'Degrees are testimonies and rewards of literary merit; and should therefore lie open to every son of science, without distinction of party, sect, or nation'.[26] As we shall see, opponents were not loath to focus upon the ulterior motives that accompanied Jebb's attempt to reform education at Cambridge.

REFORM EFFORTS

An understanding of how the University was governed is necessary in order to understand the controversy generated by Jebb's education reform proposals. Any regulatory change had to pass both the Caput and the Senate. The Caput (composed of six members elected on 12 October every year) was responsible for the day-to-day affairs of the University.[27] Any proposal for a change to

---

[22] *Remarks upon ... Education*, Jebb II, pp. 279-80n.

[23] *Remarks upon ... Education*, Jebb II, pp. 261, 271, 281.

[24] Henry Taylor to Ann Jebb, [Feb 1773?], CUL Taylor papers.

[25] 'No Petitioner, but a Friend to the Petitioners' [AJ], *Whitehall Evening Post*, 23 April 1772.

[26] *A Letter to Sir William Meredith* (1772), Jebb I, p. 260.

[27] The Caput consisted of the Vice-Chancellor, three doctors (representing each faculty: Law, Divinity, and Medicine), and two MAs (one from each house of the Senate).

university regulations had to be presented to the Caput as a 'grace' (like a bill in Parliament). It was usual for the Caput to approve every grace and pass it on to the Senate. The Senate consisted of all MAs and Doctors who had their names on the college books or were resident in Cambridge (they amounted to about four hundred individuals in 1772). These were divided into the Regents House (MAs of less than five and Doctors of less than two years standing who wore white hoods) and the Non-Regents House (the senior academics who wore black hoods).[28]

In response to the Vice-Chancellor's failure to act, Jebb busied himself with trying to gather support for his proposals in April and May 1773 (at the same time as Lindsey was establishing his Unitarian Chapel in London). On 21 April he published a second edition of his *Remarks* with a postscript signalling his intention to introduce a grace containing his proposals. In an attempt to lessen opposition Jebb decided to introduce only the proposal for annual university examinations, to which he added a grace recommending the appointment of a committee to draw up guidelines for the implementation of exams. At this time the Caput included Samuel Hallifax, William Powell (master of St John's College) and Edmund Law.

On 8 May they rejected the grace, with Powell claiming that annual *university* examinations would undermine the authority of the colleges, and that as the Caput did not fairly represent the colleges, it could not allow the grace to go before the Senate. After consulting with Law, Jebb wrote to the other members asking them to alter any part of the grace they thought necessary before it could go to the Senate, where it could be judged by the 'sense of the University'. He resubmitted his grace on May 12. During the ensuing debate he was summoned in person and told that the Vice-Chancellor, owing to a lack of adequate time to consider its merits and implications, was rejecting it. Prepared for this, Jebb produced another two graces with minor alterations. Becoming increasingly angry, Powell proposed a grace that would prevent Jebb from submitting any more, but aware that Law would veto this he 'thought it most prudent to change the subject'.[29] Nevertheless, Powell and Cooke had succeeded in preventing Jebb's proposals from being considered by the Senate.

Ten days after Jebb left the University for the summer, Cooke selected a thirty-six-member committee or 'syndicate' to consider the general issue of academic reform, and report by January of the following year. He called a meeting in October, while many of the tutors were away in their country parishes, and the Syndicate voted fourteen to nine against the idea of pursuing academic reform. When Jebb returned to Cambridge, he condemned the Syndicate's actions in a *Continuation of the Narrative of Academical Proceedings* (4 November 1773). He concluded this pamphlet with the observation that should his efforts fail, he was at least paving the way for future

[28] Jebb provided his readers with this outline of the University's constitution at the start of his 'Narrative of Academical Proceedings' (20 Dec 1773), Jebb II, pp. 309-35.
[29] *Remarks upon ... Education*, Jebb II, p. 316-23.

reformers.[30] It is worth remembering that in August Jebb had first indicated to friends that he would resign from the Church, and in September he had confronted Archdeacon Goodall at his parish church in Flixton.[31]

Continuing unruly student behaviour lent weight to calls for reform. The Cambridge Dissenting minister Robert Robinson (1735-90) published a sermon on *A Becoming Behaviour in Religious Assemblies* (1773). Raised in poor circumstances by a deserted mother, Robinson became the Baptist minister at Cambridge in 1761 and revived a flagging congregation. A strong supporter of the Dissenting petition against subscription, he was acquainted with Jebb and Tyrwhitt. Robinson complained to the University that 'we scarcely ever meet without interruptions from the undergraduates', hurling the 'same insults as in a bawdy house'. 'Is there a vacuum in nature?' he asked in his sermon, 'It is in the brain of him who behaves ill at divine worship'.[32] Dissenters were not the only targets of student abuse. According to Jebb, during November 1773 one of his academic colleagues preached a 'papistical sermon' in which 'he attacked the Latitudinarians vehemently, and maintained that the liberty of private opinions rent the Church of Christ'. This provoked vocal criticism from some students, and when the Vice-Chancellor ordered that their names be taken down, 'there was a general hiss and many rushed out before the door could be secured'. With the Bishop of Peterborough trying to block the way, they broke the church door off its hinges. Jebb saw this as proof of the need for academic reform, as 'they will have riots upon riots, unless some scheme is thought of to employ the active spirits of young men'.[33] Conservatives no doubt saw such rebellious behaviour as a result of the disrespect for authority cultivated by the likes of Jebb.[34]

The hopes of those disposed to reform were raised when a new Caput was elected, with the reputedly fair-minded Dr Lynford Caryl as Vice-Chancellor. While Samuel Hallifax remained along with Dr Thomas Brown, it also contained Plumptre and Hughes, both of whom were on good terms with Jebb. Writing in the *Whitehall Evening Post*, John Disney expressed concern that Hallifax remained in a position to block any proposals from going before the Senate. While traditionally the power of veto had been exercised with the

---

[30] Jebb reflected that the Vice-Chancellor 'appears to me to have ... permitted himself to be directed by the counsels of a person [Powell], who has always manifested a hostile disposition to the proposed establishment, and whose conduct in the committee forbids us to suppose, that he would have ever have permitted the preceding grace to have passed the Caput, unless he had been convinced, that it contained in itself the seeds of its own inevitable destruction'. Jebb II, p. 327-32n, at 329.

[31] See chapter 5.

[32] Graham W. Hughes, '*With Freedom Fired': the story of Robert Robinson, Cambridge Nonconformist* (1955), pp. 7, 16, 42, 21-22. Jebb and Robinson both preached in the parish of St Andrews.

[33] 'Life of Jebb', pp. 57-58.

[34] One of the young men involved in the riot was Gilbert Wakefield, who went on to become a noted Unitarian and radical. Gilbert Wakefield, *Memoirs of the Life of Gilbert Wakefield* (2 vols., 1804), p. 94.

'greatest caution', Powell and his assistant 'in acts of tyranny and insolence – Dr Hallifax' had allowed personal resentment to govern their decisions.[35]

Jebb's opponents also aired their views in the newspapers. Writing in the *St James's Chronicle* in late December, a fellow of St John's anonymously praised the rejection of Jebb's grace as 'in itself utterly tending to the Destruction of the University, and resulting entirely from the infernal and diabolic Malice which Mr Jebb is well known to be fraught with'. He stated succinctly his principal objection: annual university examinations would deter parents from sending their children to Cambridge, because 'either conscious of the child's inability to undergo it, or sensibly supposing, that if Nature had bestowed uncommon Talents upon them, without uniting with it at the same Time a most consummate Share of Impudence, the natural Diffidence of Youth would have such an effect upon them, that pre-supposing their Ability, they would be unable to perform the task'.[36]

This less-than-convincing argument drew a reply from a correspondent in Newington Green, who asked that Jebb's 'malice' be demonstrated, and observed that diffidence was unfortunately not a characteristic of students 'in this Age'.[37] 'Anti-Jebbite' in turn claimed that because of the disappointing response to his proposals, Jebb 'has changed his good will toward the University (supposing him once possessed of it) into the most implacable Venom and Spite against all Members thereof; and is willing to show his Teeth, (though he can't bite) and harass by innumerable Absurdities the respectable Senate'.[38] A correspondent in Essex replied that Jebb's character was good, and observed that he would never teach a student 'Bigotry and irrational Prejudice; in which principles this hot-headed writer seems to be immersed'.[39]

On 14 December 1773 Jebb brought forward a grace to have the report of the Syndicate overturned as not expressing the will of the majority of its members. This grace passed the Caput, but was rejected by the Non-Regents. Excited that the new Caput was willing to allow his grace to go before the Senate, in February 1774 Jebb proposed that a new Syndicate be appointed to consider all undergraduate courses. He recommended a list of members that balanced some notable opponents such as Richard Farmer and Samuel Hallifax against a majority 'well disposed to the good work'.[40]

---

[35] 'Socio Coemensalis' [J. Disney], *Whitehall Evening Post,* 4 December 1773.

[36] 'Anti-Jebbite' in Cambridge, *St James's Chronicle,* 23 December 1773. The 'most consummate Share of Impudence' would be a veiled reference to Jebb and his friend Waring who were second and first respectively on the honours list when they graduated together. Powell had savagely criticised Waring's appointment as Lucasian Professor of Mathematics at a young age.

[37] 'A Lover of Truth' in Newington Green (this could have been either Richard Price, James Burgh or someone associated with their circle), *St James's Chronicle,* 25 December 1773.

[38] 'Anti-Jebbite, or in plain terms A Fellow of St John's', *St James's Chronicle,* 18 January 1774.

[39] 'A Moderate Petitioner', *St James's Chronicle*, 20 January 1774.

[40] Jebb's Syndicate was composed of Dr Cooke, Dr Plumptre, Dr Barnardiston, Dr Richard Watson, Dr Samuel Hallifax, Dr Edward Waring, Beadon, Collier, Lambert,

A few days after Jebb's proposal passed through the Caput and both houses of the Senate, the Chancellor (the Duke of Grafton) visited the University and personally urged upon the Vice-Chancellor the need for an improved education of the noblemen and fellow commoners. At the first meeting of the Syndicate on 16 March the Vice-Chancellor read out a letter from Grafton expressing his sentiments. After the first three meetings it was resolved to recommend that noblemen and fellow commoners be examined annually in classics, algebra, geometry, natural philosophy, Locke's *Essay*, natural law and modern history. Jebb was delighted and wrote to a friend on 16 March: 'The Vice-Chancellor (Dr Caryl) gives general satisfaction by his very candid behaviour, and able manner of doing business.... You cannot imagine how greatly certain spirits are alarmed with the disposition there appears to do something effectual. Dr Powell, and the Emmanuel men, and Dr Hallifax, labour to spoil, what the friends of literature and good morals are mediating to establish'. The vehemence of the opposition was a response to Jebb's own forceful manner and status as the leading exponent of heterodox opinions at Cambridge. He realised this, writing that 'I endeavour to keep out of sight as much as I can, as I find my presence occasions jealousies, and heart-burnings; and, for every reason, I am desirous that the work may appear to be done by others, as I see whatever I propose, would be objected to.' Jebb was confident that the Syndicate was composed of men who would 'determine for the best: I am only afraid, that the clamours of the discontented, may intimidate them'.[41]

Despite the 'vehemency of Dr Powell, and Mr Whisson', and the efforts of Hallifax and Farmer to 'obstruct and distress their brethren', by the end of the month a list of nineteen resolutions were drawn up to be presented to the Senate.[42] Ann Jebb told readers of the *Whitehall Evening Post* that 'it is said that the greatest Politicians are so fully satisfied of the utility of the proposals which the syndics have agreed upon, that they are very anxious for their success'.[43]

A week before the resolutions were to be presented to the Senate, an unsigned 'Letter to Mr Jebb' appeared on the front page of the *Lloyd's Evening Post*. This was clearly designed to remind all concerned that Jebb and his religious radicalism lay behind the proposed reforms.[44] The continual presenting of graces, the writer observed, suggests Jebb 'must have a high conceit of the infallibility of his judgement, as well as something very Quixotic in his constitution'. While Dr Cooke was at first favourable to the proposal, the writer

Willgress, Dealtary, Longmire, Joannes Hey, Richard Farmer, Gould, Gardnar, William Paley, Squire, Arnald, and Pearce. 'Life of Jebb', pp. 59-60. Jebb listed as the most strenuous supporters: Longmire, Lambert, Collier, Hey, Beadon. 'Life of Jebb', p. 64.

41 'Life of Jebb', pp. 61-2.

42 JJ to [?], 28 March 1774, 'Life of Jebb', p. 64.

43 'Y.Z'. [AJ], *Whitehall Evening Post*, 9 April 1774.

44 He cites Jebb's professed desire that students develop a 'system of faith and practice' in accordance with an enlightened understanding of Christianity. *A Short Account of Theological Lectures*, p. 26; [?], 'A letter to Mr Jebb', *Lloyd's Evening Post*, 11 April 1774.

alleged, he 'grew at last cool and reserved – teased and tired, I presume, by your importunity'. Defeat owed much to personal animosity fostered by the controversy over Jebb's lectures, which implied that he had some 'more perfect System of Theology' to impart. The writer conceded that annual exams would promote more study, but claimed they were unfair to modest students who do not excel in public disputation – as Jebb should know, having been a university moderator five times. In a dig at Jebb's own high undergraduate achievements, he declared that medals and prizes only encourage 'mercenary souls'. The colleges, he argued, are best able to oversee and regulate the instruction of students, and the University should confine itself to appointing competent and independent lecturers. He criticised Jebb for a tendency to 'represent things in extremes' and students as 'either sluggish Door-mice, or soaring Eagles'; detected that 'the advancement of Theological Knowledge is, I presume, the grand object of your plan'; suggested that Jebb not be so 'splenetic, indecent, if not scurrilous' toward the bishops; and, with tongue firmly in cheek, recommended that Jebb

> imitate your Friend, the author of the D—e L—n [William Warburton, *The Divine Legation*?], who, when a torrent of abuse was poured upon him … retire[d] till Time, which draws Truth from the well, ripens the Understanding, subdues Prejudice, and opens the eyes of Bigots, may reconcile your Opponents to your schemes of *Reformation in Theology* &c. and you will then break forth from behind a cloud, with redoubled lustre.

A supporter of the reforms responded quickly, defending Jebb's character and conduct, and claiming that theology had nothing to do with annual examinations.[45] But in vain did such efforts attempt to counter the identification of academic reform with calls for religious and political change.

The resolutions were gathered together and presented to the Senate on 19 April 1774 in the form of three graces proposing annual examination of the nobles and fellow commoners, appointment of university examiners and examination of other undergraduates in classics and mathematics at the end of their second year. Each of the proposals was narrowly defeated in the Non-Regents house (by 4, 7 and 11 votes respectively), to 'the real astonishment of both sides' according to John Disney.[46] The following day Dr John Gordon moved 'for an examination of the nobles and fellow commoners without any particulars specify'd'. But this was rejected by seven votes. Robert Plumptre attributed the defeat to a fear that college autonomy would be undermined, the sons of the aristocracy turned away from the University, and a 'general disinclination to innovation and reformation, which has been shown by mankind in all ages'.[47]

The Jebbs, however, remained in good spirits, and thought they had been unlucky in that 'two of the friendly Heads, and two of the Syndicate were

---

[45] [?], 'Reply to a Letter to Mr Jebb', *Lloyd's Evening Post*, 15 April 1774.
[46] 'Life of Jebb', p. 64.
[47] Robert Plumptre to Lord Hardwicke, 25 April 1774, BL Add. Mss. 35,628:191.

absent' from the vote. 'I believe the enemy thought themselves in great danger', Ann wrote, 'for a report was industriously circulated on Monday, that the A—B— of C— was against the resolutions, and trembled for the fate of the University; and it is supposed by some that this report had the intended effect. Certain it is, however, that some persons appeared in the opposition, who were expected to have been neuter'.[48] In a private letter, John Jebb revealed that the opponents, in particular Samuel Hallifax and the Dean of Ely, Dr Thomas, cited 'objections to the person who moved the question'. He claimed that half of those who voted against the reforms 'in the main, approved what they opposed by their suffrage. I speak not from presumption, we have it from their own confession'.[49] Nevertheless, the prospect of future success was bolstered when, in response to the defeat, Grafton wrote to the members of the Syndicate to praise their proposals and express the hope that 'at some future period it would have a more favourable event'.[50]

In light of the narrow defeat, and Grafton's encouragement, Jebb printed another 'plan for public examinations' on 11 May 1774 before retiring to Bungay for the summer.[51] In this modified proposal he tried to minimise the threat to college autonomy by allowing that the examinations be based upon the 'settled lectures of the Tutors'.[52] At the end of the month Ann Jebb again wrote to the *Whitehall Evening Post*, claiming that half the professors did not lecture, and that those who did were ill attended. 'Maintaining the *attention* of students is the problem that must be addressed', she argued, like many who attend Church, they '*yawn*, or *sleep*, or whisper, or entertain themselves with anything rather than pay any real *attention*'. 'Let me ask', she continued, 'whether those Gentlemen who keep their horses, and run them *for fifty guineas*, are likely to attend any lectures to any purpose?' Could the opponents of reform honestly deny that 'calling upon these Gentlemen every year, to give some account of their proficiency in learning, would not make them *find more time to read*, and *less* to think of HORSE-RACING, or any other kind of dissipation?'[53]

In August Jebb himself published *A Proposal for the Establishment of Public Examinations in the University of Cambridge with occasional remarks*, which outlined his intention to resubmit the modified proposals in the form of twenty separate graces, so that each could be accepted or rejected upon its own merit. Jebb restated his main arguments: annual examinations were necessary as a 'remedy for that early dissipation, which the utmost diligence of the tutors hath hitherto been unable to prevent'. The fellow commoners should be treated differently because their 'views and pursuits' were 'materially different from those of an inferior degree'. The fear that fellow commoners would avoid the University or be academically humiliated was unfounded, as they came to Cambridge 'better prepared in classical knowledge' and with a 'higher sense of

[48] 'Y.Z'. [AJ], *Whitehall Evening Post*, 23 April 1774.
[49] JJ to [?], 23 April 1774, 'Life of Jebb', pp. 70-71.
[50] Cited in Gascoigne, *Cambridge*, p. 203.
[51] 'Life of Jebb', p. 73.
[52] 'Life of Jebb', p. 76.
[53] 'Y.Z'. [AJ] *Whitehall Evening Post*, 31 May 1774.

honour'. Fellow commoners were examined along with other students at St John's College with 'no inconveniences, but, on the contrary, great advantages'. As students study Latin prior to entering university, examination in the classics would not sap so much of their energies as to undermine the study of mathematics. Jebb pointed to the method of conducting examinations in the Senate House to answer the criticism that not all students were equally fit to 'stand the terrors of a public examination'. Seldom more than six students at a time were examined at the moderator's table. 'The examination by the other members of the Senate is still more private, the examiner and student always retiring to a place by themselves'. This method 'provides for eliciting the most latent merit of the student ... I believe scarcely a single instance can be produced of a person, who failed in obtaining the degree of credit he deserved'.[54]

The revised proposals, set out as twenty separate graces, were presented to the Senate on 28 October. Two days prior an anonymous *Letter to the Author of the Plan for the Establishment of Public Examinations* appeared. 'Written in a candid manner', it warned that the proposals would be difficult to implement, and if they failed, would ruin the University.[55] This letter was attributed to Powell, and its uncharacteristic moderation indicates how worried the opponents of reform were. In the event, through what Ann Jebb called 'great, and I may say *unaccountable* misfortune', the first grace was defeated by one vote, and the rest rejected without a division.[56] Such a narrow defeat was all the more frustrating because it was widely believed that the reforms would have passed the Regents House by eleven votes.[57]

A friend hoped the narrow defeat would encourage Jebb's supporters to persevere with a program 'so evidently pregnant with national Emolument'.[58] For his part, Powell felt compelled to publish an anonymous tract in which, in the words of D.A. Winstanley, 'the tutorial big drum was beaten extremely loudly'.[59] It was a deliberate attempt to cast 'our warm Reformer' as a dangerous and ambitious innovator who believed that there was some fundamental 'defect in our institutions'. He claimed that the '*candid* Author (as it is the fashion to call him)' had overstated the disciplinary problems at Cambridge, and that 'inattention at lectures is not a general fault among our Pupils'. Many students sought private instruction, and, in implicit criticism of Jebb (who was a prominent private tutor), Powell observed: 'It seems indeed to be the general opinion, that some of these private Instructors go forward too

---

[54] *A Proposal for the Establishment of Public Examinations in the University of Cambridge, with occasional remarks* (Cambridge, August 1774), Jebb II, pp. 351-55, 368-69.

[55] 'Life of Jebb', p. 81.

[56] [AJ], *A Letter to the Author of an Observation on the Design of Establishing Annual Examinations at Cambridge* (Cambridge, November 1774), p. 4.

[57] 'Life of Jebb', p. 80n. What is more, Dr Robert Plumptre, a strong supporter of reform, was not present at the vote. Robert Plumptre to Lord Hardwicke, 10 November 1774, BL Add. Mss. 35, 628: 206.

[58] Thomas Dalton to JJ, 1 January 1775, manuscript letter in the interleaved DWL *Illustrated Life of Priestley* mss. 12.79.265.

[59] Winstanley, *Unreformed Cambridge*, p. 327.

hastily, and aim at conducting their Pupils to the more difficult parts of science, before they are prepared by an acquaintance with the easier'. This was to be expected if a student separate from his 'principal Tutor, and choose another Instructor unknown and unconnected with him'. Powell contrasted the traditional paternal care and discipline afforded by the college tutors with the 'bold and dangerous experiment' of education under the direction of 'Examiners, hired at the mean price of ten guineas yearly, and chosen anew every year, who must be wholly strangers to most of the Pupils, to their abilities, their previous education, the professions or stations, for which they are designed'. And, despite Jebb's modifications, the college tutors would find themselves having to change their lectures each year 'according to the fancies of these Examiners'.[60]

Ann Jebb was quick to reply to Powell's tract, reiterating her argument that attendance at lectures did not necessarily mean students were *paying attention* or pursuing '*useful literature*'; having private tutors did not mean that the fellow commoners actually used them; and widespread support for the reform proposals among the college tutors testified that they wanted more university '*rules* and *regulations*' to make the students '*ambitious* of acquiring *every manly attainment*'. Far from scaring off wealthy students, she assured Powell, annual examination of the fellow commoners would spur them to become 'distinguished according to their merit' and equal 'the Pensioners in *every* literary attainment'.[61] It is clear that Jebb's reform proposals challenged traditional paternalistic college-based education in the name of a more uniform, meritocratic, university administered system.

Powell died in January 1775, but with the Feathers Tavern petition also dead and buried, and conflict with the colonies escalating, any prospect of Jebb successfully introducing education reform was fast waning. As John Gascoigne has observed, the debate over education reform at Cambridge took place in a 'politically highly charged atmosphere'.[62] Writing about a young Jacobite and High-Church friend he had introduced to Jebb, Thomas Blackburne (son of Francis) observed: 'I have frequently taken the liberty of a friend in attempting to corrupt his civil and religious principles.... I fear I have shocked his Orthodoxy by taking great liberties with his Royal Martyr Charles the First ... [which] I fear, has interrupted the confidence and intercourse that I intended should subsist between us'. 'I dare say', he continued, 'he abhors the scheme of your lectures, which he will not be untaught at Emmanuel. Athanasius has him by the right hand and A-Bp Laud by the left. I wish you may be able to make anything of him'.[63]

The association of Jebb and his closest supporters with religious and political dissent ensured a solid core of opposition to their proposals for

---

[60] [W.S. Powell], *An Observation on the Design of Establishing Annual Examinations at Cambridge* (Cambridge, 14 November 1774), pp. 3-7, 10-11.

[61] [AJ], *A Letter to the Author of an Observation*, pp. 12, 15, 20-21.

[62] Gascoigne, *Cambridge*, p. 205.

[63] Thomas Blackburne (in Richmond) to JJ, 14 October 1774, DWL Blackburne correspondence.

educational reform. 'We know', Powell wrote, 'that when any bold Pretender publishes his bills, he usually gains an audience, even though he has nothing to offer them, but trite objections to the Religion or Government of their country'. He likened Jebb to 'the Architect, who, dissatisfied with our *old buildings*, proposed, about the middle of last century, *to pull them all down, except King's College Chapel*, and to erect in their stead one ample and *uniform* structure, *such as it behoveth an Academy to be in a* FREE AND WELL ORDERED COMMONWEALTH'.[64]

Following Powell's death, Jebb asked the Vice-Chancellor and heads of colleges whether he should resubmit the reform proposals. In March he was advised to leave the issue alone until 'there was a prospect of a more general concurrence in favour of the plan than appeared at present'.[65] Nevertheless, on 22 March 1775 he printed 'An Address to the Members of the Senate' as a broadside, proposing the formation of a Syndicate composed of the Vice-Chancellor and heads of houses, which should request direction on the issue of education reform from the Chancellor. Jebb soon realised, however, that most did not approve of the measure. He retracted the proposal in *An Address to the Members of the Senate of Cambridge* (29 March 1775) and deferred any new motions until the following winter.[66]

RESIGNATION

With battle joined in North America, Jebb travelled north to Harrogate, and visited Francis Blackburne at Richmond. He returned to Cambridge via Leicestershire, where he spent time with his relation Lord Harborough at Stapleford, and then at Ann's hometown of Huntingdon. On 29 September he formally resigned his vicarage and rectory near Bungay in Suffolk (in the diocese of Norwich). 'My situation', he confided in a private letter, 'I thank God, and a good friend, will not be distressing, though it will be precarious.... I am easy in the thoughts of being delivered from what I esteem worse than Egyptian bondage'.[67] He sent a letter to Philip Yonge, the Bishop of Norwich, which he published as *A Short State of the Reasons for a Late Resignation* (October 1775). In this, as outlined in the preceding chapters, he rejected orthodox theology, argued for an improved understanding of the Scriptures and advocated a more rational and utilitarian established church/federation of churches.

Jebb remained at Cambridge and, while pondering how to make his way in the world, decided to resubmit his education reforms. After the last vote, William Cole observed that as Jebb 'will always have the last blow, and his associates are indefatigable, it is probable that their restless spirits will bring it in

---

[64] [Powell], *Observation*, pp. 5, 12.
[65] Cited in Winstanley, *Unreformed Cambridge*, p. 328.
[66] 'Life of Jebb', 89-91; *Address to the ...Senate of Cambridge*, Jebb II, pp. 371-90.
[67] 'Life of Jebb', pp. 97-104. He wrote a letter from Newark to Dr Chambers on 16 July, visited Richmond on 26 July, and wrote from Harrogate 4 August.

again in some mode or other'.[68] But success had become almost impossible, owing to his resignation from the Church and the appointment of Richard Farmer as Vice-Chancellor. Nevertheless, in late October Jebb wrote three forthright public letters to prepare the way for his next grace.

He restated his argument in favour of directing the youthful 'spirit of emulation' toward academic pursuits via competitive examinations. Four hundred young men, he argued, populated Cambridge, free from the restraints imposed at school and all trying to 'appear well mounted at Newmarket', 'surpass each other in expensive cloaths, and expensive entertainments', and every 'fashionable mode of dissipation'. Jebb implied that some parents were providing their students with far too much pocket money, and argued that directing youthful passions and ambitions toward literary pursuits would decrease the cost of maintaining a student at university.[69] He lamented that ethics was little taught at Cambridge, and 'the incomparable Locke' was 'now almost as little honoured, at the public time of trial, as real science is said to be at our sister university'.[70]

Examining 'with candour' the new Vice-Chancellor's opinion that annual exams would 'shake the constitution in both church and state', Jebb declared that the universities could be either abolished or entirely reformed without causing 'any violent alteration ... in the constitution of this kingdom'. 'The logic of Burgersdicius prevailed at Cambridge in the memory of our fathers. The barbarous sounds of Darii and Felapton now no longer grate upon our ears; the constitution nevertheless flourishes: and although the Principia of Newton have shaken down, what was supposed to be the philosophy of Moses, and swept away the vortices of Des Cartes, the Church of England still stands.' The proposals defeated on 28 October 1774 contained no 'new mode of study', not even 'a competent knowledge in the Greek Testament'. Rather, they only sought to 'secure the attention of the student to the present course of public lectures'. He called upon the Vice-Chancellor to support a statement which, 'in the judgement of many, appears extraordinary'. 'Let argument be opposed to argument; and let the sense of Cambridge reject, or establish, by its suffrages, as truth, and reason, and expedience shall decree'.[71]

Jebb expressed frustration with the existing governing procedures at Cambridge in a revised *Short Address* (20 December 1775). Any member of the Caput could reject a grace without justification, a grace that passed had to go before the Senate without modification, and if defeated in the Senate it could not

---

[68] BL Cole mss. 5873:70.

[69] Jebb reviewed the basic cost of life at college: the average annual allowance for a sizar was 40-50 pounds per annum; for a Pensioner it was 90-100 pounds per annum, which included payment to the butler of 30 shillings, hairdresser 12s, laundress 20s, bed-maker 10-12s per quarter; a fellow commoner *should* need no more than 200 pounds per annum plus perhaps 100 pounds for a servant, private tutor, and horse; to the expenses of a nobleman 'I assign no bounds'. 'Chiron' [JJ], [a London newspaper], 24 October 1775, Jebb III, pp. 261-68, at 263-64, 266-68.

[70] 'Chiron' [JJ], [a London newspaper], 28 October 1775, Jebb III, pp. 268-77, at 271.

[71] 'Chiron' [JJ], [a London newspaper], 11 November 1775, Jebb III, pp. 278-82.

be resubmitted in the same term. In late February 1776 Jebb prepared to resubmit the reform proposals, but confessed to a friend: 'I have had great vexation, and expect more; but every principle requires me to go on with the business. I must make this last trial, though the adversary hopes to bring me to great shame, and has managed the congregations accordingly; and our friends, who are a clear majority, will probably desert me; but I will retire from the question with an easy mind, whatever be the event.'[72]

While Jebb was preparing for his symbolic final confrontation, Farmer intimated that his academic qualifications could be suspended owing to his resignation from the Church. According to Jebb, when he appeared before the Caput,

> the Vice-Chancellor made no objection ... he behaved like a Tory, and I gave him a dressing, and publicly charged him with his intolerant declaration about my degree.... We had many altercations. I was pretty well fatigued, and am glad that the business is so near to completion. Lambert is very indignant at the unparalleled ill treatment I have received from the friends of the cause. The bishops were never hearty; they fell in with the language of the public when with us, and when the public grew tired, they turned to their natural temper and abhorrence of reformation.

Jebb's persistence had clearly alienated some former supporters. Farmer allowed the graces to pass, confident that the Senate would overwhelmingly reject them. While Edmund Law, Richard Watson and Robert Plumptre continued to show their support for reform, Jebb saw, at the instigation of Richard Hurd (recently appointed Bishop of Lichfield), the full weight of episcopal displeasure bearing down on the vote. 'The dastardly friends' of reform, he wrote 'are running out of the university as if from a plague'.[73] Voicing the prevailing view prior to the vote, the young nobleman Philip Yorke observed that Jebb 'is so obnoxious a person in himself that every plan or proposal, however good in itself, provided it comes from him, is sure to be rejected'.[74] In the event, Jebb was left with the support of twenty-five votes against thirty-nine in the Non-Regents house. Examination reform would not be seriously debated again until the 1820s, at which time 'Jebb's plans were brought in evidence by both sides in the dispute'.[75]

Jebb's resignation from the Church had deprived his reform proposals of much support, and left him marginalised in university circles. His Greek New Testament lectures had ceased owing to a lack of students, and Francis Blackburne was told Jebb would 'find difficulties in contriving how to live'.[76]

---

[72] JJ to [?], 22 February 1776, 'Life of Jebb', p. 113.

[73] JJ to [?], 27 February 1776, 'Life of Jebb', pp. 114-15. James Lambert (1741-1823) was a fellow of Trinity College and a strong supporter of Jebb. He had been elected unopposed as Professor of Greek in March 1771 and developed Arian views.

[74] Winstanley, *Unreformed Cambridge*, p. 329.

[75] Searby, *A History of Cambridge University: volume III*, p. 166.

[76] Blackburne to Lindsey 19 Nov 1775, DWL mss. 12.52.103.

Lindsey reported that if Jebb 'does not succeed with pupils at Cambridge, which I much fear he will not, he thinks of coming to London where I have no doubt but he will succeed as he deserves'. Yet he was disappointed that Jebb 'seemed to decline continuing in the ministry', and would not join him as a Unitarian minister at Essex Street.[77]

Not surprisingly, the mass resignation from the Church that Lindsey had hoped for did not eventuate. The heterodox clergy were clearly a minority, and government policy rewarded religious and political orthodoxy.[78] The American conflict drew calls for obedience and respect for authority from an increasing number of clergymen.[79] And social and employment security was also a powerful incentive for heterodox clergy to continue living as Latitudinarians. Christopher Wyvill talked of resigning, but did not follow through.[80] The delay and reluctance that accompanied Jebb's resignation underlines what a difficult step it was for even the most heterodox Real Whig.

Resignation also involved implicit criticism of friends who remained within the Church. William Chambers (c.1724-77), Rector of Thorpe Achurch in Northamptonshire, was a close friend of Lindsey and Jebb. He experimented with Unitarian readings of the *Book of Common Prayer*, and seems to have declined the offer of a 'considerable preferment' in London because of his unwillingness to re-subscribe the Thirty-Nine Articles.[81] Jebb was at pains to assure Chambers that 'many persons who hold similar opinions to mine, can continue in the Church with great advantage to the cause of Christianity; acting at the same time in perfect conformity to conscience'. His own resignation stemmed from 'circumstances peculiar to myself': unable to continue reading the Anglican service while openly professing Unitarianism in his lectures, he had ceased performing his clerical duties in late 1773, and the morally compromised nature of his position had provoked much anxiety and ill-health.[82]

Jebb's resignation did not go unnoticed – at least by the religious-minded. The Evangelical Hannah More wrote that:

> Being one day in a large company, who all inveighed against Lindsey, and Jebb, and other Socinians who had deserted the Church, because they could not subscribe to the Articles, I happened to say that I thought sincerity such a golden virtue, that I had a feeling bordering on respect for such as had apostatized upon principle: for when a man gave such an unequivocal proof of his being in earnest, as to renounce a

[77] Lindsey to Tayleur 19 Oct 1775, JRL Lindsey-Tayleur correspondence; Belsham, *Memoir of Lindsey*, pp. 99, 114.
[78] Ditchfield 'The Subscription Issue'; Clark, *English Society*, p. 314.
[79] Langford, 'English Clergy and the American Revolution', in Hellmuth, *Transformation of Political Culture*, pp. 275-308.
[80] C. Harrison to William Turner, 3 April 1774, DWL Lindsey-Turner correspondence.
[81] G.M. Ditchfield, 'The Revd. William Chambers, D.D. (c.1724-77), *E&D*, 4 (1985), pp. 3-12.
[82] JJ to William Chambers, 21 October 1775, 'Life of Jebb', p. 106.

> lucrative profession, rather than violate his conscience, I must think him sincere, and of course respectable.[83]

But the impact of such resignations was limited. The Unitarian Samuel Kenrick lamented that while Lindsey, Jebb, Evanson and Tyrwhitt had resigned on account of their Unitarianism, 'we have a multiplying sect called Methodists, who profess the most minute belief in doctrinal parts of the articles'.[84] Also, many sympathisers disapproved of Jebb's course of action. Francis Blackburne had implicitly criticised Lindsey's resignation with a published defence of those who chose to remain Church of England clergymen.[85] The latter reported that he had seldom seen Joseph Priestley 'more hurt than he expressed himself to be' upon perusal of the tract, declaring that 'upon the principles of it, he did not see how the Reformers, the Nonconformists of 1662, &c. &c., could be defended'.[86] A year later Blackburne told Lindsey:

> I am obliged to be totally silent on our friend Jebb's secession. You and he have *obliged* the Balguy's and Randolph's by your integrity, but none else, tho' more may commend. It has been the utter ruin of the plan of the Petitioners. For no regard will be paid by such people as the Bp of Norwich to the line he draws between the case of the petitioners and his own. I know not whether I am right, but I put the whole to the account of a man much inferior to either of you.[87]

After a long break, Ann Jebb and Henry Taylor resumed their correspondence in the wake of Jebb's resignation from the Church. Taylor wished that he had the opportunity to advise against an action that betrayed a conscience 'too squeamish and nervous'. Reading the liturgy could be left to a curate, he argued, and 'such notions as are wrong' could be undermined in sermons. He did, however, concede that he was speaking in his own defence rather than finding fault 'where virtue is to be found PERHAPS in a superior degree'.[88] Even closer to home, Jebb's parents were incensed by this end to an imprudent clerical career – 'approving his principles but disapproving his conduct'- and withheld financial support.[89]

A few pamphlets were written in response to Jebb's resignation. Anthony Temple, an Arian and one of Blackburne's circle, agreed that while defended by the 'watchful military of the establishment', the doctrine and liturgy

---

[83] Hannah More to Walpole, *Correspondence of Horace Walpole*, v 31, pp. 328-29.

[84] Samuel Kenrick to James Wodrow, 13 February 1778, DWL Wodrow-Kenrick correspondence.

[85] Francis Blackburne, *Four Discourses* (1774), in Blackburne, *Works*, IV, pp. 261-404.

[86] Theophilus Lindsey to William Turner, 2 February 1775, DWL Lindsey-Turner correspondence.

[87] Blackburne to Lindsey 13 October 1775, DWL Blackburne correspondence. When John Disney (another son-in-law) resigned in 1782 to join Lindsey at Essex Street, Blackburne bitterly complained that 'my disciples have strangled me'. DWL 'Memoir of Disney', pp. 56-8.

[88] Henry Taylor to AJ, [1775/76], CUL Taylor papers.

[89] McLachlan, *Letters of Theophilus Lindsey*, p. 102.

of the Church of England were a farce, and far from reflecting the principles of genuine Christianity. He lamented that the difficult task of preaching to an apathetic public was being hindered by a both obscure and exclusive theology, and by driving out some of the most devout and able clergy. Demanding 'plain, positive and substantial proof' of the Trinity from the orthodox instead of commands not to scrutinise mysteries, he reflected that the clergy should not receive a liberal education if they were not intended to use it. Temple was convinced of the need for a national church but wished it to be based on Scripture only, and he hoped that Jebb's resignation would spark protest within the Church that would lead to revision of the liturgy. In the tone of frustration typical of the heterodox clergy, Temple reflected that a forgiving and sympathetic God would judge fairly those who chose to continue fulfilling their clerical obligations, and laboured under conscience rather than plunge with their families 'into the miseries of life' without an income.[90]

According to Disney, Jebb was attacked from the University pulpit.[91] Yet it seems that the prelacy thought best to ignore Jebb's resignation, with one substantial tract issuing forth from the orthodox ranks, written by Edward Tew, fellow of King's College Cambridge. This (as noted in chapter 3) argued that Jebb's *Short State of Reasons for a Late Resignation* deserved no more than the standard dismissal of Socinianism as an attempt to 'reduce the whole of Religion to practical piety and Virtue'; and criticised his belief that the empirical method applied to nature could be used with similar success in comprehending the revelation contained in Scripture. Tew argued that freedom of expression brought both advantages and 'inconveniences', and that in the 'present age ... we have tempted both Religion and Liberty in their extremes'. 'A truly conscientious man', he argued, 'will be satisfied with enjoying his opinions in private; it is the furious Zealot and Dogmatist alone, who wishes to impose them on others'. Tew concluded with the lament that to the 'confessed ... VIRTUES of the MAN' Jebb had not 'been happy enough to add the FAITH of a CHRISTIAN'.[92]

Robert Robinson, an Arian Baptist at Cambridge, congratulated both Jebb and Lindsey for their conscientious resignations. Yet he sought to defend the divinity of Christ as a plain truth, eschewing learned arguments because it was unnecessary to 'suffer his mind to be bewildered in Greek and Hebrew characters'. With St Paul, he argued, 'we walk by *faith*, and not by *Sight*', and must believe Jesus to be more than just 'a good man'.[93] In a private letter Robinson expressed the 'highest opinion of the learning of Mr Jebb', and

---

[90] Anthony Temple, *A Letter to the Rev. John Jebb M.A. Occasioned by his Short State of the Reasons for a Late Resignation* (1776), pp. 1-22.

[91] 'Life of Jebb', p. 118.

[92] [Edward Tew], *Resignation No Proof*, pp. 33, 13, 19, 67.

[93] Robert Robinson, *A Plea for the Divinity of our Lord Jesus Christ: in a pastoral letter addressed to a congregation of Protestant Dissenters at Cambridge* (1776), pp. 6-11, 28. Francis Blackburne thought that the Socinians had not been able to answer 'the excellent Mr Robinson's' *Plea*. Francis Blacburne to Reverend J. Wiche, 9 September 1783, DWL Letters of Lardner &c.

confessed that 'our sentiments, much as they seem to differ, may after all differ less than they appear'. Jebb thanked him for the 'truly Christian temper' of his pamphlet and 'generous sentiments respecting religious liberty'.[94] The two seem to have been reasonably well acquainted. Of humble origins and largely self-educated, Robinson was an inspiring preacher. Steeped in the writings of Locke and Milton, 'he was extraordinarily well read, getting access through his friends to the rich stocks of the University Library, to which his own considerable output was eventually added'.[95] Robinson tended to dismiss theological dispute as superfluous and of less consequence than the price of wheat, suggesting that pamphlets with titles such as *A High Heeled Shoe for a Dwarf in Christ* and *An Effectual Shove for a Heavy-Arsed Christian* were needed in order to combat religious complacency. He became increasingly interested in politics, and was inspired by Jebb to write his *Political Catechism* (1782) in an effort to teach the lower orders basic political principles (Robinson himself had been apprenticed as a hairdresser).[96]

After resigning from the Church Jebb informed a friend that Cambridge 'swarms' with Tories, unopposed by 'prostitute' and 'slumbering Whigs'.[97] Such comments betray more than frustration with the failure of his education reforms, or even of the campaign against subscription. In 1775 Real Whigs like Jebb were confronted by a surge in loyalist support among the gentry and the Church in response to the American rebellion.[98] The increasing polarisation of opinion was vividly demonstrated by the reaction to Vice-Chancellor Farmer's proposal for a loyal 'Address' in support of the King's policy. While Jebb and Richard Watson described Farmer as a Tory, to William Cole he was 'such a Whig as those who placed King William on the throne; and, of course, deemed a violent Tory by our present Republicans, of whom, to say the truth, he could hardly speak with temper'.[99] Despite resistance by Lord Rockingham and the Duke of Grafton, the 'Address' was carried with the influence of Lord Sandwich, Lord Hardwicke and the Archbishop of Canterbury. The mild-mannered Robert Tyrwhitt was outraged by the political turn of the University, and refused to hand over the key to the university seal. The Vice-Chancellor proceeded to break the chest open and the 'Address' was delivered to George III.[100] This incident underlines the degree to which public debate had become dominated by the argument between Parliament and the Colonies over political rights.

---

[94] Robert Robinson to JJ, 5 February 1776;, and JJ to Robert Robinson, 7 February 1776, cited in George Dyer, *Memoirs of the Life and Writings of Robert Robinson* (1796), pp. 117-19.

[95] Searby, *A History of the University of Cambridge: volume III*, p. 405.

[96] Dyer, *Memoirs of Robinson*, pp. 120-21, 225.

[97] JJ to [?], 26 October 1775, 'Life of Jebb', p. 109.

[98] Eliga H. Gould, *The Persistence of Empire: British political culture in the age of the American Revolution* (Chapel Hill, N.C., 2000), pp. 140-52.

[99] Gascoigne, *Cambridge*, p. 206.

[100] Robert Plumptre to Lord Hardwicke, 27 November 1775, BL Add. Mss. 35,628:228.

7

Unitarian Doctor in London

After casting aside his clerical robes, Jebb began to attend anatomy lectures at Cambridge in February 1776.[1] His decision to pursue a medical career was made with the support of his cousin Sir Richard Jebb, an eccentric lifelong bachelor and well-known wealthy doctor who became 'physician extraordinary' to George III's family.[2] William Cole thought it fitting that Jebb was following the advice of his cousin. Along with Horace Walpole, he had met Richard Jebb one afternoon in Paris in 1766, and found his 'whole discourse was in justification of the Deistical French Philosophers and their opinions'.[3] Another figure that supported Jebb in his change of profession was William Heberden (1710-1801). The son of an innkeeper, Heberden rose to become one of the most famous physicians in England. He had studied medicine at Cambridge and was one of the leading advocates for reform within the ranks of the conservative Royal College of Physicians. He dabbled in the critical study of the Scriptures, could read Hebrew, and in the words of William Cole was a 'great and zealous favourer' of the Feathers Tavern petition.[4] Heberden became an important patron of the Essex Street chapel (though he asked Lindsey to conceal the fact), and was a friend of Priestley and Franklin. A temperate man, the successful treatment of his patients owed much to his advice to practice moderation in all things. He was also noted for mixing political with medical advice to his patients, who included old university acquaintances Bishop Richard Hurd and

---

[1] 'Life of Jebb', p. 121.

[2] William Munk, *Roll of the Royal College of Physicians of London: II 1701-1800* (1878), p. 292.

[3] William Cole, BL Cole mss. 5873:53.

[4] Edmund Law thought him a 'worthy liberal layman, who does more service to the cause than all our bench'. Ernest Heberden, *William Heberden: physician of the Age of Reason* (1989), pp. 133, 136.

Thomas Balguy.[5] Acquainted through their common friends and interests, Heberden's signature appears second on Jebb's Royal Society nomination certificate.

In August 1776 Jebb was seen 'at the Huntingdon Races and Assembly ... dancing in a Bag Whig and Ruffles and a coloured coat'.[6] In September he left Cambridge and moved to London, where he took up residence in Craven Street.[7] Jebb immediately began attending St Bartholomew's Hospital as a pupil of Dr William Pitcairn (1711-91),[8] and thought it 'hard work, but on the whole not unpleasing'.[9] Yet he had not been in London a month when he was bed ridden for two weeks with a fever that he contracted along with Lindsey when 'a stream of cold air blew upon us' at an anatomy lecture.[10] After a protracted recovery Jebb threw himself into his medical studies,[11] and wrote to Disney: 'I am very happy in my new plan. I receive great civilities, and encouragement from several worthy persons, who may promote my interest hereafter.... I have met with so many kindnesses, that my situation has been rendered far easier than I could have hoped, and my utmost views are moderate.'[12]

Throughout 1777 Jebb's energies were entirely devoted to medical training. In March he was granted a Diploma of Doctor of Physic from the University of St Andrews in Scotland, his certificate being signed by four members of the faculty resident in London.[13] Jebb was licensed by the College of Physicians the following June, but on the advice of Richard Jebb and Richard Warren he did not begin to practice until February 1778, allowing a two-year probation period from the commencement of his studies.[14] A few months later

---

[5] Heberden, *William Heberden*, pp. 136, 158.

[6] This was related to William Cole by Sir John Cotton. BL Cole mss. 5873:70.

[7] This small street runs off the east end of the Strand down to the Thames. Benjamin Franklin's home in the early 1770s still stands in the middle of a row of town houses.

[8] Pitcairn did not publish anything, but was 'an eminently sound and successful physician. He introduced and taught in the wards of St Bartholomew's Hospital a much freer employment of opium in the treatment of disease, and especially fevers, than was customary with his contemporaries'. Munk, *Roll of the Royal College of Physicians*, p. 174

[9] 'Life of Jebb', p. 122.

[10] Lindsey to Tayleur 5 November 1776, JRL Lindsey-Tayleur correspondence.

[11] 'Life of Jebb', pp. 123, 127. As late as January 28, 1777, Lindsey observed that 'Jebb has not recovered the shock of the fever which shattered him so much, though he is able to go about his medical practice in some degree'. Lindsey to Tayleur 28 Jan. 1777, JRL Lindsey-Tayleur correspondence.

[12] 'Life of Jebb', pp. 126-27.

[13] This was a mere paper qualification. John Disney obtained a D.D. from Edinburgh in the same way. When Samuel Johnson visited St Andrews in 1773, he found that one of the three colleges had been closed, and thought 'it not without just reproach, that a nation, of which the commerce is hourly extending, and the wealth increasing, ... suffers its universities to moulder into dust'. Samuel Johnson, *Poetry and Prose*, p. 660.

[14] 'Life of Jebb', pp. 128, 135. Lindsey noted in December 1777 that 'Jebb talks of beginning to practise in a short time, or rather his cousin the Dr, and Dr Heberden wish him to do it, that they may [serve] him'. Lindsey to Tayleur 18 December 1777, JRL Lindsey-Tayleur correspondence.

Lindsey told a friend: 'we hope that Dr Jebb is beginning to come a little into business. If he has practice I have no doubt of his eminent usefulness, for no man enters the profession better informed, few with equal abilities, and none with more sincere views to serve mankind'.[15]

MEDICINE IN THE EIGHTEENTH CENTURY

Jebb was certainly justified in his belief that a medical career would guarantee him the modest income he desired. The eighteenth-century medical world was dominated by free-market principles, and the most Shrewd and talented doctors could walk 'a royal road to riches, rank and respect'. William Hunter rose through entrepreneurial skill from obscure Scottish origins to become the leading surgeon in England.[16] In his 'Introductory Lectures' (which Jebb attended soon after his move to London) Hunter urged his listeners: 'I firmly believe, that it is in your power not only to *chuse*, but to *have*, which rank you please in the world'. 'In our profession', he continued, 'it seems incontestable that the man of abilities and diligence always succeeds'.[17] Jebb felt confident that he could provide for his own and Ann's modest material needs, and in the future he could eat 'independent bread' and have 'the power of my own time, a power which I have never yet enjoyed'.[18]

There were three types of medical practitioner in the eighteenth century: physicians were gentlemen with a university degree; surgeons were often from poor backgrounds, trained as apprentices, and were considered tradesmen – notorious for their liberal use of obscenities;[19] and apothecaries were the forerunners of modern pharmacists, and ranged from dubious quacks to middle-class women such as Hannah Lindsey.[20] Jebb slotted into the first category, which was in turn divided between an Oxbridge-educated establishment centred on membership of the Royal College of Physicians, and the many Dissenters with degrees from Scottish or Dutch universities who were only licensed to work as doctors.

The primary role of the College was to regulate the practice of medicine in London, and membership guaranteed a busy private practice. As a result, few College fellows were motivated to engage in difficult or time-consuming medical research. They also tended to remain content with classical Galenic medicine, which considered every illness as stemming from an imbalance in the humours and unique to the patient who contracted it. As the

[15] Theophilus Lindsey to William Tayleur, 26 July 1778, JRL Lindsey-Tayleur correspondence.
[16] Roy Porter, 'William Hunter: a surgeon and a gentleman', in W.F. Bynum and Roy Porter eds., *William Hunter and the Eighteenth-Century Medical World* (Cambridge, 1985), p. 9; Dorothy and Roy Porter, *Patient's Progress: doctors and doctoring in the eighteenth century* (Cambridge, 1989), chapter 7.
[17] Cited in Porter, 'William Hunter', p. 13.
[18] 'Life of Jebb', pp. 123, 126.
[19] George Qvist, *John Hunter 1728-93* (1981), p. 6.
[20] Cathrine Cappe, *A Small Tribute to the Memory of Mrs Lindsey* (York, 1812).

normal state of the humours depended on the individual's constitution, it was argued, treatment required an intimate knowledge of the patient that only a classically trained doctor could provide. Such an approach did not encourage the physician to think about treating illness on a mass scale in large groups of people, as each illness was specific to each individual. It followed that professional medical treatment was by its nature usually only a privilege available to wealthy individuals, and young gentlemen graduated from Oxford and Cambridge with the aim of serving wealthy patients in London or the prosperous regional towns. Classical medicine mirrored aristocratic society, and its practitioners looked down on the work of surgeons and apothecaries. The former were only supposed to treat external or 'local' ailments, and the latter were considered quacks whose remedies required no knowledge of the patient, but only of the symptoms.[21]

Roy Porter has questioned the traditional assumption that the Enlightenment led to medical 'progress' in eighteenth-century England. Most medical practice remained traditional, reformers tended to come from various Christian sects, little changed in the social structure of medical practice, and many innovations probably stemmed from necessity rather than any conscious enlightened plan. Arguing that 'in England Enlightenment attitudes grew in a soil of political and cultural individualism', Porter detects three broad changes in the evaluation of health and medicine: a secularisation of the understanding of sickness and cure, an expansion of medical institutions, and an increasingly hedonistic view of health. These changes were the manifestation of an Enlightenment ideology that represented the interests of literate and propertied polite society.[22] Jebb supports this characterisation of the medical Enlightenment in England. He worked in a socially stable medical free-market and relied upon traditional practices, was interested in new approaches to medical knowledge and institutional reform, and saw the practice and improvement of medicine as intimately connected to the cause of moral reformation.

RATIONAL RELIGION AND MEDICINE

Why did Jebb refuse to become a minister at Essex Street and allow his religious studies to take a back seat to medicine and politics? Upon commencement of his medical training, he was at pains to assure friends that he was not abandoning religious studies. He still devoted each Sunday to God's word and remained committed to the cause of religious liberty.[23] On a loose leaf of paper in his theological manuscripts Jebb wrote: 'I dictated these Heads in 12 lectures of one hour and a half long to Mr R. Smith in the month of December 1776. I must enlarge these Heads and complete the References and make them the basis of a

---

[21] Margaret DeLacy, 'Influenza Research and the Medical Profession in Eighteenth-Century Britain', *Albion*, 25 (1993), pp. 41-42.
[22] Roy Porter, 'Was there a Medical Enlightenment in Eighteenth-Century England?', *British Journal for Eighteenth-Century Studies*, 5 (1982), pp. 49-63.
[23] Jebb II, p. 126.

system of Practical Christianity; this on Sundays, agreeably to my resolutions in November.'[24]

But despite such intentions, study of the Scriptures would never again be the central focus of Jebb's energies. Up until 1780 his time was absorbed in medical studies, and from then on his political activities took over. Lindsey would frequently lament that Jebb's busy medical practice and political activities prevented him making good his promise to write in defence of Unitarianism.[25] When conveying Jebb's theological maxims to Disney for insertion in the posthumous *Works*, Lindsey reflected that 'amidst so much political manoeuvre, one regrets all along the time lost that might have been spent to such lasting account in better subjects'.[26]

Even when goaded Jebb did not produce a substantial exposition of his Unitarian theology. Robert Findlay highlighted the assertion in Jebb's *A Short State of the Reasons for a Late Resignation* that Christians had no more right to 'address' Jesus than to pray to the Virgin Mary. As there was no argument to support this, Findlay proceeded to devote his entire pamphlet to refuting Lindsey's Socinian interpretation of Scripture.[27] This forced Jebb to publicly explain why he had not published a detailed defence of his Unitarianism. He argued that 'the proper unity of God, and the unlawfulness of addressing prayer to Christ are very different questions', and that he only referred to Lindsey's *Apology* for proof of the former. Jebb claimed that his *Short State* was only designed to declare his reasons for leaving the Church, not to provide arguments supporting his theological opinions. If he had intended to do the latter he would not have contented himself with referring to Lindsey's publication, but rather have unfolded – 'perhaps very largely' – his own arguments drawn from the Bible. He proceeded to plead engagement in his new profession as an excuse for not entering into the controversy.[28] 'How vain a subterfuge, and how intellectual a shift, is this!' Findlay exclaimed in response to Jebb's fine distinctions; arguing, with justification, that Jebb 'must wholly blame' himself for giving the impression that he disapproved of the worship of Jesus. Findlay argued that Jebb should publish a detailed explanation and justification of his theological

---

[24] DWL Jebb mss. VI, loose paper.

[25] Lindsey to William Tayleur 10 December 1782 and 28 June 1784, *Letters of Theophilus Lindsey*, pp. 103-04. Lindsey thought Jebb was the best suited to write an 'Address to Unitarians', but he 'was entirely swallowed up with his new profession as to have no time'. Lindsey to William Tayleur, 23 January 1778, JRL Lindsey-Tayleur correspondence.

[26] Theophilus Lindsey to William Tayleur, 9 June 1787, JRL Lindsey-Tayleur correspondence.

[27] Robert Findlay, *A Letter to the Rev Mr Jebb with relation to his Declared Sentiments about the Unlawfulness of all Religious Addresses to Christ Jesus* (1778). Granville Sharp, the abolitionist and orthodox Anglican who became a familiar acquaintance of Jebb through their common political interests, corrected the manuscript of Findlay's *Letter*. Robert Findlay to Granville Sharp, 30 September 1778, GRO Sharp papers 13/1/f14.

[28] 'A Postscript by Dr Jebb to the Author of a Letter &c', attached to Theophilus Lindsey, *Two Dissertations* (April 1778), pp. 146-52.

opinions.[29] He was not alone. A recent convert to Unitarianism hoped that Jebb and Tyrwhitt would follow Lindsey's example and explain their 'sentiments to the world'.[30] Nevertheless, despite such encouragement Jebb's only subsequent contribution to public religious debate was the short outline of the unsuccessful 'Society for Promoting the Knowledge of the Scriptures'.[31] And it is revealing that he failed to make a single contribution to Priestley's *Theological Repository*.[32]

Jebb approached medicine as a profession that appealed to his developing materialism and belief in the harmony between science and religion.[33] As noted in chapter 4, upon recovery from illness at the end of 1776 Jebb vowed to spend every Sunday in 'sacred study', reading 'Hartley, Taylor and other books in which the spirit of piety prevails'.[34] A set of written resolutions made after completing his medical training indicate the intimate connection between Jebb's rational piety and his practice of medicine:

1. To forgo every advantage and every prospect of success in my profession, rather than act contrary to the three principles laid down by Dr Hartley as the basis of right conduct, viz. piety, benevolence, and the moral sense.
2. Never to make a difference between the rich and poor, but so far as relates to cure, to consider myself in equal manner, the servant of both, being very careful to manifest the same courtesy, mildness of speech, and manners, to every individual I may be called upon to assist.
3. To guard continually against deflecting from the proper line and duties of my profession through attention to ornamental branches of knowledge; yet in all points, to act in perfect consistency with my former conduct, not abating in my zeal for civil or religious liberty; nor sacrificing my principles, even for a moment, through any views of interest, of whatever nature they may be, considering the transitory scene I am engaged in.[35]

---

[29] [Robert Findlay], *Remarks on Mr Lindsey's Dissertation upon Praying to Christ, with a Second Letter to Mr Jebb* (1781), pp. 6, 8. Granville Sharp also corrected the manuscript of this tract. Robert Findlay to Granville Sharp, 3 September 1779 and 12 May 1780, GRO Sharp papers.

[30] John Watson to Theophilus Lindsey, 2 January 1777, DWL Lindsey-Turner correspondence.

[31] *Sketch of the ... Society for Promoting Knowledge of the Scriptures*, Jebb II, pp. 237-54.

[32] See Lindsey's list of twenty contributors to the *Theological Repository*, DWL Lindsey letters. To this can be added the fact that in the period covered by John Disney's diary (January 1783-May 1784) there is no mention of Jebb acting as guest preacher at Essex Street, while Priestley did so frequently.

[33] 'Dissenters played an important role in the numerical growth of the profession, and their idealism contributed greatly to the progress of medical knowledge'. William Birken, 'The Dissenting Tradition in English Medicine of the Seventeenth and Eighteenth Centuries', *Medical History*, 39 (1995), p. 215.

[34] 'Life of Jebb', pp. 124-25.

[35] 'Life of Jebb', pp. 136-37.

According to his former student and friend Capel Lofft, Jebb prayed for the success of all his treatments, and medicine allowed him to engage in 'what he ever valued most, usefulness to others in their sufferings and dangers'.[36]

The justified lay suspicion of medical practitioners is well known. Henry Taylor wrote to Ann: 'I hope that the Dr goes on with his new business with the same success as General Howe. How is that you'll say', he jested, 'why, I mean, that he does not kill so many as might be expected'.[37] Not surprisingly, improvement in medicine was considered central to the Enlightenment ideal of maximising temporal happiness.[38] Physicians were literally following Pope's dictum that 'the proper study of mankind, is man'. David Hartley, arguing that there was a close relationship between the study of medicine and the study of the mind, had urged physicians and philosophers to join together and follow in the footsteps of Locke and Newton.[39] Also, John and Ann had their fair share of ill health (even by eighteenth-century standards) and this no doubt helped stimulate an interest in medicine. Priestley urged Jebb to follow the same path as 'our revered master, Dr Hartley', and allow his medical studies to lead him to the 'further investigation of the phenomena of the human mind'. Such study would show 'how admirably is the whole system of revealed religion adapted to the nature and circumstances of man'.[40]

Jebb had written in his theological manuscripts around 1770 that 'the Surgeon, Physician, Anatomist, Chemist, and Natural Historian should tell us what man is – the divine what God declares he shall be'.[41] With a mind settled on fundamental theological questions, perhaps Jebb found study of 'what man is' more interesting, challenging and of greater benefit to the world than further theological researches. Medicine provided the opportunity to study the 'human frame' and help preserve and improve the quality of numerous lives – in short, it enabled him to practice and express a 'rational piety'.

ENLIGHTENMENT AND MEDICINE

John Disney's diary reveals that Jebb regularly attended to the health of his family. The few references Disney makes to actual remedies shows that Jebb, like all doctors of the time, was still largely reliant on traditional practices to a large extent. When 'Confined to my house by a complaint in my eyes', Disney wrote, 'Dr Jebb visited me, and by his direction I was bled by leeches on my temples, and in the evening blistered'. Three days later Disney was still confined to his house when 'Dr Jebb called upon me', and in the spirit of Heberden's practice, 'earnestly exhorted me to attention in my diet as the preventative of

[36] Capel Lofft, 'Biographical sketch of Dr Jebb', 'Life of Jebb', p. 244.
[37] Henry Taylor to Ann Jebb, [?] 1777, CUL Taylor papers.
[38] Peter Gay, *The Enlightenment: an interpretation* (2 vols., 1967-70), II, pp. 12-13.
[39] Hartley, *Observations*, pp. 264-67; Spadafora, *Idea of Progress*, p. 152.
[40] 'Life of Jebb', pp. 133-34; reprinted in J.A. Passmore ed., *Priestley's Writings on Philosophy, Science and Politics* (1965), p. 173.
[41] Jebb mss. IV.

disease'.[42] When Disney was afflicted with a persistent headache, Jebb put him on a prescription of rhubarb, and when his wife fell ill she was prescribed 'bark'.[43] Such traditional practices do not contradict the claim that Jebb embraced new developments in medical science. Whatever their broader attitude to medicine, all doctors relied upon conventional therapies such as blistering, purging, induced vomiting, and bloodletting, along with the increasing range of commercially available drugs.[44] While these few references show Jebb 'instructing' the 'blistering and bleeding' of his patients, it is clear that he was looking beyond traditional Galenic medicine. Jebb's interest in modern medical developments is evident from his training and desire to improve medical knowledge and reform public health institutions.

Surgeons were very much outsiders to the medical establishment. They tended to be from poor backgrounds and, as mentioned above, many physicians considered their form of knowledge inferior. Thus, it is not surprising that many medical innovators were drawn from their ranks. It is worth noting that most of Jebb's education was received from some of the most respected surgeons, and his practice revealed their influence. From 1777 to 1779 Jebb attended lectures by William Hunter, who signed his nomination to the Royal Society. Hunter provided arguably the best anatomy lectures in London and spoke in a lively style to audiences that sometimes exceeded a hundred, relating anecdotes and commenting on politics (making clear his support for Lord North's administration).[45] He charged seven guineas for 112 lectures whose 'importance can hardly be overestimated ... [as] they covered the whole of what may be described as the science part of contemporary medicine'.[46] Edward Gibbon, at times accompanied by his friend, Adam Smith, attended Hunter's series of lectures from February to April in 1777 (which Jebb attended) as a relief from his historical research. He observed that the lectures 'opened a new and very entertaining scene within myself' and at the end of every lecture he personally thanked Hunter for the pleasure and instruction that he received.[47] Hunter had two main draw-cards: he only conveyed his knowledge through lectures, and through 'contacts' he was able to secure a plentiful supply of corpses (enabling each student to practice dissection).[48] In stark contrast to his scholarly theological and philosophical studies at Cambridge, Jebb's eyes were now often fixed upon dissection of the human body.

---

[42] Disney, 'Diary', 11-14 January 1783. The same remedy was also used on his son: 'John was bled with leeches on his temples to relieve his eyes'. 22 March 1783.

[43] Disney, 'Diary', 13-15 April, 9-18 June 1783.

[44] Porter, *Patient's Progress*, pp. 153-72.

[45] C. Helen Brock, 'The Happiness of Riches', in Bynum and Porter, *William Hunter and the Medical World*, p. 49.

[46] They were held in the afternoon six days per week for three months. Roy Porter, 'Medical Lecturing in Georgian London', *British Journal for the History of Science*, 28 (1995), p. 94. Combined with reading and work at the hospital, we can appreciate why Jebb found little time to write to his friends or publish on religious matters. 'Life of Jebb', p. 126.

[47] Qvist, *John Hunter*, p. 6.

[48] Porter, 'William Hunter', p. 23.

In 1778 Jebb attended lectures by John Hunter, William's talented, industrious and witty brother. The man whom David Hume thought the greatest anatomist in Europe was driven by a desire to fathom general principles that extended through all of Nature. In sentiments with which Jebb would have agreed, John Hunter observed with reverence the harmony of Nature: 'It should be remembered that nothing in Nature stands alone; but that every art and science has a relation to some other art or science, and that it requires a knowledge of those others, as far as this connection takes place, to enable us to become perfect in that which engages our particular attention.' He believed that 'every property in man is similar to some property, either in another animal, or probably in a vegetable, or even in inanimate matter'.[49] John Hunter was the first to attempt to co-ordinate diseases through study of their pathology. He also argued that it was necessary to understand the workings of a healthy body in order to appreciate the effects of a disease.[50] That Jebb appreciated his approach is evident from a note he penned in the year he attended John Hunter's lectures: 'I see every day more and more, that the art of physic may be simplified like divinity, and that the names of diseases must in time be forgotten, and the whole of the disorder be considered as a derangement in some part of the system, generally by inflammation, its adjuncts and consequences.'[51]

One of Jebb's most influential teachers seems to have been Percival Pott (1714-88) the Senior Surgeon of St Bartholomew's Hospital. In 1782 Jebb dedicated his *Select Cases of the Disorder commonly termed the Paralysis of the Lower Extremities* to Pott, and thanked him for pointing out 'the path to substantial science' at 'an early period of my medical studies'.[52] Pott was better educated than most of his fellow surgeons and developed one of the most lucrative practices in London. He combined this with a commitment to research and lent his name to a number of medical conditions, while his publications exercised a great influence on the development of surgery. A skilful teacher, his classes at St Bartholomew's attracted students from Scotland, Ireland and the Continent. Pott emphasised the need to make treatment of patients as painless as possible and he tried to improve on the complex and clumsy nature of eighteenth-century surgical instruments. He wrote: 'The merely curing of diseases is not all; that was done (sooner or later) while surgery and anatomy were in their most imperfect state, and while every branch of medicine laboured under many inconveniences which are now happily removed; but the different methods in which chirurgical disorders are treated, or their cures attempted, will make so considerable a difference in the sufferings of the patient, as to be worth attending to.'[53] A liberal and humane man who often assisted fellow

[49] Qvist, *John Hunter*, p. xiv.
[50] Qvist, *John Hunter*, p. xi.
[51] 'Life of Jebb', pp. 139-40. Jebb also attended the lectures of Dr Higgins in 1778, and of Dr Keir and Da Costa in 1779.
[52] *Select Cases of the Disorder commonly termed the Paralysis of the Lower Extremities* (1782), Jebb II, p. 393.
[53] Cited in Jessie Dobson, 'Percivall Pott', *Annals of the Royal College of Surgeons of England*, 50 (1972), p. 57.

practitioners who had fallen on hard times, Pott was clearly one of the main figures who assisted Jebb's transition from clergyman to physician.

The voluntary hospitals of eighteenth-century Britain depended upon doctors and surgeons donating their services. They were willing to do this for the fringe benefits, foremost being the prestige that would attract wealthy private patients. It also provided earnings from teaching and the opportunity to pursue research.[54] Jebb's political stance undermined his attempts to obtain a hospital position and he was forced to rely entirely upon developing a private practice. In 1779 he spent three months attending Richard Jebb's patients in London, which can only have helped his own fledgling practice. In 1783 he stopped charging John Disney for the frequent visits he was paying to his family, which suggests that he was at least not hard-pressed financially.[55] While Jebb would have benefited professionally from a hospital appointment, he was also motivated by a desire to pursue medical research and help improve public health.

According to John Disney, if appointed as a doctor at one of the hospitals Jebb planned to pursue two ideas for advancing medical knowledge. First, he wanted to record the symptoms and treatment of every patient who passed through the hospital. Second, he would have delivered a regular course of lectures over a period of six to eight weeks, designed to provide young gentlemen and clergymen with basic medical knowledge which they could take back to rural areas where 'professional assistance is very sparingly scattered'.[56] Unable to obtain a hospital position, Jebb presented the former idea to the public in his *Select Cases of the Disorder commonly termed the Paralysis of the Lower Extremities*. This tract was written as a supplement to Percival Pott's 1779 treatise on disease of the spine – to 'confirm his theory' and explain his practice.[57]

Many of the cases Jebb relates were under the management of Pott, and Jebb wrote the *Select Cases* as an example of how research should proceed. He followed the practice of Heberden in keeping notes on all his patients and entering them in a book under the headings for the various diseases.[58] Jebb praised William Cullen's practice of pointing out instructive cases to his students, and having them meet to discuss their investigation of the symptoms and the success or failure of their treatment. Doctors should also draw up 'regular and well digested histories' of the cases both they and their students treat, which could be inserted in a hospital record of all cases that would build up to serve as 'authorities, and as evidences of nature's powers, and of nature's laws'. Jebb also urged that the study of those who died in hospital could be improved considerably. The physician with the aid of a surgeon should make a minute examination into the cause of death. 'The appearances, submitted to the

[54] W.F. Bynum, 'Physicians, Hospitals and Career Structures', in Bynum and Porter, *William Hunter and the Medical World*, pp. 109, 118.

[55] 'Life of Jebb', p. 143; Disney, 'Diary', 6 January 1783.

[56] 'Life of Jebb', p. 158.

[57] Percival Pott, *Remarks on that kind of Palsy of the Lower Extremities which is frequently found to accompany a Curvature of the Spine* (1779).

[58] 'Life of Jebb', p. 138; William MacMichael, *Lives of British Physicians* (1830), p. 200.

view of the students, and accurately reported, should be properly authenticated, and inserted in the opposite page of the history of the symptoms and the mode of treatment'. Such a practice, Jebb thought, would establish 'the art of medicine upon a solid, because truly philosophical, foundation'.[59]

The *Select Cases* reveals the extent to which Jebb became immersed in medical studies and work. Under the supervision of Percival Pott, he tended patients, took notes, observed dissections and sought to pinpoint the causes that lay behind symptoms. His tract seeks to demonstrate that a protuberance of the spine is often the cause of paralysis, and that this was best treated by a local application of 'caustics' rather than more general and traditional treatments to the body as a whole. His accounts of various case studies vividly reveal the experimental nature of eighteenth-century medicine. For example, one young man presented with a protuberance and a range of complaints that included pains and numbness in his abdomen, legs and feet and 'a numbness of the sphincter ani, costiveness, and a want of consciousness when his faeces were ejected'. Jebb outlined the process of treatment instituted by Pott: 'Before the application of the caustics he made a trial of the cold-bath, mercurial frictions, tinctura sacra, volatile liniment, a strengthening plaister to the loins, and the screw-chair, without any good effect whatever. The cold-bath and screw-chair were evidently hurtful.' With caustics applied to the protuberance, however, the patient made a 'not very rapid' recovery over 'many months' – but a complete recovery nonetheless.[60]

A far cry from scholarly life at Cambridge, medicine brought Jebb into close contact with people from the lower orders. At St Bartholomew's hospital he carefully examined patients who had suffered all manner of accidents while labouring, such as falling from a hay loft, slipping on a ladder while carrying a sack of oats, being crushed between two carts or hit in the loins by a stone. At the bedside he listened to patient's histories, probed their bodies, saw pain and death, and witnessed the effects of healing. One patient 'lay in bed with wonderful patience for eighteen weeks' with no improvement, until 'at length, upon one of my visits to him, he informed me with strong expressions of joy, that on that day, for the first time, he found himself able to move one of his toes.'[61] Experiences such as this fuelled Jebb's commitment to promoting greater 'enlightenment' in order to alleviate human suffering.

There is no hint that Jebb was interested in the 'individual constitution' of his patients. He wanted to investigate the 'external' and general causes of paralysis by comparing a large body of cases:

> In conformity to the principles upon which the inimitable nosology [disease classification] of Dr Cullen is founded, I will, in the history of these cases, confine myself solely to evident symptoms, and the patient's narrative; being fully satisfied, that to describe disorders according to the forms in

---

59 *Select Cases of ... Paralysis*, Jebb II, p. 398.
60 *Select Cases of ... Paralysis*, Jebb II, pp. 399-402.
61 *Select Cases of ... Paralysis*, Jebb II, p. 412.

> which they really evidence themselves to the senses, with a careful attention to the patients feelings, is the most likely method of acquiring both a knowledge of their causes and of their cure.[62]

As in religion, Jebb saw medical orthodoxy as being challenged by the application of empirical method. His reference to Dr William Cullen (1710-90) is significant. After beginning his career as a surgeon, Cullen became famous as a teacher of medicine at the University of Edinburgh during the height of the Scottish Enlightenment. He rejected Galenic humoralism and presented an account of the nervous (rather than the vascular) system as central to the functioning of the human body. For Cullen, 'the fundamental physiological fact was that life consisted in a state of nervous excitement produced by environmental stimuli. These produced sensations (some conscious, some not) which provoked irritable tissues in the organism'.[63] This view chimed with Jebb's Hartlean philosophy and its notion of the mind being formed by external sensations conveyed to the brain via vibrations in the nervous system.

Nowhere is the challenge to received opinion more evident than in debate over the nature of disease. Traditional Galenic medical practice sought the causes of disease in the constitution of the individual's humours. It had long been thought by many, however, that disease was caused by environmental miasma – that 'putrid' fevers were the product of poisonous exhalations arising from rotting flesh, vegetation and stagnant water. In the late seventeenth century fellows of the Royal Society for the Advancement of Science turned their attention to the question of whether 'invisible emanations' from within the earth might affect the atmosphere, and thus cause epidemics. In 1692 John Locke 'sent out questionnaires to his correspondents all over the world requesting information that could be used to correlate mortality, meteorological statistics, and disease'.[64] Locke's belief that knowledge derived from the external world encouraged a belief that disease derived from nature and could be discovered and understood by a collective empirical research programme. In the eighteenth century the Royal Society's interest in medicine declined, but doctors in the Scottish universities carried on its approach.

Early in the century some writers suggested that disease resulted from a physical entity that was transmitted from one person to another. This had been believed by many lay people since ancient times, but was frowned upon by the medical profession as incompatible with both the humoural and miasmatic theories of disease. Owing to the efforts of John Fothergill and his associates, however, the idea that some diseases were contagious became accepted within the medical mainstream.[65] This was a profound development, as it 'enabled

---

[62] *Select Cases of ... Paralysis*, Jebb II, p. 399.

[63] Roy Porter, *The Greatest Benefit to Mankind: a medical history of humanity from antiquity to the present* (1997), p. 260.

[64] DeLacy, 'Influenza Research', pp. 42-43.

[65] John Fothergill (1712-80) was a Quaker from Yorkshire, educated at Edinburgh. Jebb noted with approval his instruction to proceed 'with faith in physic'. 'Life of Jebb', p. 136. John Disney was acquainted with Fothergill, Disney, 'Diary', 1 October 1783.

these physicians to see disease as a 'thing' rather than as an 'imbalance', [and] the adoption of contagionism led to a particular 'construction' of distinct 'diseases' out of a bewildering welter of symptoms and to a greater distancing of the disease from an individual symptom.'[66] In his *First Lines in the Practice of Physic* (1778-79), William Cullen used both miasma and contagion in his analysis of the various forms of disease. Published as Jebb was completing his medical training, this work became the most Influential attempt to provide an explanatory framework for disease in the English-speaking world.[67]

This new approach to disease had wide implications for reform in the field of public health, particularly in relation to hospitals and prisons. Compared with the Galenist belief that illness was rooted in and confined to the individual constitution, contagionism made illness a community problem. Under the traditional view, prisons, hospitals and slums could be neglected as the just deserts of individual poor and criminals. However, contagionism implied that such areas could be breeding grounds for disease that could in turn spread to the rest of society.[68] At the very least, it meant the ill-health that manifested itself in such places should not be blamed on the poor themselves, but rather on the policy of those who governed, or rather failed to govern them.

The new approach to disease tied in with calls for moral and social reform.[69] Intended primarily for the poor, eighteenth-century hospitals were crowded, unsanitary and plagued by drunken and unruly behaviour among the patients. Concern that disease was spread by the putrid air that resulted from dirty, overcrowded conditions led to an emphasis on the need for cleanliness. It has been noted that before the eighteenth century dirt was frowned on for aesthetic reasons, but 'increasingly during the Enlightenment, dirt was stigmatised as having a harmful physiological action ... this new concept, the pathological action of dirt, was coupled with stress on the *moral* qualities of cleanliness'.[70] Champions of enlightenment came to see doctors as policing the public health that they thought underpinned the moral and political health of society.

Jebb's concern for the moral reform of the poor is evidenced by his involvement in the establishment of a workhouse in his Suffolk parish. In 1785 he wrote *Thoughts on the Construction and Polity of Prisons* in support of the reforms prescribed by his fellow Dissenter John Howard. Jebb advocated moving prisoners out of the 'melancholy mansions' that fostered disease and

---

[66] DeLacy, 'Influenza Research', pp. 50-51; Ronald Rees, 'Under the Weather: climate and disease, 1700-1900', *History Today,* 46 (January 1996); Roy Porter, *Disease, Medicine and Society in England, 1550-1860* (1987).

[67] Porter, *Greatest Benefit to Mankind*, pp. 260-62.

[68] The influential John Pringle argued that gaols were the 'sources of slow and malignant fevers, which generally prevail in large and crowded cities'. *Observations on the Nature and Cure of Hospital and Jayl-fevers* (1750), p. 2.

[69] Lizabeth Haakonssen, *Medicine and Morals in the Enlightenment, John Gregory, Thomas Percival and Benjamin Rush* (Amsterdam, 1997).

[70] Christopher Lawrence, 'Priestley in Tahiti: the medical interests of a Dissenting chemist', in Anderson, *Science, Medicine and Dissent*, p. 6.

misery, into new buildings that would allow in air and light. Prisoners could only be reformed if they lived in a healthy, disease-free environment.[71] The general attitude of those interested in medical reform is summed up by the Liverpool Unitarian, Dr James Currie, who wrote that the labouring poor 'demand our constant attention. To inform their minds, to repress their vices, to assist their labours, to invigorate their activity, to improve their comforts – these are the noblest offices of enlightened minds in superior stations'.[72] Jebb's political and religious ideals envisaged a society of free, rational and independent individuals regulated by moral self-restraint. As Ivan Illich has written, 'the Enlightenment, which discovered the liberties, also invented the disciplines'.[73] It is not surprising that Jebb's commitment to political and religious liberty was matched with an interest in medical and penal reform designed to encourage the formation of rational, autonomous, self-regulating individuals.

POLITICS AND MEDICINE

Dissenting physicians were more likely to be interested in medical, religious and political reform. Denied membership of the Royal College, they sought professional respectability through membership of the Royal Society, or one of the various medical societies established in the second half of the century.[74] Those not eligible for membership of the Royal College of Physicians fell into four main categories: the mass of surgeons and apothecaries; Scots who had moved to England; Anglican English and Colonial students educated at Scottish universities; and Irish and English non-conformists. Jebb was among the last group, which tended to include the most radical, in particular the Quakers and Unitarians.[75] By 1765 the number of those licensed as physicians exceeded that of members of the Royal College, and the former were paying heavy fees to an institution of which they could not become members. In 1767 the licensed practitioners formed a Society of Collegiate Physicians and William Hunter led a number of them into a meeting of the Royal College. Hunter threatened to run his sword through anyone who attempted to eject him while a demand that the College relax its membership requirement was read out. Their demands, however, were unsuccessful, and as Margaret DeLacy has observed, 'in the decade before the American Revolution, "no taxation without representation" was a slogan with great personal resonance for the licentiates'.[76] Excluded from

[71] *Thoughts on ... Prisons*, Jebb II, pp. 555-68.

[72] Cited in Porter, 'Was there a Medical Enlightenment?', p. 57. Currie purchased a copy of Jebb's *Works*. 'Life of Jebb', p. xiv.

[73] Ivan Illich, *Limits to Medicine: the expropriation of health* (Harmondsworth, 1976), p. 39.

[74] DeLacy, 'Influenza Research', pp. 37-66.

[75] DeLacy, 'Influenza Research', pp. 39-40. In late 1783 some of Jebb's friends suggested he be elected to the Royal College of Physicians, but they decided not to pursue it because of 'an apparently contrary inclination of the majority'. 'Life of Jebb', p. 187.

[76] DeLacy, 'Influenza Research', pp. 46, 47.

membership of the Royal College the outsiders sought other ways of making their reputation such as through research and publication. One of the chief alternatives that provided intellectual status was to become a fellow of the Royal Society, to which Jebb was elected on 18 February 1779, only nine months after he had commenced practice. The doctors who signed Jebb's Royal Society nomination certificate were all Dissenters or reform-minded Anglicans.[77] The support of names like Heberden, Warren, Hunter, Price and Priestley saw Jebb elected by a near unanimous vote at a meeting of over one hundred members.[78]

Politics was seldom allowed to come between patients and practitioners. In his final years Richard Brocklesby, an active member of the Society for Constitutional Information, regularly treated Samuel Johnson. William Heberden regularly attended Bishop Richard Hurd – a hammer of the clerical petitioners. However, political divisions were very important in determining the outcome of elections for public medical positions. Here again, as at Cambridge, Jebb's career suffered because of his radical opinions. He did not bother applying for a vacant position at Guy's Hospital in November 1779. On 23 June 1780, however, an election was held for the position of physician at St Bartholomew's Hospital, where Jebb had undertaken his training. He contested the election with the backing of John Wilkes and the City of London against Dr Richard Budd who was supported by the government. With Lord Sandwich and several other peers against him, Jebb was soundly defeated.[79] Soon after this he expressed interest in a position at St Thomas's Hospital in Westminster, but backed off when it became clear that political principles would again ensure defeat.[80]

Considerably disappointed, Jebb registered at Lincoln's Inn in November, with the intention of pursuing a third career as a lawyer. Yet this was no more than a passing thought, and he contented himself with a private medical practice serving his numerous acquaintances. Indeed, rather than any serious intention to pursue a legal career, Jebb's interest in the law reflects his passionate involvement in radical politics.

---

77 In order of signing they were: Richard Watson, William Heberden, Thomas Brand Hollis, Edward Waring, Richard Jebb, Richard Price, John Lewis Petit, William Pitcairn, Percivall Pott, Richard Warren, William Hunter, Samuel [Trelton], William Sharp, Edward Bridgen, Ashton Lever, George Atwood, John Smith, Joseph Priestley. Royal Society mss., 'Certificates of Election to The Royal Society', IV:6.

78 'Life of Jebb', p. 140.

79 Dr Budd held the position until 1801; he 'had rendered himself independent by marriage with the only child of a wealthy city merchant … and he was not solicitous of much laborious professional exertion'. William Munk, *Roll of the Royal College of Physicians*, II, p. 311.

80 'Life of Jebb', pp. 157-58.

8

America and Parliamentary Reform

The American war polarised the forces of reform and reaction within British politics. For those men and women who supported the colonists, the American conflict became an all-embracing drama in which the claims of liberty and authority were engaged in battle, and it fostered a sense of urgency regarding the need for moral and political reform.

Jebb readily identified the Americans as compatriots struggling against the same authoritarianism he encountered at Cambridge and in the Church. As noted in chapter 2, his opposition to the University's loyal 'Address to the King' in 1769 (which condemned rebellious elements in both Britain and America) was an early indication of radical sympathies. Jebb maintained a keen interest in American religious and political issues, and had some contact with figures such as Benjamin Franklin and John Adams. He fully indulged in an idealistic view of America as a safe haven for religious and political liberty and expressed an interest in migrating to the new nation. The American war placed enormous economic, social, political and foreign policy stresses on Britain and Lord North's government. These conditions allowed agitators for parliamentary reform to flourish.

AMERICA AND RELIGION

Religion and politics were intertwined in the fabric of the American Revolution, and it is not surprising that Jebb took great interest in American attitudes toward religion. The population of the American colonies had increased nearly ten-fold since 1700 and in response the Church of England undertook a drive to expand in the years following 1760. While the London-based Society for the Propagation of the Gospel sent many (mostly High Church) clergy to the colonies as missionaries, it was natural for some to desire the appointment of an American Bishop to enable clergy to be ordained in the colonies.[1] Yet this proposal outraged many American Dissenters and was easily mixed up with the conflict over taxation and representation.[2]

In Virginia, where there was strong anti-clerical sentiment among the gentry, an associate of Jebb came to play a prominent role in religious controversy in the early 1770s.[3] Samuel Henley (b. 1744) was educated at Caleb Ashworth's Dissenting Academy and ordained as a Dissenting Minister in 1768. He lived in Cambridge while ministering at St Neots 1768-69, and during this time cultivated the friendship of Jebb and Edmund Law, both of whom supported his successful application for Anglican ordination in 1769.[4] A Socinian, Henley believed that he could become an Anglican priest if he interpreted the articles with great latitude. Upon recommendation by the Bishop of London, Henley was elected along with Thomas Gwatkin to a chair at the College of William and Mary. They arrived in 1770, made a great impression on Virginian polite society and became closely connected with some influential gentlemen.

In the summer of 1771 a move was made to have the Virginia clergy request the appointment of a colonial bishop. As only twelve of the one hundred clergymen in Virginia attended a meeting for this purpose, Henley and Gwatkin vehemently opposed the notion that such a small group could petition in the name of the Virginia clergy. Conflict on the subject was played out in the pages of the *Virginia Gazette*, and in July the House of Burgesses thanked the protesting clergy for the 'wise and well timed opposition they have made to the pernicious Project ... for introducing an *American* Bishop; a measure by which much Disturbance, great Anxiety, and Apprehension, would certainly take place among his Majesty's faithful *American* Subjects'. Henley's active opposition was successful, and to avoid further inflaming the colonists and their supporters among the Dissenting Interest, the British government and Anglican hierarchy dropped the whole question of an American bishop.[5]

No group in the colonies provided more loyalist support for the British Crown and Parliament than the Church of England clergy; and it was widely perceived that the proposal for a bishop was part of the general conspiracy against American liberties. The *St James's Chronicle* in London explicitly stated in 1765 that 'The stamping and episcopising our colonies were understood to be *only different branches of the same plan* of power'.[6] John Adams later claimed

---

[1] Clark, *Language of Liberty*, p. 339.

[2] Sanford H. Cobb, *The Rise of Religious Liberty in America* (New York, 1968), pp. 470-74.

[3] The source for much of the following is Rhys Isaac, *The Transformation of Virginia, 1740-1790* (Chapel Hill, N.C., 1982), pp. 181-240.

[4] Fraser Neiman, 'The Letters of William Gilpin to Samuel Henley', *Huntington Library Quarterly*, 35 (1971-72), pp. 159-69.

[5] Jack M. Sosin, 'The Proposal in the Pre-Revolutionary Decade for Establishing Anglican Bishops in the Colonies', *Journal of Ecclesiastical History*, 13 (1962), p. 84.

[6] Cited in Colin Bonwick, *English Radicals and the American Revolution* (Chapel Hill, N.C., 1977), p. 56.

that fear of the Church of England 'contributed as much as any other cause to arouse the attention, not only of the inquiring mind, but of the common people, and urged them to close thinking on the constitutional authority of parliament over the colonies'.[7] There was a fear that the Church in America would wield the same influence on civil power as in Britain.

There were those, however, who were happy for the Americans to have a bishop. A leading London Dissenter, Andrew Kippis, allowed that American Anglicans could have a bishop 'as a religious officer, to ORDAIN, CONFIRM and perform the other SPIRITUAL duties belonging to that character'.[8] In 1774 Jebb was told that many Americans who were opposed to taxation did not object to the appointment of a bishop. He lamented this, and thought it 'the consequence of [Archbishop] Secker's unremitting efforts, to spread Church-of-Englandism on the other side of the Atlantic'.[9] Opposition to the appointment of a bishop dried up following independence, as there was no possibility of a political threat under the new constitution. It is ironic that when two bishops were finally appointed in 1785 one had been tutored by Jebb at Cambridge.[10]

With some powerful Virginians shocked by his openly heterodox theological opinions, Henley proceeded to attack bigotry and argue for a complete separation of church and state in a sermon before the House of Burgesses. This was a provocative move in light of the increasing popularity of itinerant Baptist preachers. Many in the Virginia establishment were offended by this lecture on religious liberty. They were even more incensed when Henley proceeded to publish the sermon with a dedication praising John Jebb as an example to the Virginians. Jebb had entered in his prime upon endeavours that 'LOCKE and NEWTON, towards the close of life, regretted they had not earlier begun'. Where Francis Bacon had tried to 'strike off the shackles from the human mind' through 'the science of Nature', Jebb was attempting to do the same 'in the study of Revelation'.[11]

The Whig gentlemen who governed Virginia were happy to use anti-authoritarian rhetoric against episcopacy, but they were still attached to the social order associated with the Church of England. Henley offended many moderate Anglicans and was subject to a 'heresy hearing' in which his Socinian

---

[7] Cobb, *Rise of Religious Liberty*, pp. 478-79.

[8] Andrew Kippis, *A Vindication of the of the Protestant Dissenting Ministers with Regard to Their Late Application to Parliament* (1772), p. 101; Bonwick, *English Radicals*, p. 55.

[9] Jebb writing on 11 December 1774, relating information from 'a correspondent in Virginia' who was most likely Henley. 'Life of Jebb', p. 88.

[10] Samuel Provost had strongly supported the cause of independence and was put forward for the position by his congregation. While in England for consecration, Provost was presented with a copy of the *Book of Common Prayer* in which John Disney had copied the deletions and revisions that Samuel Clarke had made in his own copy (preserved in the British Museum). DWL mss.

[11] Samuel Henley, *The Distinct Claims of Government and Religion, Considered in a Sermon Preached before the Honourable House of Burgesses, at Williamsburg, in Virginia, March 1 1772* (Cambridge, 1772). This pamphlet was printed at Cambridge and possibly guided through the press by Jebb. Isaac, *Transformation of Virginia*, p. 222.

views were clearly revealed. He subsequently lost an election for the position as Rector of Burton. He continued to harangue the members of the Burton Vestry for the next two years, and made himself increasingly unpopular with the Virginia establishment. His ambitions frustrated, in an ironic twist Henley sided with the British when rebellion broke out and fled the colony on a Royal Navy ship. There is no record of any contact with Jebb upon his return to England. Henley's example illustrates the complex role played by religion in the years before the war. The proposed appointment of an American bishop was identified as part of an authoritarian imperial policy. Yet most of the Virginia establishment (and thus many who rebelled) remained theologically and socially conservative.

Jebb came to see America as a bastion of religious liberty, pointing the way to a more enlightened future for the whole world. In light of the exertions of Samuel Henley in Virginia, he reflected: 'The Americans, I am sensible, have much to learn with respect to religious liberty. We have been, I trust, of service in this particular; we have bought forth the principles of their and our adversaries into full view, and have exhibited the form of true Protestantism, which they may improve by, if they please.'[12] Following the end of the conflict, Jebb praised the support for religious toleration enshrined in the American state constitutions, and in particular that of Maryland. He eagerly assumed that reality conformed to constitutional rhetoric: 'The exertions of the human intellect are there unfettered by those iniquitous restraints which dishonour European climes: every man, therefore, lives in charity with his neighbour, and the rage of proselytism is unknown'.[13]

HONEST WHIGS

In many ways the general re-positioning of Dissent into opposition to the government was the product of the American conflict. James Bradley has argued that the Dissenting laity had to be *told* that the law was oppressing them; as for the most part few had felt any sensible disadvantage under the first two Hanoverians. Men such as James Murray, Joseph Towers and Joseph Priestley readily identified with American claims that they could not be taxed by a Parliament in which they were not represented, as the majority of Dissenters in England lived in the growing towns that were disproportionately under-represented in the unreformed electorate.[14]

This shift was evident in the work of James Burgh, the Scottish schoolmaster at Newington Green and a close friend of Richard Price. His early tracts were primarily concerned with the moral laxity of the times and looked forward to leadership being provided by a 'patriot king'. By the second edition of his *Crito* (1767) he was focusing upon the corruption of the constitution and

---

[12] 'Life of Jebb', p. 96.

[13] JJ, 25 October 1783, in *Letters Addressed to the Volunteers of Ireland*, Jebb II, pp. 544-45.

[14] James E. Bradley, *Religion, Revolution and English Radicalism: nonconformity in eighteenth-century politics and society* (Cambridge, 1990), p. 58.

taxation of the colonies without representation. In the year before he died, Burgh published his *Political Disquisitions: or, an inquiry into public errors, defects, and abuses* (1774), in which he argued that a national association should be formed to over-rule Parliament and force it to reform – it was this idea that Jebb espoused in his *Address to the Freeholders of Middlesex* (1779).[15]

Joseph Priestley was also a vocal advocate of the American cause, and in 1769 outlined the ground upon which the friends of America stood. He urged that 'this dreadful and unnatural struggle' between Britain and the colonies might be prevented 'by the success of their constitutional, loyal and peaceable efforts for freedom, for securing their natural rights as men, and the civil rights which they hitherto enjoyed as Englishmen'. Priestley pointed to the prosecution of Wilkes as evidence of the assault on English liberties at home, and then outlined the greater threat of oppression that the Americans faced. The colonies should be left to govern themselves, he argued, urging that commerce would bring far more wealth to Britain than could be got by taxation.[16]

While not all Dissenters supported the rebellious colonies, in general the leading representatives of Dissent spoke on behalf of the Americans because they 'shared a more powerful sense of community with their counterparts in the colonies and had closer associations with America than any other Englishmen save Quakers'.[17] The political sentiments of many low Anglicans like Jebb followed this realignment of Dissent, as debate over the nature of political authority was added to the religious controversy that had divided Latitudinarians.

Following the partial repeal of the Townshend Duties there was relative peace between the administration and the colonies. But while the House of Commons found it convenient to forget about America, discontent continued to brew in the colonies where the Tea Duty was correctly seen to maintain the supremacy of the British Parliament. Between 1770 and 1773 the attitude of many Americans was profoundly transformed by John Dickinson's *Letters from a Farmer in Pennsylvania*, which argued that the British Parliament had a right to regulate trade, but that duties had never been imposed for the sole purpose of raising revenue. If the Parliament established the right to raise revenue from duties, they would be able to levy 'such sums of money as they choose to take, *without any other* LIMITATION *than their* PLEASURE'.[18] The Boston Tea Party destroyed the relative calm across the Atlantic in December 1773, when radicals attacked the first shipment of cheap tea from the East India Company.

---

[15] See Clara H. Hay, *James Burgh: spokesman for reform in Hanoverian England* (Washington, D.C., 1979); and 'The Making of a Radical: the case of James Burgh', *Journal of British Studies,* 18 (1979), pp. 90-117.

[16] Priestley, *Political Writings*, pp. 130, 140, 144.

[17] Colin Bonwick, 'English Dissenters and the American Revolution', in H.C. Allen and Roger Thompson eds., *Contrast and Connection: bicentennial essays in Anglo-American history* (1976), pp. 90-91.

[18] John Derry, *English Politics and the American Revolution* (1976), p. 99; Bailyn, *Ideological Origins*, p. 101; John Dickinson, *Letters from a Farmer in Pennsylvania* (Philadelphia, 1768), p. 55.

Public opinion was incensed when the news of this assault on property rights reached Britain. In March Benjamin Franklin reflected that 'I suppose we never had since we were a People so few Friends in Britain. The violent Destruction of the Tea seems to have united all Parties here against our Province'.[19]

Franklin called his favourite dining group at the London Coffee House the 'Club of Honest Whigs'. This group was an intellectual engine-room of opposition to the administration and support for America. Its members were predominantly Dissenters, with a large contingent of clergy and schoolmasters. Founded in the early 1760s by John Canton, the son of a weaver who became a well-known journalist and scientist, the core members were Richard Price, Franklin and James Burgh, while Priestley attended whenever in London. James Boswell, who attended a few times when he was interested in the Corsican struggle for independence, conveys something of the temper of the club:

> It consists of clergymen, physicians, and several other professions.... We have wine and punch upon the table. Some of us smoke a pipe, conversation goes on pretty formally, sometimes sensibly and sometimes furiously. At nine there is a sideboard with Welsh rabbits and apple-puffs, porter and beer. Our reckoning is about 18d. a head. Much was said this night against the Parliament. I said that, as it seems to be agreed that all Members of Parliament become corrupted, it was better to choose men already bad, and so save good men.[20]

It is probable that Theophilus Lindsey dined with the club when he took up residence in London, as he was closely connected with Priestley and Franklin.[21] On 17 January 1775 Lindsey related that 'I dined yesterday ... with Drs Price, Franklin, Priestley, and Mr. Quincey: no bad company you will say. We began and ended with the Americans'.[22] Did Jebb attend the Club of Honest Whigs? As noted in chapter 2, Jebb had at least some contact with Thomas Hollis's band of Real Whigs in the late 1760s. If Lindsey began attending the Club of Honest Whigs when he settled in London, it seems reasonable to speculate that Jebb accompanied him when visiting the capital. On 5 February 1775, a few weeks after he had dined with the Honest Whigs, Lindsey informed

---

[19] John Sainsbury, *Disaffected Patriots: London supporters of revolutionary America* (Kingston, Ont., 1987), p. 56.

[20] James Boswell, *Boswell in Search of a Wife, 1766-69* (Frank Brady and Frederick A. Pottle eds., 1957), pp. 318-19.

[21] Lindsey noted in May 1774 that 'Dr Priestley leaves us on Sunday night – to my great concern and distress – I have seldom missed a day seeing him ... he has been my most singular friend and promoter of my ease and interest'. Theophilus Lindsey to William Turner, 5 May 1774. Timothy Hollis took up residence near the Essex Street Chapel in late 1774 and provided a place where Lindsey could dine regularly and hear news from America. Lindsey to Turner, 3 November 1774, DWL Lindsey-Turner correspondence.

[22] Verner W. Crane, 'The Club of Honest Whigs: friends of science and liberty', *William and Mary Quarterly,* 23 (1966), p. 222; McLachlan, *Letters of Lindsey*, pp. 79.

a friend that 'Mr Jebb has been with me a fortnight', and was 'miserable in the Church trammels – never does any duty – and will quit as soon as ever he can'.[23]

Perhaps at this time (with troops drilling in Hyde Park before embarking for America) Jebb found encouragement among like-minded company on a Thursday evening at the London Coffee House. It seems likely that he began to dine each fortnight with the Honest Whigs once he moved to London. John Disney did so when he settled in the metropolis – in February 1783, he went with Andrew Kippis 'to the Club at London Co[ffee] Ho[use] which was the first time after my election. The Meeting large, and agreeable'.[24] Jebb was evidently acquainted with Benjamin Franklin, to whom he wrote a letter of introduction for two young friends who were to visit Paris. Franklin 'first inquired particularly after Dr Jebb' and later 'seemed much pleased' with Jebb's 'noble sentiments on the American war'.[25] And Jebb seems to have been fairly familiar with Richard Price, a Dissenter, philosopher and prominent Honest Whig. For example, Lindsey met Price and Jebb at Brand Hollis's in February 1779;[26] Jebb and Price convalesced at Brighthelmstone in August 1783;[27] and the two often met with John Adams in 1785.

In 1774 the Americans were hoping for a British Revolution that would reconstitute the government.[28] However, while leading Dissenters championed the cause of the colonists, there appeared to be little support in the wider British electorate. One Englishman wrote to his correspondent in America that: 'Universal Bribery and Corruption has Annihilated the little share of Liberty and Patriotism which Walpole left behind, and I'm really at a Loss to judge which is the most venal and corrupt, the Minister or the House of Commons, the People or their Representatives.'[29] Despite such pessimistic reports the Americans continued to hope for a ground swell of support in Britain. In the autumn of 1774 the Continental Congress addressed the British people, warning that the government sought control over American lives and property so that it could 'with greater facility enslave you', and expressed hope that the British people would elect a Parliament 'of such wisdom, independence and public spirit, as may save the violated rights of the whole empire'.[30]

The American cause was given a boost by an outburst of protest on both sides of the Atlantic in response to the Quebec Act. Britain's gains in Canada as a result of the Seven Years War had raised the problem of how a

---

[23] Lindsey to Turner 5 Feb. 1775, DWL Lindsey-Turner correspondence.
[24] Disney, 'Diary', DWL mss., 6 February 1783.
[25] John Baynes, 'Journal', 27 August and 15 September 1783, attached as an appendix to Samuel Romilly, *The Life of Sir Samuel Romilly* (1842), p. 447.
[26] Theophilus Lindsey to William Turner, February 1779, DWL Lindsey-Turner correspondence.
[27] Theophilus Lindsey to William Tayleur, 1 September 1783, JRL Lindsey-Tayleur correspondence.
[28] Pauline Maier, *From Resistance to Revolution: colonial radicals and the development of opposition to Britain, 1765-1776* (New York, 1973), pp. 246-63.
[29] George Peacock to William Palfrey, London, 4 March 1774, cited in Maier, *Resistance to Revolution*, p. 249.
[30] Maier, *Resistance to Revolution*, p. 249.

largely French Catholic colony should be governed. The Quebec Act of 1774 upheld French civil law, allowed the Catholic Church to collect tithes, and established a legislative council (rather than an elected assembly) to which Roman Catholics were appointed and allowed a modified oath of loyalty. As Colin Haydon has observed, granting such concessions to a colony within the Protestant British Empire represented 'a massive shift of policy' that 'also neatly illustrates the intersection between political realism and growing liberal feeling' among the governing elite.[31] This piece of enlightened policy, however, was met by a storm of condemnation. Opposition seems to have focused upon two main aspects of the Act: the fact that it not only tolerated but encouraged Catholicism; and the decision to rule through a government appointed council rather than an elected assembly. The anti-Catholicism of the streets and coffee-houses was encouraged by Commonwealthmen like Thomas Hollis and Francis Blackburne who saw in 'the Quebec bill ... the effects of a spirit of popery actuating the carcase of a Protestant government'.[32] Enlightened critics who disliked anti-Catholicism and religious persecution, such as Edmund Burke and the Unitarian politician George Savile, focused upon the constitutional dimension. 'Give them English liberty,' Burke declared in the House of Commons, 'give them an English constitution – and then, whether they speak French or English, whether they go to mass or attend our own communion, you will render them valuable and useful subjects of Great Britain.'[33] Jebb does not appear to have contributed to the anti-Catholic diatribes that were levelled at the Quebec Act. He shared Priestley's commitment to universal toleration and later (in the 1780s) argued for full citizenship rights for Catholics in Ireland. He thought the Act was a 'shame to patriotism' because it established 'an arbitrary government ... in the extensive province of Quebec' that could contribute to the 'influence of the crown' being 'enormously increased' in Britain.[34]

Toward the end of the year public opinion seemed impressed by the firmness of the American stand. Yet hopes that a new Parliament would address colonial grievances were dashed when North called a surprise election to take advantage of relatively passive public sentiment in September 1774. This election witnessed few heated contests and returned a favourable outcome for the government. Samuel Adams wistfully reflected that had the administration 'suffered the election to be put off till the spring it might have cost them their heads'.[35] Yet the election demonstrated that there was little organised support for the colonists outside of London and that most of the country treated their claims with either apathy or hostility.[36] Thomas Blackburne assured Jebb that

---

[31] Haydon, *Anti-Catholicism*, pp. 172-73.

[32] Francis Blackburne, *Memoirs of Thomas Hollis* (2 vols., 1780), I, p. 215.

[33] Cited in O'Brien, *The Great Melody*, p. 94. See also Haydon, *Anti-Catholicism*, pp. 192-97.

[34] 'Trebatius' [JJ], 2 August 1785, Jebb III, p. 387. See also 'Life of Jebb', p. 92.

[35] Samuel Adams to Arthur Lee, 14 February 1775, cited in Maier, *Resistance to Revolution*, p. 250.

[36] Sainsbury, *Disaffected Patriots*, p. 69; Gould, *Persistence of Empire*, pp. 136-47.

the new Parliament would have its work cut out dealing with America and speculated that Britain would become a province in the Empire of America.[37]

Following this election, it seemed to many Americans that if the British people were going to aid them it would have to be in the form of an insurrection. In the words of Maier, 'gauging the chances for an English uprising became a primary concern of American representatives in England'.[38] Josiah Quincey (who dined with the Club of Honest Whigs) was pessimistic, claiming that while there was support for the American cause, they could expect no help because the English were cowed by oppression and would only rise if the Americans spilt their own blood first. Many others, however, did not doubt the possibility of an imminent uprising. One report in April 1775 asserted 'that everything in London wears a strong Appearance of a speedy Rising against the present Administration'.[39] But such hopes were misplaced and based on the vocal opposition of Dissenters and radical London artisans. The broad support of propertied Englishmen seems to have rallied behind the King and Parliament once hostilities broke out in April 1775. Yet the effect of these developments in further alienating men like Jebb from the establishment cannot be underestimated.

Reflecting upon his own brushes with authority, Jebb hoped that the Americans would act forcefully. Following the 1774 election he wrote to a friend that a 'very sensible letter in the *Ledger* of yesterday, shows the absurdity of petitioning for redress; the most vigorous measures are best; the English Ministry must feel, before they will repent'.[40] A further fault of petitions, he added, was that the length of time they took to organise, submit and be discussed allowed the Ministry 'an opportunity of trying their usual arts of conquering by division'.[41] He had not yet seen the 'Address' by the Congress, but hoped the Americans would 'go the whole ground at once, and yet leave matters open for an accommodation. The only way to avoid bloodshed is for the Americans to show their resolution in the first instance'.[42] In December he reiterated his desire that the Americans pursue their demands through peaceful and legal means, such as a complete suspension of trade.[43] When the Jebbs left Cambridge in the summer of 1775 to travel north, their thoughts were preoccupied with the outbreak of war in America, which they 'supposed must be decisive of the liberties of both countries'. In July Jebb wrote of the American situation: 'I now begin to despair of an accommodation; that country however will be free, and this must go backwards, perhaps to its original state of barbarity'. On the brighter side, he reflected that the American rebellion meant that 'Liberty has an

---

37 Thomas Blackburne to JJ, 14 October 1774, DWL Blackburne-Lindsey correspondence.

38 Maier, *Resistance to Revolution*, p. 250.

39 Cited Maier, *Resistance to Revolution*, p. 251.

40 Letter dated 17 November 1774, 'Life of Jebb', p. 86.

41 'Life of Jebb', p. 86.

42 'Life of Jebb', p. 86.

43 Letter 3 December 1774, 'Life of Jebb', p. 87.

asylum on that continent', adding that 'the abominable slave trade will, I trust, be abolished'.[44]

INDEPENDENCE AND LIBERTY

It is clear that the American Revolution had both material and ideological origins. On the one hand, the conflict grew out of the logic of the imperial situation. The British government regarded North America as a source of primary produce and a market for British manufacturers; and the loudest voices in Whitehall were those of British landowners, West Indian planters, the East India Company and British governors and placemen in America. In this system, the colonies would always serve the interests of those at the centre of the Empire. Yet the social, economic and cultural dynamism of the colonies was at odds with such a system, and after decades of salutary neglect the British government's attempt to tighten its rule drove the diverse colonies into unified resistance. As a result, the Americans avoided the kind of long-term subordination of their economy suffered by Ireland and India.[45]

Nevertheless, for some years after the Declaration of Independence, British Dissenters continued to hope that some form of compromise could be reached that would preserve the Empire. In 1780 Jebb still hoped that a federal union with the American states was possible.[46] But eventually the reality of Independence had to be accepted. When the American envoy John Adams visited London and moved in radical circles in late 1783, the best that could be hoped for was the establishment of friendly relations and the swift resumption of mutually beneficial commerce.[47]

In challenging the authority of the British Parliament the Americans and their supporters drew upon natural rights arguments and the radical Whig and Dissenting traditions.[48] The American patriot Benjamin Rush wrote to an English friend in 1774: 'We are enraged at our being considered the "subjects" of the House of Commons'.[49] The right to participate in the legislative process was not a dry and unemotional notion for the likes of Rush and Jebb. The thing that distinguished English culture, they thought, was that independent men had the *right* and *duty* to make their own laws. Conflict between Parliament and the

---

[44] 'Life of Jebb', p. 92.

[45] Edward O. Countryman, *The American Revolution* (Harmondsworth, 1985), pp. 54-56. For the view that the Revolution was an avoidable 'human tragedy, for which certain men were responsible', see Ian R. Christie, *Crisis of Empire: Great Britain and the American Colonies 1754-1783* (1966), p. 114.

[46] *An Address to the Freeholders of Middlesex*, Jebb II, p. 484.

[47] McLachlan, *Letters of Lindsey*, p. 86.

[48] Steven M. Dworetz, *The Unvarnished Doctrine: Locke, liberalism and the American Revolution* (Chapel hill, N.C., 1990); Bailyn, *Ideological Origins*; Pocock, *Machiavellian Moment*; Clark, *Language of Liberty*.

[49] Benjamin Rush to Granville Sharp, 9 July 1774, in John A. Woods, 'The Correspondence of Benjamin Rush and Granville Sharp 1773-1809', *Journal of American Studies* 1 (1967), p. 8.

Colonies encouraged examination of the theory and practice of this cultural assumption.

As Caroline Robbins has put it, 'one idea ran through all the different kinds of liberty, the idea of self-direction or of self-government'.[50] The American colonies already had a relatively broad popular involvement in their governance. They confronted a stark choice between the authority of their own assemblies and that of a Parliament elected in Britain. As a result there was little need to theorise about the nature of representation during the Revolution. For the Americans it was essentially a matter of liberating themselves from the authority of the British Parliament, and then formally drafting their various state constitutions in which many (including many white males) were excluded from the franchise. Some British thinkers, however, both geographically and culturally closer to the seat of authority, were led to examine the nuts and bolts of their electoral system. In doing so, some began to advocate universal manhood suffrage in tracts that had a profound influence upon Jebb.[51]

One of the earliest and most important tracts to question the structure of the British electorate was Obadiah Hulme's *Historical Essay on the English Constitution* (1771). In the words of Gerald Newman, this book was 'a powerful polemic, resting on and drawing all its authority from a mountain of historical and pseudo historical fact'.[52] Hulme claimed that since the Norman Conquest, and especially since the Revolution of 1688, legislative innovations had caused a 'total change in the spirit and temper of our government'.[53] Government and the House of Commons had at length become captive to the interests of the monarchy and aristocracy, and thus laws were made in favour of those 'rich in land'. 'Much has been writ about patriotic kings, and patriotic ministers', he thundered, 'but give me leave to tell the good people of England, that it is all PATRIOTIC NONSENSE'.[54] The only remedy for the 'present discontents' was a return to the Anglo-Saxon constitution in which representation was more equal and Parliaments elected annually. 'Where annual election ends, there Slavery begins' he declared, arguing that 'constitutional clubs' should be formed in each parish to pass resolutions calling for the reform of Parliament.[55] As Christopher Hill has observed, the *Historical Essay* had 'a remarkable vogue' and radicals propounded its basic ideas until it became a pillar of Victorian historiography.[56]

In his *Political Disquisitions* (1774-75) James Burgh was more democratic and more precise in discussing the means by which reform could be affected. A Dissenter, schoolmaster and friend of Richard Price, he had been calling for political and moral reform since the late 1740s. Burgh had initially

---

50 Robbins, *Commonwealthmen*, p. 337.
51 Clark, *Language of Liberty*, pp. 143, 338-9, 301.
52 Newman, *Rise of English Nationalism*, p. 185.
53 Hulme, *Historical Essay*, pp. ii-iv.
54 Hulme, *Historical Essay*, pp. 79-147, 150.
55 Hulme, *Historical Essay*, pp. iii, 161.
56 Christopher Hill, 'The Norman Yoke', in *Puritanism and Revolution: studies in interpretation of the English Revolution in the seventeenth century* (New York, 1958), pp. 111-12.

placed his faith in the prospect of a 'patriot king', but with the accession of George III he became increasingly disillusioned with those who wielded political power. Like many of his contemporaries, the debate over representation occasioned by conflict between the colonists and Parliament led him to explore the radical implications of Locke's contractual theory of government. In his *Political Disquisitions* Burgh outlined three main grievances: that Parliament was unrepresentative, corrupt and that elections were too infrequent. 'Every man', he argued, 'has a life, a personal liberty, a character, a right to his earnings, a right to a religious profession and worship according to his conscience'. Thus, the franchise should be based upon personality rather than property.[57] Hulme did not address the issue of what to do if the Parliament ignored public pressure to reform. Burgh took the step of arguing that a national convention consisting of delegates from county assemblies could force Parliament to reform.[58] The *Political Disquisitions* became a basic textbook for critics of the unreformed system in the late eighteenth century, and was carefully studied by such diverse figures as Tom Paine, William Pitt the Younger, Samuel Taylor Coleridge and William Hazlitt.[59]

The arguments of Hulme and Burgh inspired the British supporters of America to maintain their rage during the first half of the American war when loyalist support was widespread. Hulme had argued that London would have to take the lead in mobilising a movement of reform associations. In the summer of 1775 the former schoolmaster Thomas Joel, a passionate supporter of the Americans and freedom of the press, formed the London Association in order to rally pro-American sentiment. George III's proclamation that the American colonies were in a state of rebellion was also aimed at suppressing such dissent within Britain. Six days after the proclamation Jebb wrote to Lindsey requesting 'facts' as to the nature and authenticity of the London Association, from which he had received a circular letter. 'I am heartily disposed to exert all my powers in support of so just a cause', he wrote, 'I think it my duty at present to argue in support of our invalid rights, regardless of a proclamation, which on all occasions and in all companies I treat with the most marked contempt.[60] The London Association was composed largely of tradesmen, and it's championing of revolution principles and the ancient constitution only succeeded in encouraging a surge of loyalist support for the government. There is no indication that Jebb became involved with this group, which maintained a 'precarious existence' until it dissolved in February 1777.[61]

While organised support for the Americans was not forthcoming, the 'friends of liberty' kept up a vocal criticism of the government. In the year when

---

[57] James Burgh, *Political Disquisitions* (1774-75), I, pp. 24, 38. Burgh took his democratic arguments from Locke and probably Priestley's *First Principles of Government*. Ian Christie, *Wilkes, Wyvill and Reform: the parliamentary reform movement in British politics, 1760-1785* (1962), p. 55.

[58] Burgh, *Political Disquisitions*, I, p. 6.

[59] Hay, 'The Making of a Radical: the case of James Burgh', p. 112.

[60] JJ to Theophilus Lindsey, 29 August 1775, DWL *Illustrated Life of Priestley* f.204.

[61] Sainsbury, *Disaffected Patriots*, pp. 106-13, at 106.

independence was declared, Richard Price published his enormously popular *Observations on the Nature of Civil Liberty,* in which he called for moral and political reform in Britain. In the same year John Cartwright published *Take Your Choice!* in which he challenged the British people to pursue a radical reform of Parliament along the lines of universal manhood suffrage and annual parliaments. Cartwright's arguments, which he tirelessly repeated in tracts, letters and speeches until his death in 1824, formed the basis of radical demands into the first half of the nineteenth century.

Radicals envisioned America as a repository of the robust, masculine, virtuous and independent spirit they thought was fading away in England. Henry Taylor was convinced that 'all our Governors are mad' and assured Ann Jebb that 'everything worth preserving is going over to America; there is a spirit in that Country superior to anything in other parts of the world'; and the mixture of religions and a flowering of philosophy would see them become 'the greatest nation in the world'. Adding that 'we have done such things of late that I am afraid to be called an Englishman'.[62] In August 1782 John Jebb wrote:

> To American resistance, I owe, under heaven, that I now enjoy the freedom of my person; ... I remember the time when I gloried in the name of Englishman. Whatever was generous, manly, and humane, seemed, by nature, associated to that much loved sound. I thought it virtue to believe, that my country was the peculiar care of heaven; and my ear hung delighted on the accents that pronounced her praise. It is, therefore, with pain inexpressible, that I now behold a nation, once ruled over by the immortal Alfred, the birth-place of Milton, an Hampden, and a Sidney, dishonoured and degraded by deeds of foul injustice; sunk in inglorious luxury and ease; unmindful of its former generous spirit; eager, at the call of despotism, to destroy the liberties of its more virtuous brethren; incapable of being roused, by the thousand dangers that surround her, and the fair example of her sister kingdom, to defend her own.[63]

The Revolution could be seen as of global importance – a point at which the English political tradition and Enlightenment universalism merged to form a model state. Jebb congratulated Benjamin Franklin on the end of 'a contest which, for seven years, agitated my mind with feelings not to be described'.[64] He thought that in the 'glorious institutions' of America 'the human species will, at last, obtain an asylum; and every individual be permitted to enjoy a larger proportion of civil and religious liberty, than hath been indulged in any age or clime'.[65]

---

[62] Henry Taylor to Ann Jebb [1776], CUL Taylor papers.
[63] 'Alfred' [JJ], 26 August 1782, Jebb III, pp. 341-42.
[64] 'Life of Jebb', p. 188. For Franklin's favourable reception of the letter see Romilly, *Life*, p. 449.
[65] 'Laelius' [JJ], [October?] 1782, Jebb III, p. 361.

After his migration to America in 1784 Walter Pollard, a young barrister and member of the Society for Constitutional Information, continued to correspond with his friend Thomas Day and pass on respects to Jebb. Pollard soon became disillusioned by the degree to which the American reality failed in comparison to his idealistic preconceptions. Day claimed to have been less 'subject to enthusiasm than some of my friends' when it came to the nature of American virtue and liberty.[66] Jebb, no doubt, was one of those enthusiastic friends. In October 1783 he pointed to the example of religious toleration in the American constitutions, and in particular that of Maryland: 'The exertions of the human intellect are there unfettered by those iniquitous restraints which dishonour European climes: every man, therefore, lives in charity with his neighbour, and the rage of proselytism is unknown'.[67]

Near the end of his life Jebb had the pleasure of frequent conversations with John Adams, the American Ambassador. The two found themselves in close agreement on religious and political matters. Adams's daughter Abigail told her brother that 'Dr Jebb, who has visited your father several times since we arrived, and who is of his opinions I believe in Politics, brought his Lady to see Mamma this morning. She is also a great Politicianess, which consequently pleased Mamma'.[68] Adams was one of the most systematic of thinkers in the republican and Harringtonian vein. He believed that a natural aristocracy would always emerge, and to deal with this he advocated that it should be planned for and provided with a function that would render it socially beneficial.[69] Adams praised James Burgh's *Political Disquisitions* when it was published in 1774, though he was unimpressed by Tom Paine's *Common Sense*, which he saw as advocating democracy, which 'must produce confusion and every evil work'.[70] Adams early but reluctantly resigned himself to the necessity of Independence, and after the war laboured hard to establish ties with Britain. Jebb told Adams that 'I regard the establishment of Liberty in America with a pleasure bordering on enthusiasm. I feel with Dr Price the ardent wish that nothing may retard the extent and influence of freedom'. He trusted that under the guidance of Providence the 'bright example' set by the Americans would

> influence the People from whence they sprang, and every other European state, to shake off the shackles of Civil and Religious despotism and enable their inhabitants more generally to become what Heaven intended men to be – virtuous, rational, wise and happy here – and consequently prepared for the enjoyment of still superior degrees of happiness in a more enduring state.[71]

---

[66] Thomas Day to Walter Pollard, 1 August 1785, BL Add. Mss. 35,655:252.

[67] JJ, 25 October 1783, in *Address to the Volunteers of Ireland*, Jebb II, pp. 544-45.

[68] Abigail Adams jr to John Q. Adams, 31 July 1785, *Adams Family Correspondence*, VI, p. 216.

[69] Pocock, *Virtue, Commerce and History*, p. 269.

[70] *The Diary and Autobiography of John Adams* (4 vols., L.H. Butterfield ed., Cambridge, Mass., 1961), II, p. 330.

[71] JJ to Adams, 13 September 1785, MHS Adams papers.

Notions of religious liberty, republican virtue, and universal political rights coalesced around the American cause and encouraged calls for political reform within Britain.

ASSOCIATIONS AND POLITICAL EDUCATION

The American conflict eventually created the political and economic conditions in which a popular movement for reform of the Parliament could flourish. British politics became more polarised following the battle of Saratoga in October 1777 and the subsequent alliance between France and the Americans.[72] While there was a surge in loyalist support, particularly in 'the old Jacobite heartlands', the relatively small number of opponents of the war kept up a vocal protest, emphasising the threat to British trade, the possibility of invasion and government corruption.[73] In 1778 John Cartwright first discussed the formation of a 'society for political enquiry', and there were suggestions in some newspapers that an 'Association' of the people should be formed.[74] Early in that year Sir Philip Jennings Clerke introduced a bill to prevent government contractors who had not won their contracts through public tender from sitting in the Commons. While this was easily defeated, it was the first hint of the Rockingham party's future 'economical reform' proposals.

By the end of the decade it seemed to many that Britain was facing impending doom. The war in America was dragging on with no sign of a satisfactory end in sight, following the entry of France on the colonists' side. The Rousseauian Thomas Day complained that Britain was faced with a choice of deaths, either by 'a desperate attack upon France' or 'the less expeditious method of dying by decay'.[75] Following the Franco-American alliance a wave of volunteer militias formed in Ireland to counter the threat of invasion; discussion at their meetings turned into calls for economic and political reform. In the summer of 1779 the North administration's morale and public support were at a low ebb, though the parliamentary opposition was little better respected. A number of duels were reported between leading aristocrats of opposing political persuasions, and as the year came to an end there were increasing calls for reform from both in and outside Parliament. The stage was set for a turbulent parliamentary session.

In November Lord North was accused of unfairly interfering in the nominations for a vacant seat in Middlesex. A gathering of the electors called on

---

[72] The following political narrative is drawn from Christie, *Wilkes, Wyvill and Reform*; John Cannon, *Parliamentary reform, 1640-1832* (Cambridge, 1973), chapter 4; Eugene C. Black, *The Association: British extraparliamentary political organization 1769-1793* (Cambridge, Mass., 1963), chapter 2.

[73] Langford, *Polite and Commercial People*, pp. 543-44.

[74] *Life of Cartwright*, I, p. 120; Christie, *Wilkes, Wyvill and Reform*, p. 68. Granville Sharp and Cartwright met at Capel Lofft's chambers in Lincoln's Inn on 3 December 1777 and 'corrected the Major's scheme of an Association for Political Reformation'. Sharp, 'Diary', GRO Sharp papers, 3 December 1777.

[75] Thomas Day to Erasmus Darwin, 29 January 1779, BL Add. Mss. 29,300:54.

22 November resolved to meet monthly and campaign against the administration. The Wilkite candidate Thomas Wood was elected for Middlesex, and by the next meeting of the freeholders on 20 December the campaign for reform was gathering momentum. In Yorkshire, the liberal clergyman Christopher Wyvill and some of his friends among the gentry began to organise a campaign to promote the 'economical reform' of Parliament. In a circular letter to MPs on November 29 they suggested that if corruption were reduced the Parliament could be so changed at the next election that 'it would be an easy matter to carry the other regulations, annual Parliaments, more county members, etc., which are thought necessary to restore the freedom of the Parliament'.[76]

Wyvill wanted to keep the Yorkshire organisation free from party politics, and while he could not prevent politicians from attending meetings, he did ensure that no Member of Parliament could join the Yorkshire Association Committee. Nevertheless, Rockingham, who was expressly opposed to electoral reform, was keen to place his party at the head of the Association movement. To this end Edmund Burke presented a bill for economical reform in December, and at the end of the month Rockingham and some supporters attended the Yorkshire Association. At this meeting more than two hundred of Yorkshire's leading gentry and clergy adopted a petition requesting 'an enquiry into the civil list to be followed by abolition of all sinecure places, of exorbitant salaries attached to efficient places, and pensions unmerited by public service'.[77] Meanwhile, Jebb had prepared an *Address to the Freeholders of Middlesex*, which was presented to the chairman and read out at their meeting on December 20. According to Herbert Butterfield, this tract contained 'the extreme statement – indeed we might say the most comprehensive statement that was made at this time – of the doctrine and programme of the Association, as the radical leaders understood it'.[78]

The failure of parliamentary reform in the early 1780s is in part explained by the inability of these three distinct political groupings to reach agreement. The Rockinghamites remained essentially conservative, interested only in limiting the government's ability to control Parliament with placemen. Anxious to retain the support of conservative Yorkshire squires, Wyvill sought a moderate reform of the system of representation, which would see more independent gentry elected to Parliament. Jebb and the radicals, however, wanted to see a broadly defined political nation force radical reform of the House of Commons. Jebb's role in the political developments between 1780 and his death in early 1786 will be examined in the final chapter. Here, however, I want to outline his contribution to the initial flurry of extra-parliamentary activity in early 1780.

As noted earlier, in response to the discontent of the early 1770s Hulme and Burgh had suggested that the people form associations and demand that the Parliament be reformed. Jebb first proposed the idea to Sir George Savile, a Unitarian and Member of Parliament, in two private letters in the spring of

---

[76] Wyvill, *Political Papers*, III, p. 151.
[77] Christie, *Wilkes, Wyvill and Reform*, p. 74.
[78] Herbert Butterfield, *George III, Lord North and the People, 1779-1780* (1949), p. 191.

1776.[79] In the *Address to the Freeholders of Middlesex* Jebb argued that petitioning the House of Commons would not effect political change. He pointed to Burke's famous claim that the MP was not bound to obey the will of his electors. 'With greater appearance of reason', he argued, Parliament could and did ignore petitions emanating from only part of the political nation. Also, as the Crown, Lords and Commons were 'free and independent' elements of the Constitution, even a unanimous Commons could not 'dictate to the Crown'.[80] It was not surprising, he observed, that previous petitions asking Parliament to dissolve itself had failed, for 'men possessed of power are not disposed to part with it'.[81] Alternatively, he proposed the formation of a movement 'founded on principles, which, like axioms in geometry, admit not of debate'. The basic principle he asserted was the 'acknowledged right of the people to new-model the constitution, and punish, with exemplary vigour, every person with whom they have entrusted power, provided, in their opinion, he shall be found to have betrayed that trust'. To such strong words Jebb added that the people could go further and overturn the established form of government.[82]

Jebb proceeded to outline his plan for a national convention formed of delegates from the county Associations. Each county should estimate its population and determine its proportionate number of delegates, which should be agreed to by the 'approved friends of liberty in the other counties'. When a majority of counties had elected corresponding committees, these should send a proportionate number of representatives to a national convention, which would pass a 'public ACT' containing reforms to be demanded of the House of Commons. The objection to petitions would thus be overcome, as 'the command would proceed from the principal to the delegate, from the master to the servant'. If this act of a national convention was ignored, then the delegates should return to their counties and propose the election of new committees with 'more important powers'. With the committees supported by a 'general association' in each county, Jebb thought 'the attention of the people will thus at length be excited' and their sense of patriotism stimulated. Past this, Jebb would 'not presume, even in idea, to anticipate' what measures may be taken 'by the concentrated wisdom of an enlightened people'. Though he did suggest that the House of Commons could be legally dissolved and a new system of representation devised by the convention. Jebb tried to temper this subversive suggestion with the requirement that any 'Act' by the convention would need the assent of the Crown and Lords to be constitutional. The threat of withholding supply of taxation revenue would ensure such co-operation.[83]

---

[79] Jebb II, p. 484n.

[80] *Address to the Freeholders of Middlesex* (4th ed. May 1782 [December 1779]), Jebb II, pp. 459-66. In the subsequent editions Jebb added notes to elaborate and explain his arguments. The following account of the *Address to Middlesex* is drawn from the original primary text, and the contents of the footnotes will be referred to in later discussion.

[81] *Address to the Freeholders of Middlesex*, Jebb II, p. 471.

[82] *Address to the Freeholders of Middlesex*, Jebb II, pp. 461, 469.

[83] *Address to the Freeholders of Middlesex*, Jebb II, pp. 472-81.

Jebb argued that reform was the only 'remedy for the increasing disorders of our distempered state', and warned that as 'the times of distress, long predicted' would soon arrive, reform of Parliament should be proposed and discussed in the 'hour of tranquillity which precedes the storm'. He stressed that the Associations should focus upon 'one constitutional point, clear, distinct, and comprehensive in its nature'. As in religion, political principles should be expressed in terms 'adapted to the understandings of all orders of men; [and] such as the intelligent and virtuous of all parties will approve'. The simple constitutional goal Jebb advocated for the Association movement was 'equal, annual and universal representation of the Commons'. If this were achieved, 'the fabric of government, reared by our ancestors, at the expense of so much blood, would appear in finished beauty; and the popular pillar of the Constitution, thus set upon its proper basis, would give security and permanency to the whole'.[84] In short, Jebb entered the extra-parliamentary arena waving the flag for annual elections and equal representation – and his proposals were, in Ian Christie's words, 'entirely revolutionary'.[85]

Those who wanted Jebb to write in support of the Unitarian cause were disappointed that his attentions had been drawn to political activism. William Tayleur told Lindsey that 'political debates on all sides, both in and out of Parliament, are carried on with so much malice, that ... I have long been sick of politics'. As such, he was 'really aggrieved to see our friend so deeply immersed in politics'. The 'temperate manner' of the *Address*, he continued, 'deserves great praise; but give me leave to tell you privately that the subject matter is of a nature much too deep and problematical, for the Middlesex freeholders, (if they be not much wiser than other freeholders), to form any solid judgement concerning it'.[86] While some of Jebb's Unitarian friends lamented his political idealism, there were new acquaintances like John Cartwright who would encourage and join him in political agitation. Reviewing his friend's tract, Paul Henry Maty observed that 'the author of this address is a close thinker, and a sound reasoner.... [His] arguments are conceived with solidity, and urged with judgement and temper'.[87]

Following the Yorkshire lead, Middlesex and several other counties adopted petitions calling for economical reform. On 8 February Sir George Savile tabled the Yorkshire petition in Parliament, declaring that while it was not presented by 'men with swords and muskets', if it were ignored, 'here I leave a blank'.[88] Burke and the opposition proceeded to produce a series of bills for economical reform, which were substantially defeated owing to Lord North's skilful parliamentary management. The best that could be achieved was the passing on 6 April of Dunning's famous but hollow motion that 'the power of the Crown has increased, is increasing, and ought to be diminished'. Nevertheless, it is clear that the political establishment had been shaken. A

---

84 *Address to the Freeholders of Middlesex*, Jebb II, pp. 482, 490, 486, 483.
85 Christie, *Wilkes, Wyvill and Reform*, p. 79.
86 William Tayleur to T. Lindsey, [1780?], JRL Mss. Lindsey – Tayleur correspondence.
87 [Paul Henry Maty], *Monthly Review* (January 1780), p. 81.
88 Cannon, *Parliamentary Reform*, p. 76.

concerned Horace Walpole informed his friend Horace Mann (the British representative in Florence) that,

> In short, I think that the Ministers must fall, and would increase their own danger every hour if they stayed. The committees in the country will be animated by this specimen of their importance ... in truth it is to be hoped that the die *is* cast. A change of men and measures may prevent that most dreadful of evils, civil war; and the longer the Court attempts to stem the current, the more destructive the deluge will be.[89]

Mann replied that 'I always thought the provincial committees, associations, and petitions would produce a flame difficult to extinguish'.[90]

Beneath the bluster of petitions and parliamentary debate Jebb was busy trying to create a popular base for radical reform. While the leading opposition magnates were trying to control extra-parliamentary politics, Charles James Fox decided to become a 'man of the people'. In the words of Ian Christie, 'impetuous, passionate, and frustrated, he was carried away by the flood-tide of popular excitement'.[91] At a meeting of 3,000 freeholders of Westminster, and flanked on the platform by Wilkes, Jebb and John Sawbridge, Fox delivered a rousing speech in which he dwelt on the principle that the people could force Parliament to reform. Pointing to the example set by the American colonists and the Irish Volunteers, he asked: 'shall the heart of the empire be tame and lifeless while the limbs are in activity and motion?'[92] Moved by 'zeal' for the cause, Jebb rose for the first time at a public political meeting and congratulated the freeholders of Westminster, 'from all ranks of the people', for taking a stand against corruption, and urged them to follow 'the glorious examples set by the county of Middlesex' and carry their future member 'without expense, to the door of the House of Commons'. His motion that Fox be adopted as the future candidate for Westminster was greeted with 'universal applause'.[93] A committee of over one hundred members was also appointed to plan the Association campaign and correspond with other committees.

Christopher Wyvill was wary of the radical thrust of the Westminster Committee and refused an invitation to attend their meetings when in London. To counter their attempt to lead the Association movement he organised a conference of deputies to meet at the St Alban's Tavern from 11 to 20 March. Delegates from seventeen counties attended, and while Wyvill failed to keep the meeting free of politicians, it also contained many dedicated to parliamentary reform. Jebb was elected to represent Huntingdon (where he held some land inherited through Ann's family), and was joined by Cartwright (Nottingham), Brand Hollis (Westminster), Rev Dr Rycroft (Kent), Alderman Brass Crosby

---

[89] Horace Walpole to Horace Mann, 22 February 1780, Walpole, *Correspondence*, 25, p. 19.

[90] Horace Mann to Horace Walpole, 11 March 1780, Walpole, *Correspondence*, 25, p. 23.

[91] Christie, *Wilkes, Wyvill and Reform*, p. 83.

[92] *The Speech of the Hon. C.J. Fox delivered at Westminster on Feb. 2, 1780*; L. G. Mitchell, *Charles James Fox* (Oxford, 1992), p. 35.

[93] 'Life of Jebb', pp. 147-49; *The Remembrancer* 9 (1780), p. 148.

(London), and Lord Mahon (Kent).[94] George Savile noted that some ridiculed this meeting as a 'little Anti-Parliament'. Wyvill and Robert Bromley (Middlesex) were asked to draft a *Memorial and Report*, which declared the necessity of one hundred additional county MPs, annual elections, equal electoral areas, and tests for candidates.[95]

Rockingham was angry that parliamentary reform was being pursued, and Horace Walpole probably spoke for many in the elite when he declared that 'such innovations dictated by deputies of thirteen counties at a tavern in London, and announced in so wretched a manner and with so little argument, can but be a joke'.[96] In spite of Rockingham's disapproval, the Yorkshire Committee adopted the plan at the end of March, except that triennial parliaments were substituted for annual.[97] Rockingham was furious that the limited aims of the original petition had given way to 'ingenious speculative Propositions'.[98] As a result, only ten of the original twenty-six petitioning counties adopted the cause of parliamentary reform. With Lord North having weathered the storm in Parliament, by the end of April the county movement was clearly waning.

Nevertheless, during this period important institutions were established, and statements made by the London radicals. Since early February, twenty or so members had attended each weekly meeting of the Westminster Committee at the King's Arms Tavern. As chairman, Fox found himself awkwardly positioned between parliamentary allies like Richard Brinsley Sheridan, and extra-parliamentary radicals like Jebb and Brand Hollis. At the start of March Jebb told Fox that he would propose a 'select committee' to examine the state of representation and ascertain 'the number of Persons, which ought to be returned' by Westminster.[99] On the 15th a six-member sub-committee was appointed with Sheridan in the chair, but it was evidently Jebb and Brand Hollis who dominated the deliberations. Jebb wrote to his lawyer friend Granville Sharp requesting some books addressing the competing claims of 'Property' and 'Population'.[100]

---

[94] The Committees represented were Yorkshire, Essex, Dorset, Sussex, Middlesex, Gloucestershire, Hertfordshire, Surrey, Westminster, Huntingdonshire, Buckinghamshire, London, Nottingham, Kent, Newcastle, Gloucester, Devonshire and Cheshire. Black, *Association*, p. 51n.

[95] Wyvill, *Political Papers*, I, pp. 427-38.

[96] Horace Walpole to Rev William Mason, 22 March 1780, *Horace Walpole's Correspondence*, 25, p. 28.

[97] N.C. Phillips, 'Country against Court: Christopher Wyvill, a Yorkshire champion', *Yorkshire Archaeological Journal* 40 (1962), pp, 595-97. Black, *Association*, pp. 50-57; Lord Mahon told Wyvill that the Middlesex Committee was also against annual Parliaments, and that 'the question of annual Parliaments or of shortening the duration of Parliaments ought to be quite left out of sight at the present … if that question is started … the cause of the people is forever gone; because opposition will be knocked to pieces. If it is not started at all … our great and good friends will be quite satisfied'. [c. 20 March 1780], cited in Christie, *Wilkes, Wyvill and Reform*, p. 94.

[98] Rockingham to Croft, [mid-July? 1780], cited in Black, *Association*, p. 57.

[99] JJ to Granville Sharp, 2 March 1780, GRO Sharp papers.

[100] 'Supposing Property to be the Rule where shall I find in a small compass what I want? Supposing Population be the rule where must I apply for authority? If you could send me

On the 20th the sub-committee reported that 'all the reasons that had been given for long parliaments might be given for making them perpetual, which would be an absolute subversion of the third "estate"'. And, they argued, the current electoral distribution failed to accurately represent either persons or property (if the latter be measured in light of the tax burden). Restriction of the franchise to forty-shilling freeholders was an unconstitutional innovation made during the reign of Henry VI. In a telling review of the composition of the electorate, the sub-committee concluded: 'a number scarcely above six thousand, being the majority of voters of a hundred and twenty nine of the boroughs, return two hundred and fifty seven representatives, which is a majority of the whole English House of Commons, and the efficient representation of above five millions of People'.[101]

On 6 April (the day of Dunning's motion) the freeholders of Westminster met, and again Jebb rose after Fox and gave an 'animated speech' displaying a 'warmth of patriotic attachment'. He urged the electors to ensure that any future candidates promise to advocate annual Parliaments and equal electorates, and then moved that the Committee be instructed to campaign for the election of Fox.[102] With his hopes raised, Jebb told Sharp that 'if the livery of London were called upon to declare [support for annual parliaments] ... and upon the plain question put decided in their favour, the cause which Yorkshire &c hath given up might yet be saved'.[103]

The following week another Westminster sub-committee was officially appointed to examine the electoral system and to draw up specific reform proposals.[104] With Brand Hollis in the chair, Jebb's radical clique dominated the sub-committee. In late May it presented a *Report* on the British electoral system to support the 'Plan of Association' published by the Association conference. The *Report* provided a clear, concise and radical statement of the principles argued for by Hulme, Burgh, Price, Cartwright, Lofft and Sharp during the late 1770s. It declared that equal electorates, annual elections and universal manhood suffrage were both natural rights and the 'birthright of Englishmen'. They were 'enjoyed in the times of the immortal Alfred; they were cherished by the wisest princes of the Norman line; they form the grand palladium of our nation'; and they provide a 'triple cord of strength, which alone can be relied upon to hold, in times of tempest, the vessel of state'. The *Report* argued that Parliaments that extend beyond one session were vulnerable to 'aristocratic domination, and regal despotism', and (taking a swipe at the Rockingham Whigs) asserted that

---

a few books with references to the parts most likely to be useful'. JJ to Granville Sharp, 15 March 1780. On the 24th Jebb thanked Sharp for the loan of some books. GRO Sharp papers. The sub-committee was composed of Jebb, Brand Hollis, Sheridan, Vincent, Vardy and Crompton, BL Minutes of the Westminster Committee, 15 March 1780.

101 BL Minutes of the Westminster Committee, 20 March 1780. The figures were drawn from James Burgh, who had calculated that 5,723 borough votes could elect 254 out of a total of 558 members of the House of Commons. *Political Disquisitions,* I, pp. 36-62.

102 'Life of Jebb', p. 150.

103 JJ to Granville Sharp, 7 April 1780, GRO Sharp papers.

104 Again Jebb wrote to Sharp asking for 'any hints or authorities likely to assist in the accomplishing of such a Plan'. JJ to Sharp, 18 April 1780, GRO Sharp papers.

any undertaking by the Parliament to reform itself 'would only be calculated to deceive and amuse the nation to its final destruction'. Rather than introducing new legislation, reform was best carried out by removing the accumulated weight of legislation regulating elections, allowing the Constitution to 'recover its energies'. A sixteen-point plan was proposed which would allow for equal electorates in which all males ('aliens, minors, criminals and insane persons excepted') would vote in a secret ballot every July. Annual parliaments would sit from November to April, with disputed electoral contests decided in court before a jury. MPs would receive a salary, and any enfranchised person could stand for election with the exception of those holding an office of the crown.

Fox delayed publishing the *Report* for as long as possible until all other avenues were closed. Eventually it was published during the conservative backlash that followed the Gordon Riots in July. In the words of Eugene Black,

> in what might be called a 'fit of absence of mind', Fox presided over the formation of the British radical doctrine. Brand Hollis, Jebb and Cartwright ... produced many articles of which Fox could never have approved; but he was too committed to retreat. The *Plan*, often reprinted, outlined the principles of radical agitation. Nothing in the program of the corresponding societies of the French Revolution, the doctrine of the Cobbett and Hunt radicals, or the Chartist points is not adumbrated in the *Plan* and sanctioned by analysis in the *Report*.[105]

Under no illusion as to the limited support for their proposals, the radical core of the Westminster sub-committee proceeded to form the Society for Constitutional Information (SCI).[106] While Jebb had read John Cartwright's tracts calling for parliamentary reform in the 1770s, there is no record of any contact between them prior to the rise of the Association movement in 1780. United in political agitation, the two became firm and close friends. Cartwright described Jebb as the 'friend of my bosom and pattern of my conduct', and his religious writings echo Jebb's Unitarianism.[107] For his part, Jebb acknowledged that 'the incomparable publications of Major Cartwright' had led him to support universal manhood suffrage.[108] While Cartwright was considered the 'father of the Society'[109] (having first suggested the idea to friends in 1778), it was sustained through the early 1780s by Jebb's tireless attendance and frequent chairmanship.[110] Among the founding members were some of Jebb's associates:

---

[105] Black, *Association*, p. 60; see also Cone, *The English Jacobins*, p. 51.

[106] For the most substantial treatment of the SCI see Black, *Association*, pp. 174-212.

[107] *Life of Cartwright*, I, p. 165; John Cartwright, *Internal Evidence: or, an inquiry how far truth and the Christian religion have been consulted by the author of 'Thoughts on Parliamentary Reform'* (1784); David Drinkwater-Lunn, 'John Cartwright, Political Education, and English Radicalism, 1774-94' (Oxford DPhil., 1970), p. 316.

[108] *A Letter to Sir Robert Bernard, Chairman of the Huntingdonshire Committee* (1781), Jebb II, p. 509.

[109] See the toasts at the 'General Audit' meeting of the Society for Constitutional Information 12 December 1780. PRO SCI Minutes I:43.

[110] *Life of Cartwright*, I, p. 120.

Thomas Brand Hollis, Capel Lofft, Thomas Day and John Churchill (the apothecary brother of the poet and veteran Wilkite, who attended the early meetings of the Westminster Committee with Jebb).[111]

Both the *Address to Middlesex* and the Westminster *Report* stressed the need for political education. Jebb wanted to see 'our fellow-citizens, of the lower classes' instructed in the true meaning of constitutional terms such as majesty, sovereign, republic, loyalty, allegiance, rebellion, prerogative and so on. The 'natural good sense, and spirit of the nation' would only be exerted, he argued, 'when the understandings, and affections, of all orders of men, are emancipated from the influence of false ideas, which ignorance, or the art of designing politicians, have annexed to these expressions'.[112] The Society began its work by publishing an *Address to the People*, which declared that 'LAW TO BIND ALL, MUST BE ASSENTED TO BY ALL'. It vowed to print pamphlets detailing the nature of the Constitution, how it had been corrupted, and how it could be reformed. The Society vowed to 'diffuse this knowledge universally throughout the realm, to circulate it through every village and hamlet, and even into the humble dwelling of the cottager'.[113]

In the long term they achieved some success. In the last months of 1791 Thomas Hardy spent his leisure hours reading over numerous short tracts published gratis by the SCI. Reading works by 'those *really* great men' such as Granville Sharp, Jebb, Cartwright and Price, Hardy became convinced that 'it was very evident that a *radical reform in parliament* was quite necessary', and he set about establishing the London Corresponding Society (LCS).[114] Involvement in politics could be a life transforming experience for members of the 'lower orders'. For the first five nights after establishing the LCS Hardy and his friends spent their time discussing whether they as 'treadesmen (sic), shopkeepers and mechanics' had any right to agitate for parliamentary reform.[115] Initially the educational efforts of the SCI were greatly restricted by the concentration of its members in London and the Home Counties, and a reasonable distribution of publications was achieved only in the 1790s.[116]

---

[111] In the early meetings Jebb and Churchill's names appear adjacent on the lists. Also, it appears that Richard Jebb may have paid for the education of Charles Churchill's son following the early death of his father. The other founder members of the SCI were Richard Brinsley Sheridan and John Frost of the Westminster Committee; the Middlesex clergyman Edward Bromley who helped Wyvill draw up the 'Plan' adopted by the first Association convention; Richard Brocklesby, a well-known doctor and friend of Edmund Burke; while Edward Brigden, James Trecothick, John Vardy and Frederick Vincent complete the list of founder members. PRO Minutes of the SCI.

[112] *Address to Middlesex*, Jebb II, p. 470n; *Report of the Westminster Committee*, Jebb III, pp. 404-05.

[113] [John Cartwright], *An Address to the Public from the Society for Constitutional Information* (April, 1780), pp. 1-2.

[114] Cited in Mary Thale ed., *Selections from the Papers of the London Corresponding Society 1792-99* (Cambridge, 1983), p. 5.

[115] Cited in Mark Philp, 'The Fragmented Ideology of Reform', in Philp ed., *The French Revolution and British Popular Politics* (Cambridge, 1991), p. 73.

[116] Black, *Association*, p. 182.

Nevertheless, owing in no small part to Jebb's efforts, from 1780 on the SCI provided a base and public face for London radicalism.

9

Political Thought

Jebb's failure to produce a significant work of political philosophy could be due to a lack of intellectual ability, time, desire or a combination of all three. It is hard to imagine that Jebb would have been incapable of writing a substantial political tract. While he may not have produced something in the order of Priestley's *Essay on the First Principles of Government* (1768) or Price's *Observations on the Nature of Civil Liberty* (1776), a vindication of the ancient constitution along the lines of Cartwright's *Take Your Choice!* (1776) or Granville Sharp's laborious *A Declaration of the Peoples Natural Right to a Share in the Legislature* (1774) could have issued from Jebb's pen. The fact that it did not would appear to be owing to a lack of time and desire. Up until 1775 Jebb's energies were absorbed by scholarly pursuits and reform activities at Cambridge, and then at the age of forty he retrained for a medical career, which clearly absorbed a great deal of time. In the summer of 1773 Jebb began to prepare a course of constitutional lectures, but perhaps owing to his increasingly marginal position at Cambridge, nothing came of this venture. In addition to the constraints of time, perhaps Jebb thought that there was no need to add another tract to a list of political works issuing from such capable writers as Price, Priestley and Cartwright. 'Political truth' needed implementation rather than further articulation.

As noted in chapter 3, Jebb was a hard-line empiricist committed to the need for all individuals to exercise their private judgement. He was primarily concerned with ensuring that others had access to 'the facts', whether in relation to science, religion, medicine or politics. Thus it is not surprising that Jebb was instrumental in seeing the SCI commission a study of the British electoral system. In June 1783 he drafted a circular letter to all of the SCI's correspondents requesting detailed information regarding the state of electoral representation. Jebb did what he could to promote the project in the years leading up to his death, and in 1792 his friend Thomas Oldfield published *A*

History of the Boroughs, which was reprinted as *The Representative History of Great Britain and Ireland*. This was the first of several research publications that nineteenth-century reformers used to support their cause.[1] Jebb seems to have thought his energies best spent as an organiser and agitator, promoting the dissemination of 'political truth' through the Association movement and the SCI. As a result, any attempt to delineate the contours of Jebb's political philosophy must necessarily rest upon a sifting of his various polemical tracts and letters, and his private notes and correspondence.

THE HISTORIOGRAPHY OF RADICALISM

It was traditionally assumed that eighteenth-century Anglo-American radicals lifted their politics from John Locke's *Two Treatises of Government* and were representatives of a burgeoning middle class.[2] This interpretation of radicalism has been restated by Isaac Kramnick, who argues that after 1760 English radicals were 'more likely to frame their arguments in terms of natural rights than of historical rights and much more likely to invoke Lockean than republican themes. They were less concerned with nostalgic country themes than with modern middle-class socio-economic grievances'. According to Kramnick this was the last stage in the historical evolution of a 'liberal vision' being shaped by Protestantism and capitalism since the sixteenth century.[3]

In contrast, since the 1960s a number of historians have argued that opposition to the British state was fundamentally conservative and couched in the backward-looking language of classical republicanism and the ancient constitution. According to John Pocock, following the financial revolution of the 1690s the Court Whigs developed a conservative ideology which included the 'monied interest' in a broad definition of 'property', and promoted the cultivation of deference, polite manners and a negative conception of liberty. With Daniel Defoe as their first spokesman, followed by the political economists of the Scottish Enlightenment, Pocock argues that until the French Revolution, appeals to commercial individualism were always made by representatives of established authority. This establishment ideology was criticised, and, he argues, *could only be criticised* by a republican civic humanism that identified virtue with active participatory citizenship. With commerce harnessed to the state-building program of the Court Whigs, the English political class became divided over a perceived dichotomy between commerce and virtue.[4]

In recent decades historians have tended to favour the republican interpretation of radicalism. John Derry has written that the thinking of radicals like Jebb 'was still linked with the old legends of Anglo-Saxon freedom, and despite their programme their modes of thought were drenched with the rhetoric

---

1 Black, *Association*, p. 204.

2 Carl Becker, *The Declaration of Independence: a study in the history of political ideas* (New York, 1942 [1922]), esp. pp. 24-79.

3 Kramnick, *Republicanism and Bourgeois Radicalism*, pp. 4-5.

4 See in particular Pocock, '*The Machiavellian Moment* Revisited'; and *Virtue, Commerce and History*.

which had descanted on the decline of the country's institutions since the beginning of the century'.[5] In her study of James Burgh, Clara Hay wrote of 'the fundamentally conservative aspiration of English radicals ... to restore some mythic yesteryears when virtue flourished and an harmonious equilibrium governed men's social and political relationships'.[6]

While an appreciation of the centrality of republicanism is essential to any understanding of eighteenth-century political dissent, it needs to be appreciated that there were many varieties of 'republicanism'. As John Adams, the American revolutionary, observed: 'There is not a more unintelligible word in the English language than republicanism', adding that 'the word republican is so loose and indefinite that successive predominant factions will put glosses and constructions on it as different as light and darkness'.[7] Particular versions of republicanism, such as that espoused by Jebb, were shaped by the influence of other ideas, values and experiences.

We should not draw a sharp line of distinction between republicanism and liberalism in the eighteenth century. John Locke, the fountainhead of liberal political theory was, after all, a Commonwealthman himself. Joyce Appleby has pointed to a developing conception of the rational, autonomous and free individual in discussions of market economics in the late seventeenth century. While there was a 'lacuna in the development of liberal theory' in the early eighteenth century, she argues, liberalism evolved alongside republicanism in opposition to the growing power of the British state. 'However much court and country disputants monopolised conventional political discourse', she writes,

> fragments of the liberal paradigm found lodging in other inquiries. The idea of a uniform human nature and the assumption that human beings have a natural tendency to think rationally about their self-interest spread, as did the larger conviction that social relations were susceptible to analysis as systems of behaviour. It is of no small importance that John Locke contributed significantly to these developments.[8]

Jebb lends support to Appleby's view. While his writings reflect republican assumptions and ideals, at base his political philosophy was liberal.

In recent years historians have become increasingly sensitive to the intellectual nuances of radicalism. H.T. Dickinson has observed that while the ancient constitution and Locke's contract theory of government 'are inherently contradictory ... this did not prevent the Whigs from appealing to both theories

---

[5] Derry, *English Politics and the American Revolution*, p. 189.

[6] Hay, *James Burgh*, pp. 104-05.

[7] Cited in Joseph J. Ellis, *Passionate Sage: the character and legacy of John Adams* (New York, 2001), p. 74.

[8] Appleby, *Liberalism and Republicanism*, p. 138; see also Albert O. Hirschman, *The Passions and the Interests: political arguments for capitalism before its triumph* (Princeton, 1977).

when it suited them'.[9] Historical arguments were favoured, but appeals to natural rights and the championing of middle-class values became more common after 1760. Iain Hampsher-Monk has rightly observed that 'an important feature of the period is radicals' attempts to accommodate their inherited patterns of thought to the new and irresistible features of society and to the aspirations of growing urban middle and lower orders'. In the process, discourses were variously mixed and matched, with a happy correspondence between natural rights, ancient English liberties, utility and providence often asserted without elaboration.[10] In doing so, figures such as Jebb constructed and championed radical interpretations of the 'English Constitution' in the light of which 'corruption' could be criticised and reform advocated.

In his criticism of the political system Jebb drew upon the Commonwealth tradition, but the influence of a version of Enlightenment rationalism and individualism is evident in his advocacy of universal male suffrage. Throughout the century opponents of government demanded a reduction in the number of placemen in the House of Commons, more frequent elections, and electoral reform. The first two were by far the most common demands in the decades prior to the reign of George III, while electoral reform gained considerable support in the second half of the century. In what follows I will first show how Jebb engaged in the traditional critique of constitutional corruption, and then explore the way his religious and philosophical disposition informed a commitment to universal manhood suffrage.

HISTORY AND ENGLISH LIBERTY

The Revolution of 1688 was instituted to remove a Catholic king of absolutist and Francophile tendencies, and in doing so it helped advance the theory and practice of parliamentary sovereignty. As consensus regarding the central role of the Parliament gradually developed during the eighteenth century, debate arose as to how 'the people' should be represented. Tension between evolving notions of popular sovereignty and the reality of aristocratic oligarchy led to vigorous debate in the eighteenth century over the relationship between civil and political liberty.

People of all political hues in eighteenth-century England tended to agree upon the existence and importance of basic civil liberties such as the right to equal justice, security of property and freedom of conscience. But there was disagreement over how much political liberty was either consistent with or necessary for the preservation of these civil liberties.[11] Conservatives argued that

[9] Dickinson, *Liberty and Property*, p. 61. Eckhart Hellmuth has warned that 'contemporary political discourse was not always sophisticated and logically consistent'. Eckhart Hellmuth, 'The Liberty of the Press in England', in Hellmuth, *Transformation of Political Culture*, p. 471.

[10] Iain Hampsher-Monk, 'British Radicalism and the Anti-Jacobins', unpublished paper, forthcoming in *The Cambridge History of Political Thought: the Enlightenment and Revolution*, p. 1.

[11] Dickinson, *Politics of the People*, pp. 161-89.

these civil liberties (and in particular the rights of property) were best protected by ensuring that the aristocracy dominated politics. Such men, it was argued, had the independence, assets and leisure necessary to make policy for the common good. They claimed that the threat of despotism had been laid to rest forever by the Revolution, which had settled the division of authority between the executive and legislature. Most politically active Englishmen agreed with the privileges accorded to property (especially in the first half of the century). Yet they were sharply divided over whether or not the House of Commons was fulfilling its proper constitutional function and that the danger of tyranny had passed.

In the absence of disciplined modern political parties, eighteenth-century governments had to work hard at securing support in the Parliament. The House of Lords, with its large number of office-holders and contingent of bishops, was more likely to support the Crown. In the House of Commons, the Septennial Act ensured that administrations would only, in theory, have to face the electorate every seven years, and the disposal of patronage was used to help obtain a working majority for the government. The prime example of this was Sir Robert Walpole, who built a long career as Prime Minister upon his skilled management of personalities, patronage, and policy. This led opponents to claim that English liberties were under threat because the Crown was effectively preventing the Commons from acting as an independent check upon government. Country and Real Whig critics drew upon Revolution principles, civic humanism and the ancient constitution in demanding moral and institutional 'reformation' to ensure the independence of the House of Commons.

Jebb and his friends were supporters of the Commonwealth tradition that can be traced back to the seventeenth-century opponents of absolute monarchy.[12] Jebb began his second political pamphlet with Algernon Sidney's declaration that 'A general presumption that kings (or ministers) will govern well is not a sufficient security to the people'.[13] John Disney proudly displayed his political stance by naming his son Algernon; Capel Lofft wrote a glowing review of Catherine Macaulay's republican *History of England*;[14] and Brand Hollis presented Abigail Adams on 'the 5th of November, the day of deliverance from Popery and Tyranny' with a set of 'three Commonwealth coins to record what England once was'.[15] During the constitutional crisis of early 1784, Ann Jebb wrote that 'I am determined if possible never to despair of the Commonwealth';[16] and in her defence of the French Revolution she declared that 'you scarce ever heard of a nation rising against its chief magistrate, till

[12] On this tradition see Robbins, *The Eighteenth-Century Commonwealthman.*
[13] *Letter to Sir Robert Bernard* (1781), Jebb II, p. 491.
[14] Capel Lofft, *Observations on Mrs Macaulay's History of England; ... from the Revolution to the resignation of Sir Robert Walpole, in a letter addressed to that lady* (1778).
[15] Thomas Brand Hollis to Mrs Abigail Adams, 4 November 1786, MHS Adams papers.
[16] AJ to John Cartwright, 22 January 1784, *Memoir of Ann Jebb*, p. 19.

resistance was become almost a virtue.'[17] John Jebb encouraged his students to study 'government, more especially as it was treated in the works of Sydney, Locke and other writers who have placed its origin on a popular basis'.[18] James Burgh listed the authors he consulted in writing his *Political Disquisitions* as 'Sidney, Locke, Harrington, Gordon, Trenchard, Bolingbroke, St Pierre, Hume, Montesquieu, Blackstone, Montague, Rymer'.[19]

Because Jebb did not write a systematic work of political philosophy, it is hard to gauge his exact sources, but they cannot have differed much from Burgh's list, and he has left direct references to Sidney, Locke, Trenchard and Montesquieu. Jebb was determined that England's brush with absolute monarchy should not be forgotten. For him the worth of a monarch was measured according to how well he or she respected the 'voice of the people'. Henry VIII was 'that tyrant',[20] and the Stuart kings provided ample evidence of absolutist tendencies. 'In the time of James the first', he reminded his fellow countrymen, 'benevolences were requested in all that soft and silken language, which kings and their ministers can at times employ. In a subsequent period they assumed a sterner form.'[21]

Commonwealthmen were deeply suspicious of anyone who wielded political power, and (as noted in chapter 2) this suspicion was provoked by George III's conduct in the 1760s. Jebb espoused the widespread Whig belief that under the new king the reins of power had fallen into the hands of a closet of Tory royal advisers. He persisted in this belief, and when the Shelbourne ministry was toying with the idea of reintroducing ship money Jebb (under the pseudonym 'Hampden') exclaimed: 'Away with those shades that veil the real substance! Lord B -- [Bute?] and Lord M-- [Mansfield?] still sway the counsels of the cabinet'.[22] In 1785 he was still complaining about the threat to reform from 'that most odious of all Parties – the Party of the king's friends'.[23] In private correspondence he criticised the King himself. Following the resignation of Lord North's ministry Jebb asked an Irish friend the rhetorical question: 'though a North and a Sandwich no longer surround the Throne, do different passions prevail in the possessor of the crown?'[24] This fear of an authoritarian executive lay behind all the various parliamentary reform measures proposed throughout the century.

In tandem with the corruption of Parliament the seventeenth-century experience led patriots to fear the growth of a standing army. A well-regulated citizen militia was held up as the alternative. Jebb cited Fortescue, Bracton and Queen Elizabeth to support his argument that all Englishmen were obliged to

---

[17] AJ, *Two Penny-worth of Truth* (20 December 1792), p. 12.
[18] DWL 'Memoir of Disney', p. 9.
[19] Burgh, *Political Disquisitions*, I, p. vii.
[20] Jebb III, p. 294.
[21] 'Mentor' [JJ], 16 September 1782, Jebb III, pp. 352-53.
[22] 'Hampden' [JJ], 'To the Inhabitants of London and Westminster', 10 August 1782, Jebb III, p. 314; Jebb referred to the power of 'the closet'. Jebb III, p. 338.
[23] JJ to John Forbes, 18 May 1785, NLI Bourke collection.
[24] JJ to Frances Dobbs, 25 January 1782, NLI Dobbs papers.

bear arms.[25] It appears that Jebb himself kept a musket and powder at the ready, as he congratulated the SCI for being attentive to the obligation 'incumbent upon the members of every well regulated state, to be skilled in the use of arms', and praised William Jones (the lawyer and orientalist) for stressing the constitutional obligation to bear arms.[26] Jones declared that the English would 'never be a people, in the majestic sense of the word' until a 200,000-strong volunteer militia could be called into the field within twenty-four hours.[27]

In 1785 the SCI and Jebb were urging the public to resist the establishment of a police force.[28] Jebb was suspicious of naming regiments after counties, thinking it an attempt to make the existence of a standing army more palatable.[29] Rather than pay ship money, Jebb suggested that the men of Suffolk follow the Irish example and spend their money on guns and training as a volunteer militia, while reducing the size of the army could raise additional funds for the navy.[30] With all this emphasis upon a citizen militia, it is not surprising that military metaphors recur throughout Jebb's writings. When the fortunes of the reform movement were at low ebb, he wrote that 'the troops' were becoming dispirited; William Meredith was the parliamentary 'general' of the clerical petitioners; and Jesus was the 'captain of our salvation'.

The central tenet of civic humanism was that the preservation of liberty was as much dependent upon the existence of a virtuous and vigilant citizenry as it was upon institutional arrangements. As noted in chapter 2, many saw the corruption of politics as a reflection of a wider moral degeneration caused by the spread of luxury, particularly among the elite. This led to calls for a 'moral reformation' of both the elite and the wider nation. The independence of the House of Commons, it was argued, could not be secured unless there was a widespread revival of a sense of virtue and patriotism that would see both electors and elected transcend self-interest. It was in light of this that the existence of a voluntary militia was accorded great importance. Jebb declared that 'the constitutional strength of England exists in the voluntary exertions of the virtue of its free-born sons, armed with their elective franchises, to guard

---

[25] 'Hampden' [JJ], 23 August 1782, Jebb III, p. 331.

[26] *Letter to the Secretary of the SCI* (1784), Jebb III, p. 363; William Jones, *An Inquiry into the Legal Mode of Suppressing Riots* (1781), and *The Principles of Government in a Dialogue between a Scholar and a Peasant* (1782).

[27] William Jones to John Cartwright, 23 May 1782, *The Letters of Sir William Jones* (Garland Cannon ed., Oxford, 1970), p. 547.

[28] 'Trebatius' [JJ], 12 July 1785; 'Trebatius' [JJ], 2 August 1785, Jebb III, pp. 383-84, 388.

[29] 'A standing army ought to be an object of perpetual jealousy to the English people'. 'Mentor' [JJ], Jebb III, p. 351. Attaching army regiments to various counties, and thus linking them to 'the free constitution of England', was an idea 'full of danger to everything Britons should hold dear', Jebb III, p. 360.

[30] 'Alfred' [JJ], 9 August 1782, Jebb III, pp. 308-11; 'Alfred' [JJ], 26 August 1782, Jebb III, pp. 336-37. For an assessment of Sandwich's very capable administration of the navy see Rogers, *The Insatiable Earl.*

against internal enemies; and adorned with the habiliments of war, for the purpose of resistance against external foes'.[31]

Radicals drew upon the defenders of republican Rome whose texts championed virtue, independence and participatory citizenship. Jebb's writings are peppered with the language of classical republicanism. He would address his 'fellow-citizens', and Granville Sharp was that 'very excellent citizen'.[32] While English citizens could not play a direct role in their political assembly as in classical times, Jebb repeatedly urged that greater popular participation in politics would see a rekindling of 'public spirit ... in the glowing heart of every English citizen: "patriae decus et tutamen" should appear resplendent upon his martial brow'.[33]

There was near universal disapproval of 'party' or 'faction' in British politics. Most wanted a patriotic king and ministers who would govern in the interests of the whole nation. Patriotism developed as a means of legitimating opposition to government under the first two Hanoverians. As Quentin Skinner has expressed it, the eloquent Tory Lord Bolingbroke stole some of the Whig ideological armour (fear of crown influence and a standing army) and reinforced it with the cloak of patriotism.[34] Politicians like Pitt and Bolingbroke claimed to be patriots defending the interests of the country against a corrupt government. Such claims to virtuous independence were often undermined by a willingness to take office and act according to their true nature as career politicians. The astonishing successes of the Seven Years War and his continuing appeals to popular support ensured that many patriots revered William Pitt, despite his obvious flaws and failings. Yet as Derek Jarrett has observed, during the 1740s and 1750s many discerned that 'a Patriot rewarded was a Patriot destroyed'.[35]

With the evident failure of moral reform to produce a revolution in the conduct of politicians, calls for institutional reform became more vocal. All proposals for parliamentary reform were designed as means to attain the end of forcing MPs to conduct themselves in a patriotic manner. In this spirit Jebb declared (echoing Algernon Sidney) that 'the happiness of Englishmen ought not to depend upon the precarious virtue of the minister of state'.[36] This cynicism was only increased by the political gymnastics that accompanied the various political crises of George III's reign. The radicals repeated Cato's complaint that 'Caesar has friends, and Pompey has friends; but none are friends of Rome' during the political instability that followed the death of Rockingham in 1782.[37] The lesson they drew was that the people must not place their faith in

---

[31] 'Mentor' [JJ], 16 September 1782, Jebb III, p. 355.

[32] Jebb III, p. 388; *Address to the Freeholders of Middlesex*, Jebb II, p. 462n.

[33] *Address to the Freeholders of Middlesex*, Jebb II, p. 476; 'Letter to the Secretary of the SCI' (1784), Jebb III, p. 363.

[34] Quentin Skinner, 'The Principles and Practice of Opposition: the case of Bolingbroke versus Walpole', in Neil McKendrick ed., *Historical Perspectives* (1974), pp. 93-128.

[35] Derek Jarrett, 'The Myth of "Patriotism" in Eighteenth-Century English Politics', *Britain and the Netherlands* 5 (1975), p. 127.

[36] *Address to the Freeholders of Middlesex*, Jebb II, p. 460.

[37] John Cartwright, *Give Us Our Rights!* (1782), p. 1; AJ to John Cartwright, 21 December 1783, *Memoir of Ann Jebb*, p. 17.

politicians, but rather act themselves to make the House of Common more accountable. The shift in radical politics is evident in the career of James Burgh. In the 1740s he espoused Bolingbroke's utopian vision of a country ruled by a patriot king. Yet, like many other Real Whigs, when the ideal of patriotic leadership failed, Burgh's attachment to Locke's political principles led him advocate popular control of government.[38]

Jebb's concern to ensure the independence of public officials is evident in his correspondence with the American John Adams on the issue of providing salaries for politicians. The Westminster Committee had proposed the payment of elected representatives. This reflected John Cartwright's view that MPs should receive 'no higher emolument at most than reasonable wages'.[39] But Jebb clearly had reservations. In a personal discussion with Adams he had expressed approval of the 36th Article of the Pennsylvania constitution. It declared that:

> As every freeman to preserve his independence (if without sufficient estate), ought to have some profession, calling, trade or farm ... there can be no necessity for, nor use in establishing offices of profit ... but if any man is called into public service, to the prejudice of his private affairs, he has a right to a reasonable compensation. And whenever an office ... becomes so profitable as to occasion many to apply for it, the profits ought to be lessened by the Legislature.[40]

Adams objected that the phrase 'offices of Profit' was ambiguous, and that the article was contradictory. On the one hand it seemed to be saying that 'all who serve the Public should have no Pay'. He thought this was inspired by 'vulgar Avarice', and argued that as 'Public offices in general require the whole time and all the attention of those who hold them ... they must then starve with their Families unless they have ample fortunes'. Without salaries for public service, Adams argued, 'the Poor and Middling ranks would be excluded and an Aristocratical Despotism would follow'. On the other hand, the article allowed for the granting of 'reasonable compensation', which left the system open to corruption because it would encourage politicians through 'the Hypocritical Pretence of Disinterestedness' to 'excite Enthusiasm among the People' for granting them rewards. Adams was in favour of establishing reasonable and regulated salaries. 'Mankind will never be happy', he wrote, 'nor their Liberties secure until the People shall lay it down as a fundamental Rule to make the support and reward of Public offices a matter of justice and not gratitude.'[41] Adams suggested that the 'dangerous enthusiasm' for George Washington had been stimulated by his serving without pay, whereas he should have been paid for his services like the other generals – 'the People should have too high a sense of their own Dignity even to suffer any Man to serve them for nothing'. As an illustration of the dangers involved, he suggested that Lord Chatham was a 'striking example' of a politician who had 'preserved the character of

---

[38] Hay, 'Making of a Radical', p. 96.
[39] Cartwright, *Internal Evidence* (1784), p. 25.
[40] *The Constitution of Pennsylvania*, 28 September 1776, Article 36.
[41] John Adams to JJ, 21 August 1785, MHS Adams papers.

disinterestedness but imperfectly'. All this led Adams to 'think that it has been the People themselves who have always created their own Despots'.[42]

Jebb replied that the Pennsylvania article was not contradictory, but seemed to be saying that where an individual could perform his public duties without 'any considerable detriment to his private fortune, or injury to his family, no recompense is due'. His position was close to that of the Pennsylvanian Benjamin Franklin, who in expounding the virtues of the 36th article to a friend of Jebb's declared: 'Persons will play at chess by the hour without being paid for it.... Deciding causes is in fact only a matter of amusement to sensible men'.[43] Jebb took issue with Adams's claim that public offices *in general* consume all the time and attention of those who hold them. Positions such as Justices of the Peace, the lower magistracy, and officers in the militia required no prior training and could be fulfilled in addition to the citizen's usual employment. He conceded that the 'Governor' should be granted a 'very honourable allowance ... during his continuance in office'. For a member of the 'House of Assembly', he thought that 'Independency of fortune is ... certainly a proper requisition, yet I agree it ought not to be required by law'. But he was confident that 'Free Citizens will naturally elect independent characters to represent them'. Jebb considered the 'nature of the office, and mode of appointment' to be important factors and he had no objection to 'reasonable emoluments' being attached to 'such offices as are necessary in a well constituted state'. These would include the judiciary, bureaucracy and armed forces, but the pay should not be so great as to draw too many men away from the agriculture and commerce that provide the nation's wealth.[44]

Adams suggested that Jebb's view was close to David Hume's ideal political system composed of a salaried administration and unpaid magistrates and elected representatives. But Adams continued to insist that in addition to the executive all members of the legislature and the magistracy should be provided with a salary in proportion to their duties, as 'one of the best securities to Liberty and Equality'.[45] To some extent, no doubt, this difference of opinion reflects the fact that one man was a practicing doctor who devoted his spare time to political agitation, while the other was fully employed as an appointed representative of a new nation. Yet it also reveals how committed Jebb was to seeing the British state governed by virtuous and independent citizens. He hoped to awaken his fellow Englishmen to a realisation that, while it was an obligation imposed 'by the Law of Nature' that a man 'pursue the means of acquiring an independent income, yet it is also every freeman's duty to bear his portion of the Public burdens, and in either just rotation, or according to other prescribed rules to perform those services which the welfare of the state requires'.[46]

Jebb was intensely proud of his heritage. At times he signed his public letters 'An Englishman', and a desire to encourage patriotism pervades his

---

[42] John Adams to JJ, 10 September 1785, MHS Adams papers.
[43] Baynes, 'Journal', 27 August 1783, in Romilly, *Life*, p. 447.
[44] JJ to John Adams, 13 September 1785, MHS Adams papers.
[45] John Adams to JJ, 25 September 1785, MHS Adams papers.
[46] JJ to John Adams, 13 September 1785, MHS Adams papers.

writings.[47] Yet the interest in reform displayed by 'the people' waxed and waned. At times during the fluctuating fortunes of the Association movement, Jebb lamented a general 'languor of patriotism'. He attributed this to a cynicism fostered by the duplicitous and Machiavellian conduct of the leading politicians. The only remedy, he believed, was education and exposure to 'political truth'. Jebb clung to the belief that deep down the English were naturally committed to liberty as a result of their history and geography.

It would seem that this faith was encouraged by his participation in popular political meetings and celebrations. Sharing the platform with the eloquent and inspiring Charles James Fox at public meetings in Westminster must have been an exhilarating experience. Jebb displayed a 'warmth of patriotic attachment' in a speech in Westminster on 6 April 1780.[48] A year after the Gordon Riots he defended the 'general disposition' of 'my fellow-citizens' by reminding his readers of the public response to the trial of Admiral Keppel. When the government prosecution failed and a jury acquitted Keppel, Jebb reminisced that every 'English breast' was filled with 'sentiments of more than Roman virtue'. If the English people could respond so warmly to the 'injured virtue' of an individual, Jebb argued, it could be hoped that the nation would soon rise to defend itself against a corrupt government.[49] He continually tried to talk-up the 'naturally open and honest spirit of the English people'.[50]

Jebb's patriotism led him to join contemporaries such as John Brown and James Burgh in expressing concern that widespread indulgence in vice and dissipation was eating away at English patriotism. It was to counter this that he pursued religious and educational reform, as he believed that institutional and moral reform were co-dependent. This was one of the ways Jebb's religious concerns had a direct connection with his politics – political and moral reform must go hand-in-hand. Thus, he noted that 'I am more and more persuaded that the evils of government and the want of felicity among the governed, as well as a deficiency in true patriotism, arise from the want of a moral and religious principle'. His answer was to 'push on the combined causes of a diffusion and right arrangement of political power, and a philological knowledge of the scriptures'.[51]

Radicals appealed to the myth of an ancient Anglo-Saxon constitution in which electorates had supposedly been more equal, elections more frequent and, consequently, the House of Commons more independent. Jebb told the freeholders of Middlesex that every citizen was authorised and encouraged by 'the genius of English liberty' to freely 'examine the defects of the constitution, the errors of government ... and as freely to censure'. 'I wish to see', Jebb

---

[47] *Letter to Sir William Meredith*, Jebb I, pp. 225-262. There is a strident letter in support of the Feathers Tavern petition signed 'An Englishman', *General Evening Post*, June 30, 1772. Authorship is attributed to Jebb in John Disney's collection of newspaper cuttings in DWL.

[48] 'Life of Jebb', p. 150.

[49] *Letter to Robert Bernard*, Jebb II, pp. 515-16n.

[50] 'Hampden' [JJ], 2 September 1782, Jebb III, p. 345.

[51] 'Life of Jebb', p. 189.

wrote, 'the ancient spirit of my countrymen revive; I wish to see them a nation of politicians'. Through the means of a national association he urged them to reconstitute the 'Common's House of Parliament, in exact conformity to the primeval principles of the constitution of this country'.[52] Jebb's commitment to the ancient constitution is demonstrated by his undertaking the study of Anglo-Saxon law and history in his last year of life.

The notion of an ancient constitution had a long history, and had been appealed to frequently in the seventeenth century.[53] The eighteenth-century conception of the ancient constitution reflected contemporary concerns regarding corruption of the House of Commons. Jebb argued that annual elections and a wide franchise had been ancient practice and if re-established would lead to removal of the Crown's ability to buy support. He pointed to the Septennial Act as the root cause of the 'numerous and substantial evils' such as the American conflict.[54] With an independent House of Commons functioning according to the 'primeval principles' of the constitution,

> it would never be in the power of an abandoned administration, with its dependent tribes of placemen, pensioners and contractors, to riot unrestrained in the public plunder; sacrificing, with unbounding prodigality, at the shrine of despotism, the resources of the present generation, and the just inheritance of millions yet unborn; while discontent, distress, and disgrace prevail, in every part of this once glorious, happy and extensive Empire.

A reformed House of Commons would protect the public from 'the treachery and insults OF ITS OWN SERVANTS'.[55] It was in this spirit that Jebb rejected Burke's argument that the MP is elected to exercise his independent judgement in parliamentary votes, and to act as a representative for the interests of the entire nation.[56] Jebb argued that the MP is a proxy for his district and 'should consider himself as the organ of their will, in every instance where that will is positively declared'. If an MP wished to vote contrary to the wishes of his constituents, then he should resign.[57] Annual elections, it was argued, were the only way to ensure that MP's obeyed the dictates of their constituents.

In an age that revered the past, Jebb, Cartwright and other reformers sincerely argued that they were restorers rather than innovators. 'If the people call for a reform in the commons house of parliament', Jebb wrote, 'the cry of innovation is violent and immediate, although it is evidently the intention of the

---

52 *Address to the Freeholders of Middlesex*, Jebb II, pp. 464-5, 486.

53 J.G.A. Pocock, *The Ancient Constitution and the Feudal Law: a study in English historical thought in the seventeenth century* (Cambridge, 1957); Christopher Hill, 'The Norman Yoke'.

54 Jebb III, p. 385.

55 *Address to the Freeholders of Middlesex*, Jebb II, p. 487n.

56 Sutherland, 'Edmund Burke and the Relations between Members of Parliament and their Constituents', pp. 105-21.

57 *Address to the Freeholders of Middlesex*, Jebb II, p. 462n.

friends of that necessary measure not to innovate, but restore'.[58] Jebb wanted to restore what he *imagined* the English constitution to have been, and as such he acted as an 'historical folklorist'.[59] As James Vernon has written, it is impossible to determine precisely when the constitution replaced the monarch 'as the sacred centre of English political culture'.[60] But that process was underway in the late eighteenth century, and it was contributed to in a significant way by Jebb and the Society for Constitutional Information, who promoted a radical interpretation of the 'English Constitution'.

UNIVERSAL MANHOOD SUFFRAGE AS A NATURAL RIGHT

As Paul Langford has observed, 'the respect which attended property was a striking feature of the mental landscape of the eighteenth century'. When Thomas Burnet described the apocalyptic destruction that would precede the establishment of paradise on earth, he took time to assure his audience that this would not necessarily involve any change in the existing distribution of property.[61] Supporters of the eighteenth-century constitution claimed that it conformed to reason and natural rights, striking a balance between individual liberty and the rights of property. The common law, it was argued, protected the rights of individual liberty and security, while the political system was designed to afford due influence to the landed wealth of the kingdom. The Parliament was expected to represent various 'interests'. This reflected the structure of a society in which the individual was defined by his or her membership of a corporate group such as the Church, the aristocracy, the City of London or the East India Company. Apologists for this Parliament of the propertied sought to put it beyond the reach of reform by popular pressure. They argued that the Glorious Revolution had settled the division of labour between executive and legislature, and preached the supremacy of Crown-in-Parliament. This view was given textbook statement by William Blackstone, who argued that Locke had been wrong to assert that the people retained the supreme power to 'remove or alter' Parliament. 'So long as the constitution lasts', he wrote, 'we may venture to affirm that the power of Parliament is absolute and without control'.[62]

The radicals challenged this doctrine of parliamentary supremacy and claimed that the constitution had become unbalanced, arguing that it was the ancient constitution that conformed to reason and natural rights. Cartwright thought it in 'perfect harmony and correspondence' with 'the great constitution of moral government, called the law of nature'.[63] For Jebb, the jurisdiction of the

---

[58] 'Mentor' [JJ], 16 September 1782, Jebb III, p. 351.

[59] Newman, *Rise of English Nationalism*, p. 183.

[60] James Vernon, 'Notes Towards an Introduction', in Vernon, *Re-Reading the Constitution*, p. 1.

[61] Langford, *Public Life*, pp. 1-3.

[62] William Blackstone cited in R.R. Palmer, *The Age of Democratic Revolution: a political history of Europe and America, 1760-1800: volume 1, The Challenge* (Princeton, N.J., 1959), p. 63.

[63] *Life of Cartwright*, p. 90.

House of Commons was defined by 'reason and the constitution'.[64] He constantly talked in terms of 'justice and the constitution', 'the ancient generosity and humanity of our nation', 'the constitution and the reason of things'.[65] Cartwright, whom Jebb regarded as his political mentor, clearly based his politics upon an appeal to historical precedent. Yet it is clear that his conception of the ancient constitution was profoundly influenced by a commitment to natural rights. 'A title to the liberty of mankind', Cartwright wrote, is not to be looked for

> among the cobwebs of the causists brain ... it is the immediate gift of God, and the seal of it is that free will which he hath made the noblest constituent of men's nature. It is not derived from anyone, but is the original in everyone; it is inherent and inalienable. The most ancient inheritance cannot strengthen this right, the want of inheritance cannot impair it. The child of a slave is as free-born according to the law of nature, as he who would trace a free ancestry up to the creation.[66]

In contrast to the eighteenth-century political system, Jebb and Cartwright thought the ancient constitution laudable primarily because it gave accurate expression to the principle of popular sovereignty. All Englishmen, they argued, had historically exercised natural political rights.

As Gunter Lottes has noted, among the mainstream radicals of the 1770s and 1780s Jebb came closest to the idea of popular sovereignty.[67] While he mouthed conventional praise for the *form* of the English constitution in which Crown, Lords and Commons were independent of each other, he argued that this system could be altered if it failed to give proper expression to the will of the people. For Jebb, the monarch and aristocracy were granted political privileges only out of expediency. Taxes were a 'gratuitous act of the commons', given the assent of the landed nobility, and the 'consent of the king is required for no other purpose than to expedite its equitable collection'.[68] If the Crown or Lords abused the important role granted to them by the constitution the people could in principle alter their status. In the *Address to Middlesex* Jebb warned that the people could 'new-model' the constitution and entirely alter their form of government. 'Widely different from the present', he warned, 'would be my argument ... were I treating of that solemn hour, when the delegates of a state, chosen according to forms, which not law and custom, but necessity and expedience shall prescribe ... shall sit in awful judgement upon the traitorous invaders of their rights'. Only in such an assembly would 'the sovereign power reside' and to which could 'the tremendous name of majesty ... be attributed'.

---

[64] *Address to the Freeholders of Middlesex*, Jebb II, p. 466.
[65] *Address to the Freeholders of Middlesex*, Jebb II, pp. 457, 484n; *A Letter to the Secretary of the Society for Constitutional Information* (July 1784), Jebb III, p. 362.
[66] Cartwright, *Life of Cartwright*, pp. 65-6.
[67] Gunter Lottes, 'Radicalism, Revolution and Political Culture: an Anglo-French comparison', in Philp, *British Popular Politics*, pp. 82-84.
[68] 'Hampden' [JJ], August 1782, Jebb III, p. 323.

Compared with the 'imperial jurisdiction' of such a body, the prerogative of the Crown, privileges of the Lords, and authority of the Commons, 'either separately considered, or combined, are less than dust upon the scale'.[69]

In this spirit, when defending the French Revolution Ann Jebb assured her readers that Jesus had given no 'directions about forms of government, and, therefore, we have a right to please ourselves'.[70] In a private letter to John Adams in late 1785 John Jebb gave a candid insight into his mature political thought: 'I am of opinion with Dr Price', he wrote, 'that those states are happy which know not Bishops, Peers, or Kings, and are strangers to those Offices and Honours falsely so called, which owe their existence to those fantastic monuments of human folly'.[71]

In addition to arguing that the people could force reform upon the political system, Jebb advocated a dramatic expansion of the electorate. Indeed, it was the issue of universal manhood suffrage that ultimately separated Jebb and his fellow radicals from moderates like Christopher Wyvill. The Westminster sub-committee went out of its way to justify the inclusion of universal manhood suffrage among its reform proposals on the grounds of both right and utility. 'The doctrine that representation and taxation are inseparable' is a truth, the *Report* declared, that had been obscured by the traditional privileges accorded to property. 'Every man has an interest in his life, his liberty, his kindred, and his country', and without direct representation these interests ('which are as substantial, as land or money') are at the mercy of those 'possessed of property, the grand enchantress of the world'. The argument that the unpropertied lacked independence was skirted: while the poor man may occasionally vote 'without a proper regard to its importance', at times of 'public calamity' a suffering nation would elect the 'real friends of humanity and their country'. The restoration of universal political rights and responsibilities, the *Report* asserted, would capture the attention and reform the manners of a wayward younger generation. With all males obliged to serve in the militia, it asked, 'is it generous, is it politic, to treat him as an alien in the community at the moment he may be ornamenting it by the powers of his understanding, or defending it by his arms?'[72]

Some historians have claimed that John Locke's impact on eighteenth-century politics has been greatly exaggerated. To some extent this may be true for the first half of the century. Yet Locke's political influence cannot be gauged simply by a survey of the degree to which the *Two Treatises* was left on shelves and referred to rather than read.[73] On the one hand, the contractual view of

---

[69] *Address to the Freeholders of Middlesex*, Jebb II, pp. 469-70.

[70] AJ, *Two Penny-worth of Truth* (20 December 1792), p. 12.

[71] JJ to John Adams, 13 September 1785, MHS Adams papers.

[72] *Report of the Sub-Committee of Westminster* (1780), Jebb III, pp. 403-23, at 410, 415, 417, 420-23, 412-14. See also S. MacCoby ed., *The English Radical Tradition, 1763-1914* (1952), pp. 34-38. This argument had been put forcefully by James Burgh, *Political Disquisitions*, I, p. 38.

[73] John Dunn, 'The Politics of Locke in England and America in the Eighteenth Century', in Yolton, *John Locke: problems and perspectives*, pp. 56-62.

government was popularised by polemicists like Benjamin Hoadly. On the other, Locke's religious and philosophical legacy encouraged an emphasis upon the importance of individual rights and duties. While theological heterodoxy proved a point of conflict with the establishment and encouraged political radicalism, it was often a symptom of a deeper philosophical evolution which saw men like Jebb confine moral authority and responsibility to the rational and autonomous individual. This led to a view of society in which the individual was the basic unit, rather than corporate bodies. Jebb complained: 'One maxim, which will be found to predominate, more or less, in the minds of individuals in every corporation, consists, in an overweening opinion and extravagant zeal for the interest of that body, to which, as it is often expressed, they have "the honour to belong".' He thought that 'this corporation-spirit' was most evident in the army, the East India Company, the Society of Jesus and the Church of England.[74] This view was no doubt encouraged by Jebb's conflict with two of the central institutions of unreformed England (the Anglican Church and Cambridge University) before entering into the field of free-market commerce that was eighteenth-century medicine. It was in opposition to a political system built around corporate interests that Jebb invoked his conception of the ancient constitution. Thus Jebb declared that the British House of Commons should be 'representative of persons, not of property; of men, not of things'.[75]

Locke's theory of government was open to radical interpretation because he passed over some key issues such as defining 'the people' and the mechanism by which they should participate in politics. D.O. Thomas has argued persuasively that because Locke left such questions open we should assume that he did not intend for there to be any diminution of the political power of the landed class. Quite the contrary in fact, as his intention was to justify the actions by that class in carrying out the Revolution of 1688.[76] Locke was helping to fight a late seventeenth-century conflict between aristocracy and monarchy rather than the late eighteenth-century debate over the franchise. Nevertheless, whatever Locke's own intentions might have been, his espousal of popular sovereignty profoundly influenced eighteenth-century radicals. Nowhere was this more evident than among Jebb's associates: the *Two Treatises of Government* was the first book Francis Blackburne read upon entering Cambridge; Edmund Law published an edition of Locke's works; and John Disney declared that he 'owed much to Mr Locke – more, probably, than to any other individual person'.[77]

The radical influence of Locke was recognised by Josiah Tucker, Dean of Gloucester, friend of Bishop Warburton, and opponent of the Feathers Tavern petition. As John Pocock has noted, if Tucker had thought a conservative reading of Locke possible he would have offered one.[78] Instead, he sought to

---

[74] Jebb III, pp. 170-71; Langford, *Public life*, p. 210.

[75] *Letter to Sir Robert Bernard* (1781), in Jebb II, p. 500.

[76] D.O. Thomas, 'Richard Ashcraft on Locke's *Two Treatises*', *E&D*, 14 (1995), pp. 128-54.

[77] Cited in 'John Disney', *BDMBR*, p. 126.

[78] Pocock, *Virtue, Commerce and History*, chapter 9.

refute Locke's political philosophy by drawing upon Scottish economic and historical theory. A measure of the seriousness with which he approached the task is the fact that he had a small number of his tract printed for criticism by friends before publication. The response by radicals was predictable: where Tucker claimed that 'subordination and government' followed from natural human inequality, William Jones thought that human sociability tended naturally toward 'a system of perfect *equality*, and would produce a *pure republic*, the only rational form of government, where manners and circumstances render it practicable'.[79] Thomas Day entertained the idea of attacking Tucker's book because it was 'written with all the contractedness, ignorance and dogmatical impertinence of an orthodox divine'.[80] Though Day did not get around to it, Joseph Towers, an active member of the SCI, issued *A Vindication of the Political Principles of Mr Locke* (1782).

Jebb himself was an obvious adherent of Locke's theory of government. At the beginning of the American Revolution he lamented: 'I did not think that despotism was so much resolved on.... Locke has shewn me who are the real rebels, in a contest of this kind; they are those, who, by unjust oppression, renew that state of war, which laws and society had banished'.[81] When he condemned all alterations to the constitution since the time of Alfred he was not revealing an uncritical reverence for the past: 'even the act of Henry the sixth, which deprived so many hundred thousand citizens of their right of suffrage, is an innovation. But were it otherwise [i.e., of ancient origin], that detestable act would be equally unconstitutional; ... were the limitations of that act in use since the time of Julius Caesar, they would not be legal, as being contrary to natural right'.[82] While some may have simply attached Locke's name to add authority to their views without having read the *Two Treatises of Government*, Jebb was clearly not one of them.

Universal manhood suffrage was a controversial issue and source of division among the reformers. Many who wanted to expand the franchise nevertheless wished to exclude servants and the labouring poor. Priestley suggested 'that those who are extremely dependent should not be allowed to have votes in the nomination of the chief magistrates', and later wrote of 'the lowest and most illiterate of our common people, who can never have any degree of influence in the state'.[83] Granville Sharp took a highly legalistic approach to political reform and based his arguments for annual parliaments primarily upon historical precedent. On the issue of universal manhood suffrage he observed that 'we know not what would be the effects of it; *probably they would be good*: but we ought to walk in a trodden path, and build on sure

[79] William Jones to Viscount Althorp, 31 March 1781, *Letters of William Jones*, pp. 462-63.

[80] Thomas Day to Erasmus Darwin jr., 29 January 1779, BL. Add. Mss 29300.57. Paul Langford, 'Thomas Day and the Politics of Sentiment', in R.F. Holland and G. Rizvi eds., *Perspectives on Imperialism and Decolonisation* (1984), pp. 57-79.

[81] Letter, 3 December 1774, 'Life of Jebb', p. 87.

[82] 'Mentor' [JJ], 20 September 1782, Jebb III, p. 358.

[83] Priestley, *Political Writings*, pp. 15, 60.

foundations'.[84] Benjamin Franklin displayed a similar caution. When told that 'Dr Jebb was for having every man vote: he said he thought Dr Jebb was right, as the all of one man was as dear to him as the all of another. Afterwards, however, he seemed to qualify this by expressing his approbation of the American system, which excludes minors, servants, and others, who are liable to undue influence'.[85] Social prejudice ensured that most reformers recoiled from the ideal of granting universal political rights and sought refuge in appeals to expediency. In addition to demanding universal manhood suffrage as an historical and natural right, however, Jebb argued that it was also justified on utilitarian grounds.

THE UTILITY OF UNIVERSAL MANHOOD SUFFRAGE

The issue of representation needs to be viewed in light of debate over the relationship between civil and political liberty. As noted above, conservative Whigs argued the common good required that politics be confined to the propertied elite, a large church and state be maintained, and some restrictions be imposed upon religious liberty. In opposition to this, Lockean liberals were primarily concerned to limit the power of the state to intrude upon the rights of the individual. In particular, they demanded free inquiry and communication of ideas in order to facilitate material and cultural progress. A broadening of political rights was usually thought to be a necessary means toward attaining the ends of greater civil liberty and progress.

The views of Richard Price and Joseph Priestley regarding political liberty have considerable historical significance, and provide a context within which to consider Jebb's position.[86] Price declared that 'Civil Liberty is the power of a *civil society* or *state* to govern itself by its own discretion', and that such a state was '*free* or *self-governed* ... more or less so in proportion as it is more or less fairly and adequately represented'.[87] Yet Price, like most eighteenth-century liberals, drew back from endorsing universal manhood suffrage, arguing that prudence dictated the franchise should be restricted to those capable of independent judgement.[88]

While Price argued that political rights were an inherent element of civil liberty, Priestley drew a careful distinction between civil and political liberty. He defined civil liberty as the power an individual retains over his own actions, and political liberty as the power an individual has over the actions of others. Priestley was primarily concerned to maximise the former, and argued that it was possible that small government and extensive civil and religious liberty could exist in an absolutist state, concluding with Alexander Pope that 'those governments which are best administered are best'. Yet if civil liberty did

[84] Cited in 'Granville Sharp', *BDMBR*, p. 435.
[85] Baynes, 'Journal', 27 August 1783, in Romilly, *Life*, p. 447.
[86] John Rawls, *A Theory of Justice* (1971), p. 201.
[87] Richard Price, *Observations on the Nature of Civil Liberty* (1776), pp. 3, 9-10.
[88] D.O. Thomas, 'Introduction', *Richard Price: Political Writings* (Cambridge, 1991), p. xix.

not by definition include political liberty, Priestley nonetheless believed that the granting of broad political rights was the best way to secure civil liberties and justified on utilitarian grounds. 'Without a spirit of liberty, and a feeling of security and independence', he argued, 'no great improvements in agriculture, or anything else, will ever be made by men'.[89] Though Priestley often appealed to natural rights, a version of 'utilitarianism' formed the basis of his political philosophy.[90]

The difference between Price and Priestley's conception of political liberty can be traced back to their differing moral philosophies. Price defended the exercise of private judgement as an end in itself, because he considered free will to be a defining aspect of human nature. This stance underpinned his definition of political liberty as an integral element of civil liberty. As a necessarian, however, Priestley was primarily interested in the exercise of private judgement as a means to uncover and disseminate truth – political liberty was an instrument to hasten the revelation of truth.[91]

Jebb knew Price and praised his defence of the Americans. Yet (as chapter 4 has demonstrated) like Priestley, Jebb espoused a determinist and hedonist moral philosophy derived from David Hartley. Jebb was primarily interested in political reform as a means of facilitating progress, happiness and the spread of truth. He was impressed by Cesare Beccaria's influential work *On Crimes and Punishments* that, along with Priestley's essay on government, has been cited as the source of Bentham's principle that policy should promote the greatest happiness for the greatest number.[92] Jebb was not a secular Utilitarian like Bentham (who rejected natural rights). Rather, he believed that utilitarian measures would naturally follow from a full recognition of political rights, and that this would help fulfil the intention of Divine Providence that everything be brought to perfection. Priestley and Jebb confidently believed that greater happiness and progress were dependent upon civil equality and greater intellectual liberty. They evaded the problem of conflict between right and utility by assuming that there could never be a clash between natural rights and the common good. Yet as Thomas has pointed out: 'An insidious consequence of supposing that all interests are harmonised in one over-arching public good, is that it obscures the possibility that there may be real clashes of interest, and leaves the individual defenceless against those who are alleged to represent the public interest.'[93] Priestley himself did just this in claiming that it was prudent to deny political liberty to the lower orders. On this point, at least, Jebb was more

---

[89] Priestley, *Political Writings*, pp. 29, 32-36; Alexander Pope, *Essay on Man*, Ep.3.303.

[90] As D.O. Thomas has pointed out, Priestley 'evades difficulties that arise whenever natural rights may be thought to conflict with considerations of the public good, by supposing that natural rights have their foundation in the public good and cannot conflict with it'. D.O Thomas, 'Progress, Liberty and Utility: the political philosophy of Joseph Priestley', in Anderson, *Science, Medicine and Dissent*, pp. 73-79, at 79. See also James J. Hoecker, 'Joseph Priestley and Utilitarianism in the Age of Reason', *E&D*, 3 (1984), pp. 55-64.

[91] Fitzpatrick, 'Toleration and Truth', pp. 1-31.

[92] *Address to the Freeholders of Middlesex*, Jebb II, p. 482.

[93] Thomas, 'Progress, Liberty and Utility', p. 79.

generous, consistent and optimistic in arguing that universal manhood suffrage was not only a natural and historical right, but should be granted on the grounds of utility. In arguing thus we can see a direct connection between Jebb's Hartlean conception of the mind and his political thought.

Jebb placed great faith in the power of political education to enlighten the masses and guide their conduct. He thought that poor education was no more a barrier to understanding the basic principles of politics than it was to understanding the basic principles of Christianity. Jebb believed that the common people were ill prepared for political activity because (as in the case of religion) they were deceived and fed false notions by the establishment. He constantly bemoaned the 'dark contrivance' of successive administrations to manipulate and delude public opinion. 'Were the film of prejudice removed, so that truth could attain an admission to the uncorrupted mind, we should be disposed, with unanimous voice, to hail the triumph of liberty in every clime, and clasp the defenders of that choicest gift of heaven to man, to our kindred breasts, with more than fraternal love.'[94]

Jebb applied the same optimistic rationalism to politics as he did to religion. He believed that 'political truth' was simple and could be discovered and agreed upon like the principles of geometry. When his motions for annual parliaments and universal manhood suffrage were greeted with silence at the second Association convention, Jebb justified his singular behaviour by stressing the need for everyone to freely state what they saw to be the truth. 'Many doctrines now universally received', he argued, 'were at one period, the opinions of a few private individuals, which though for a time opposed by the combinations of interest, an open appeal to the good sense of the community, at length hath carried into effect.'[95] Jebb's radicalism in politics was underpinned by a belief that he was acting a part in universal political progress, and he assured Christopher Wyvill that annual parliaments and universal manhood suffrage would eventually be attained. 'The constitution of the Commons house of parliament can never be restored by gradualism', he asserted, 'nor by any other power than that to which it owes its existence; I mean, the power of the people, whose proper weight and authority in the scale of government, is now rising in every part of Europe.'[96] Jebb was supremely confident that if political equality were established, agreement would follow on all-important issues. 'Measures of extensive utility are generally plain and simple', he wrote, 'and immediately approve themselves to the general sense of mankind; with respect to such, therefore, unanimity may be expected'.[97] As with religion, even an unlettered labourer could understand the basics of politics and contribute to the political process. It was for this reason that Jebb devoted his time and energies to political education.

It became commonplace during the Enlightenment to argue that the passions could be regulated by the interests. A popular critique of capitalism

---

[94] 'Trebatius' [JJ], 22 August 1785, Jebb III, p. 392-93.

[95] *Letter to Sir Robert Bernard*, Jebb II, p. 514.

[96] JJ to Christopher Wyvill, 7 August 1781, 'Life of Jebb', p. 167.

[97] *Address to the Freeholders of Middlesex*, Jebb II, p. 487.

since Marx involves the claim that it stifles development of a rounded personality and causes alienation. Yet as Hirschman has pointed out, this is exactly what eighteenth-century exponents of commerce expected and wanted it to achieve – to tame the passions by channelling them into 'innocent' and socially beneficial moneymaking.[98] In the wake of the South Sea Bubble of 1720, some patriot critics of Walpole attacked commerce as undermining Britain's moral fabric. Yet while Jebb supported calls for moral reform, he joined in the widespread praise for the benefits of commerce. He followed Montesquieu in arguing that commerce promotes wealth, social harmony and (by thus strengthening civil society) also acts as a natural counterbalance to despotism. While Jebb was deeply influenced by the republican notion of participatory citizenship, he shared none of that tradition's belief that commerce inherently undermines a civic virtue based upon landed independence. Jebb clearly believed that the spread of liberty and commerce were inextricably entwined, declaring that 'liberty, public virtue, national honour, commerce, and internal prosperity' would flourish following radical parliamentary reform.[99]

Jebb's hedonistic moral philosophy emphasised the regulation and right direction (rather than repression) of ambition and self-interest. This was the source of his approval of commerce, and it underpinned his commitment to parliamentary reform. Jebb concluded that corruption and deceit is fostered by political inequality, as concentration of political power and patronage in the hands of some encourages either obsequious conduct or resentment on the part of others. Far better, Jebb argued, that the political process act as a socially useful outlet for the ambitions of all men. As ambition and the pursuit of self-interest was natural, he argued, these desires were better put to use in a community of freely acting, morally guided individuals, rather than relying upon authoritarian restraint and repression of natural desires. Individuals should not be oppressed, but rather be allowed to let their rational, moral selves point the direction to 'true happiness' (under the guidance of education). Jebb suggested that if the Parliament became more accessible and elections more frequent, then more young men of 'spirit and ability' would be drawn in by the 'prospect of flattering distinction'. This echoes the associationist psychology that inspired his education reforms. Young men would come to 'disdain each meaner gratification' as their ambitions were satisfied by applause for patriotic and virtuous conduct in Parliament.[100]

Jebb's belief that political activity could act as a constructive outlet for the ambitions of all men is indicated by an argument he employed in defence of freedom of the press. When a bill was passed in Ireland to restrain the liberty of the press, Jebb observed that a free press helped prevent political assassinations. His reasoning provides a revealing insight into the way his view of human psychology informed his liberalism:

> A man conceives resentment; the press affords an opportunity of venting his passion; the present feeling is gratified; the

[98] Hirschman, *Passions and the Interests*, pp. 132-35.
[99] Speech in Westminster Hall, 14 February 1784, 'Life of Jebb', p. 193.
[100] *Address to the Freeholders of Middlesex*, Jebb II, p. 482n.

> resentment is no more. But, if he is restrained from the opportunity of pouring forth complaint into the breasts of his fellow-citizens, the passion conceives fresh fury from confinement, and dark resentment affects its purpose by a more fatal and surer process.[101]

Jebb's understanding of human nature also influenced his stance toward the aristocracy at the level of practical politics. He consistently refused Christopher Wyvill's pleas to moderate his radical stance in the interests of forming an alliance with the Rockingham Whigs. Jebb believed that the aristocracy would naturally defend their self-interest, and ally only with the middle and lower orders in a time of extreme national danger.[102] The parliamentary opposition, he argued, would support substantial reform only if a widespread popular movement left them with no choice (in which case their participation would be only an ornament to the movement). Rockingham's opposition to electoral reform is understandable. In his famous 1776 speech on parliamentary reform John Wilkes had declared that abolishing rotten boroughs would lay 'the axe to the root of corruption and treasury influence, as well as aristocratic tyranny'.[103] Jebb suggested that the aristocracy would be great beneficiaries of parliamentary reform, declaring that the nobility would side with a national convention because any 'diminution of the present enormous influence of the Crown, tends to restore, to that illustrious order of our fellow citizens, its proper dignity and constitutional importance'.[104]

Yet Jebb was under no illusions as to the power of aristocratic vested interest and believed that it must be firmly opposed by the 'Friends of the People'. Privately he told Wyvill 'that class' [the Rockinghamites] would only support substantial reform if 'we make it in their interest to unite with us'. The aristocracy would never accept 'what we term a reasonable compensation for borough interest, until ... compelled by the power of the people'.[105] In the course of reforming the electoral system a 'proper compensation' would be paid, and if some aristocrats were initially reluctant to go along with the process, Jebb suggested that 'such persons would probably not continue to oppose the wish, when they reflected, that the power they enjoyed was utterly inconsistent with the people's undoubted right to an equal representation, whenever they might think proper to assert it'. As the aristocracy were bound to pursue their self-interest, so must the 'agents of the democratical part of the Constitution'.[106] This belief drove his conduct as an agitator for reform, as indicated by his warning to the Volunteers of Ireland that if electoral reform were left to the Parliament 'the

---

[101] 'Life of Jebb', p. 206n.
[102] *Letter to Sir Robert Bernard*, Jebb II, p. 512.
[103] Cited in E.N. Williams, *The Eighteenth-Century Constitution* (Cambridge, 1960), p. 217.
[104] *Address to the Freeholders of Middlesex*, Jebb II, p. 481.
[105] JJ to Christopher Wyvill, 7 August 1781, 'Life of Jebb', p. 165.
[106] *Letter to Sir Robert Bernard*, Jebb II, p. 512.

aristocratic interest, united with the regal, like a blight from the east, will assuredly blast every hope of harvest'.[107]

Jebb also used the language of associationist psychology to explain how political institutions and states should interact in order to produce progress and happiness. Walpole had argued that the Crown, Lords and Commons were interdependent rather than independent, and as such, the use of influence was necessary to preserve a balance.[108] Jebb, on the other hand, thought 'the passions incident to human nature, when placed in certain circumstances' ensured that the Crown, Lords and Commons would both work together and remain independent if the constitution were established in its perfect state. The three branches of government would be regulated by 'those moral causes' that 'in a state of political liberty, with restless energy, though frequently silent and unobserved, control, direct and modify the actions of mankind'.[109] The exertions of groups of men could be understood as reflecting the 'restless energy' of the human affections writ large. The ancient constitution was laudable because the ambitions and interests of Crown, Lords and Commons were balanced against one another. In like manner he wanted Irish independence and free trade in order that Britain and Ireland should be 'united by the indivisible bonds of interests and affection'.[110]

UNIVERSAL PROGRESS

Jebb's moral philosophy tempered his patriotic chauvinism and saw him become a pioneering advocate of the universalism that became a prominent feature of British radicalism during the French Revolution. As noted in chapter 2, patriotism was an evolving and contested concept in late eighteenth-century Britain. In the decades (and even centuries) prior to the American Revolution, patriotism was extremely chauvinistic and generally associated with opposition and radicalism.[111] Newman has argued that a surge of radical patriotism in the middle of the eighteenth century developed into what he calls a clearly defined 'English nationalism' in the 1780s and 90s.[112] Radical patriotism initially reflected a challenge to the cosmopolitan values of the ruling aristocracy. Yet in response to the American and French Revolutions, the British elite adopted the language of 'middling sort' patriotism and harnessed it to the constitution of King-in-Parliament and Anglican Church. While the Seven Year's War and the French Revolution 'served to unite a Protestant Britain pursuing imperial aims',

---

[107] *Letters Addressed to the Volunteers of Ireland, on the subject of parliamentary reform* (1784), Jebb II, p. 532.

[108] W.A. Speck, *Stability and Strife: England 1714-1760* (1977), p. 23.

[109] *Address to the Freeholders of Middlesex*, Jebb II, p. 468n.

[110] JJ to Francis Dobbs, 27 April 1782, NLI Dobbs papers.

[111] Christopher Hill, 'The Norman Yoke'; Hugh Cunningham, 'The Language of Patriotism, 1750-1914', *History Workshop Journal* 12 (1981), pp. 8-33.

[112] Newman, *Rise of English Nationalism*. While Newman's book is a valuable and stimulating study, it is flawed by a failure to adequately examine how English identity interacted with an emerging *British* nationalism.

the process was by no means a smooth one, and at the end of the century nonconformists and radicals remained in opposition to the establishment.[113] Reformers continued to draw on the patriotic tradition with its ideal of preserving native English liberties.

Radical ideas and organisations evolved in conjunction with a developing sense of the British nation, for which reason the government did not pursue a systematic encouragement of nationalism. Linda Colley has questioned the degree to which nationalism became a conservative force, pointing out the way nationalist ideas in Britain could be used by lower class people. Yet, as John Dinwiddy has reaffirmed, during the French Revolution nationalism in England became 'overwhelmingly a conservative force', and if the government did not *systematically* promote nationalism, 'the prevailing view of the authorities was that national feeling was something to be encouraged rather than opposed'.[114] British radicals became hamstrung in their appeals to patriotism by their association with French and cosmopolitan republican ideals. If anxious during the tumults of the late eighteenth century, loyalists at least became increasingly unified and vocal in their support for 'Church and King'. Radicals, on the other hand, had to deal with a tension between patriotism, and the cosmopolitan and universal ideals of the Enlightenment and the American and French Revolutions.[115]

The chauvinism of the English during the eighteenth century was notable, and even the supposedly 'enlightened' upper classes were characterised by prejudice against foreigners. The most scathing condemnation was directed at the Welsh, Irish and Scottish. Even the cosmopolitan Lord Shelburne told Richard Price that Scotland was 'composed of such a sad set of innate, cold-hearted, impudent rogues that I sometimes think it a comfort when you and I shall be able to walk together in the next world ... we cannot possibly then have any of them sticking to our skirts'.[116] This sense of English superiority was characteristic of the circles within which Jebb moved. Thomas Brand and his friend Thomas Hollis travelled to the Continent at mid-century and returned intensely patriotic, with the latter scorning 'vain Frenchmen, trucking Dutchmen, [and] fame lost Danes'.[117] When Joseph Priestley travelled to the continent with Lord Shelburne he found little to admire among the customs or ideas of the French and retreated into study of his Bible.[118] Samuel Romilly

---

[113] Murray G.H. Pittock, *Inventing and Resisting Britain: cultural identities in Britain and Ireland, 1685-1789* (1997), p. 129.

[114] Linda Colley, 'Whose nation? Class and national consciousness in Britain 1750-1830', *Past and Present* 113 (1986), pp. 97-117; John Dinwiddy, 'England', in Otto Dann and John Dinwiddy eds., *Nationalism in the Age of the French Revolution* (1988), pp. 53-70, at 69; see also David Eastwood, 'Patriotism and the English State in the 1790s', in Philp, *French Revolution and British Popular Politics*, pp. 146-68.

[115] Martin Fitzpatrick, 'Patriots and Patriotisms: Richard Price and the early reception of the French Revolution in England', *Studies on Voltaire and the Eighteenth Century,* 335 (1996), pp. 211-29.

[116] Langford, *Polite and Commercial People* p. 328.

[117] Robbins, 'Strenuous Whig', p. 420.

[118] Priestley, *Works*, I, pp. 255-57.

(who had frequent contact with Jebb when he returned from the Continent) best summed up the prevailing attitude toward the Continent when he reflected: 'it is astonishing how much the French are disposed to refine, to account for everything that happens in an extraordinary way, and to find deep design and contrivance in the most simple transactions'.[119]

Jebb was intensely proud of his Englishness. Yet he was also at the forefront of those patriots attracted to the cosmopolitan ideals of the Enlightenment. This is illustrated by his attitude toward the Celtic fringe. Jebb thought the Scots had been unfairly represented as favourable to despotism, and that, quite to the contrary, they were an enlightened people who had produced many advocates for liberty.[120] Jebb's optimistic blend of natural rights and utilitarian argument is probably best illustrated by his request that the Irish Volunteers include the rights of full citizenship for Catholics in their reform platform. To overcome their reservations he pointed to a possible future when, with the absence of religious intolerance and 'under the influence of mild and equal laws, human industry shall be generally excited and encouraged'. In such a climate, he asked, 'is it not reasonable to conclude, that religious prejudices will also give away, and truth extend her salutary empire over the minds of men, in proportion as the light of science ... shall prevail?' Politicians of the day would fail in their 'bad purposes, through false conceptions of the human character', and it was a natural tendency toward virtue that had led the Americans to assert their independence when threatened by a corrupt regime. In this spirit, Jebb assured the Irish that 'Compliance with the obvious rules of justice, by allowing free scope to the virtuous energies of the mind, enables us to overcome obstacles apparently insurmountable, and leads to peace and happiness.'[121]

Jebb thought that the international community and a federal British Empire (preferably with the inclusion of the American states) should operate in the same way that he wanted to see a society of individuals function. The path to universal peace lay in having strong, independent, self-governing nations engage in free trade. Jebb thought it 'uncharitable' of Shelburne to style France and Spain 'the natural enemies of England'.[122] He was critical of the oppressive form of government imposed on India by British interests.[123] And he thought that both Ireland and Scotland should be able to build their own navies, under the control of their own representative assemblies, to defend their own trade. He wanted to

[119] Romilly, *Life*, II, p. 424.

[120] Jebb inserted an extract from *An Historical Account of the Ancient Rights of the Parliament of Scotland* (1703), in the Society for Constitutional Information's collection of *Tracts*, II, pp. 59-62, and wrote: 'It has been, too much, the custom to represent the inhabitants of a neighbouring kingdom [Scotland], as friendly to despotism, as insensible to the genuine feelings of patriotism.... The following quotation and authorities ... speak the sense of free parliaments and a gallant people'. 20 July 1784, Jebb III, pp. 362-68. He claimed that Scotland had been the 'scourge of tyrannical power in many a former generation', 'Trebatius' [JJ], 22 August 1785, Jebb III, p. 392.

[121] *Letters to the Volunteers of Ireland*, Jebb II, p. 547-48.

[122] 'Laelius' [JJ], [October?] 1782, Jebb III, p. 361.

[123] Speech in Westminster Hall, 14 February 1784, 'Life of Jebb', p. 193.

see 'that long oppressed country [Scotland] once more respectable, and owe its security to the native virtue and valour of its sons'.[124] Jebb constantly promoted the idea that a prosperous and independent Ireland would benefit Britain.[125] He wrote to a correspondent in Belfast,

> O let the friends of freedom throughout the Globe be friends to each other also! Tyrants are leagued against them everywhere, and nothing under Providence but generous sentiments of civil and religious liberty, fully diffused ... arming of the People, free commerce, and an unreserved communication of every species of sound Political knowledge and mutual animation of each other can long preserve the friends of freedom from their dark designs.[126]

Far from seeing a conflict between nationalism and international peace, Jebb clearly believed that universal harmony and prosperity would follow promotion of a rational patriotism. Death spared him the pain of divided loyalties experienced by radicals during war between Britain and revolutionary France.

Religious, philosophical and political progress was inextricably entwined in Jebb's mind. As noted in chapter 2, Jebb was spared doubts about the coherence and consistency of his heady mixture of natural rights and utility by an unflagging faith in Divine Providence. He assumed that God would not have designed a universe in which right and utility were not in harmony. In addition, Jebb's faith in the coming millennium led him to believe that universal progress was inevitable. History had witnessed many setbacks in particular times and places, and he often thought that his own country was heading for ruin. Jebb concluded his *Address to the Freeholders of Middlesex* with the suggestion that 'the times of distress, long predicted' would soon arrive, and a plan to reform Parliament should be prepared 'in that hour of tranquillity which precedes the storm'.[127]

Jebb believed that Providence would work through natural means (chiefly the mechanism of the human mind) to ultimately and inevitably undermine established institutions and spread true religion in preparation for the Second Coming. He saw himself as a conscious and positive instrument of God's will. That is why he wanted to 'push on the combined causes of a diffusion and right arrangement of political power, and a philological knowledge of the scriptures'.[128] And it gave him the confidence to brush aside prudent concerns about the consequences of radical reform. The millennium was coming one way or another. As noted in the previous chapter, he viewed the outcome of the American conflict in cosmic terms. And as chapter 11 will show, he held fast to his ideals through the ebb and flow of the Association movement's fortunes. Time and again he rebuffed Wyvill's pleas for moderation with assurances that

---

[124] Jebb III, p. 310.
[125] JJ to Francis Dobbs, 5 October 1783, NLI Dobbs papers.
[126] JJ to Henry Joy, [September 1785?], LHL Joy papers.
[127] Jebb II, p. 90.
[128] 'Life of Jebb', p. 189.

if the reformers would only hold fast to their demands, then time and Providence would see their goals attained.

Jebb would no doubt have greeted the French Revolution with the same enthusiasm as his Rational Dissenting friends (for many of whom it heightened expectations that Christ's return was near). It is worth noting that an acquaintance of Ann Jebb's in her last years was Joseph Lomas Towers (the son of Dr Joseph Towers, an early member of the Society for Constitutional Information). His *Illustrations of Prophecy* (1796) welcomed the French Revolution as fulfilling biblical eschatology through the 'overthrow of tyranny' and 'restoration of the people to their rights'.[129] Nevertheless, prior to the French Revolution at least, Rational Dissenters were generally unwilling to set a date for the Second Coming. Thus it was with Jebb – while no man might know the hour or the day, all were duty bound to work toward the coming kingdom of God through promoting liberty and progress.

[129] Harrison, *Second Coming*, p. 76.

10

Gentlemen Dissenters and the Law

It was the extent of its extra-parliamentary nature that marked the radicalism of the 1760s as a new departure. This reflected a considerable expansion of urban culture that gained pace in the second half of the century, and involved the establishment of many voluntary societies and professional associations, which allowed the middling sort to escape the constraints of patrician control.[1] The result, however, was not a cohesive middle class united in its opposition to the aristocratic establishment. As Wilson has argued, 'eighteenth-century urban culture embodied the status, material, and aspirational divisions within the middle classes and even encouraged divergent political principles, so that as some of the bourgeoisie became entrenched in the interstices of Old Corruption, others were in the vanguard of a radical assault on it.' She suggests that 'urban culture may have been more important in promoting a *political* consciousness that, transcending nascent class formations, united members of different social groups, such as, in the case of radical politics, intellectuals, professionals, middling retailers and artisans'.[2]

The importance of Rational Dissent is magnified in this view of politics and society, because it provided a political and intellectual elite and a congregational base, which could articulate and support an ideology of political dissent. It is here that we can see some correlation between opposition politics and a body of self-consciously middle-class people. As John Seed has argued, the rationalism of Rational Dissenters was 'linked to the experience and

---

[1] John Brewer, 'The Commercialization of Politics', in Neil McKendrick, John Brewer and J.H. Plumb, *The Birth of a Consumer Society: the commercialisation of eighteenth-century England* (1982), p. 200.

[2] Kathleen Wilson, 'Urban Culture and Political Activism in Hanoverian England', in Hellmuth, *Transformation of Political Culture*, p. 184.

"common sense" of a prosperous bourgeoisie'.[3] While political alignments cut across social groups, prior to the French Revolution most of the leading radicals were clergy, professionals and gentlemen of liberal religious disposition. In light of this, we need to examine Jebb's social context and ethos in order to understand the limitations of his radicalism.

SOCIAL ATTITUDES

Rational Dissenters and reform-minded people were often closely associated and even interrelated. Catherine Cappe found visiting the Lindseys in London very different to when they had been living in Catterick. She was quite intimidated: 'surrounded as they were by persons of the first talents, and attainments in literature – the Priestleys, the Franklins, the Jebbs, the Lees, the Prices, the Sergeants, etc., my society could add nothing to them; but was on the contrary, an encumbrance'.[4] Rational Dissenters and reformers were a middle-class intellectual elite interconnected by a web of familial, religious and professional associations. Of the 411 subscribers to Jebb's posthumous *Works* that Robert Webb has been able to identify, most were professionals or provincial clergy. These include 36 physicians and surgeons, 60 lawyers, 45 businessmen, and at least 40 present or future MPs (mostly Whigs and radicals); there is a handful of radical peers, and the 50 or so identifiable gentlemen are 'drawn less from the traditional gentry than from merchant wealth of a generation earlier'; and there were 38 predominantly Unitarian Dissenting ministers. There were also 150 clergymen (including dons and schoolmasters) of the Anglican Church, 'most but not all of them from Cambridge and most in parochial rather than academic careers'.[5] This analysis further demonstrates that Rational Dissent was largely a religion of those involved in commerce and the professions. It also supports Seed's argument that the elite of Rational Dissent were socially and politically well connected.[6]

Jebb thought equality of religious and political rights possible, however, he did not believe (and had no reason to believe) that economic and social equality was possible or desirable. Jebb assumed that material inequality was an inherent feature of the natural order, and his primary concern was how to ensure that all those strung out along the social hierarchy understood and performed their rights and duties. One way was to encourage the propertied (broadly defined) to take an enlightened approach to their self-interest. For example, Jebb suggested that the brutal management and conditions of prisons encouraged 'riot, insurrection and escape'. To ensure that they operated in a more humane and reformist manner, prisons should be supervised by 'such persons as are most interested in the peace and good order of the district', with

---

[3] Seed, 'Gentlemen Dissenters', p. 324.
[4] Cappe, *Memoirs*, p. 185.
[5] Webb, 'Emergence of Rational Dissent', p. 39.
[6] John Seed, 'A set of men powerful enough in many things': Rational Dissent and Political Opposition in England, 1770-1790', in Haakonssen, *Enlightenment and Religion*, pp. 140-68.

the various 'justices, gentry and tenantry of the county' rotating through a series of committees.[7] In his sermon on Acts 10:34, 'God is no respecter of persons', Jebb asked why Providence allowed an evident inequality between animals and men, and within human society? And why had the English been favoured with a geography, climate and exposure to the Gospel that had encouraged the spirit of liberty? He replied with a paternalist answer that had a utilitarian spin: the sum total of happiness is greater if 'imperfect creatures be classed in various ranks and orders, with various powers and capacities of improvement, than if there were only one class, possessed of an absolute equality of endowments'.[8] According to this view, the greater one's knowledge and privilege, the greater one's responsibility and duty. An academic had a solemn duty to research and instruct, and a wealthy aristocrat was morally bound to set an example of noble patriotism.

While Jebb praised 'patriot' noblemen like the Duke of Richmond, he was generally critical of the aristocracy. As noted in previous chapters, from the middle decades of the century there were increasing calls for a reformation of manners by writers such as James Burgh, David Hartley, John Brown and Richard Price. These writers criticised both the perceived luxury and profligacy of the wealthy and the laxity of the lower orders. There is plenty of evidence that Jebb and his associates participated in the social rituals of polite society. Jebb met his future wife at a ball in Huntingdon, and after he resigned from the ministry he was seen dancing at the Huntingdon ball and assembly.[9] Likewise, Theophilus Lindsey was happy to attend the Lincoln races.[10] Yet middle-class reformers like Jebb clearly thought that they were morally superior to a social and political elite for whom time and money were an inducement to indulge in vice. In this vein, James Burgh declared that the 'bourgeoisie' (his term) have the education and 'behave as the nobility and gentry' should.[11] Jebb's proposed education reforms were primarily aimed at instilling a middle-class sense of morality and duty in the sons of the aristocracy and gentry. Ann Jebb observed that 'A king can make a lord, but cannot make a gentleman'.[12] The American Abigail Adams, who greatly enjoyed the company of the Jebbs, thought the English nobility were 'totally depraved' in comparison to the 'virtue and morality' that could be found in the middle class.[13] Jebb praised the nobility in print, but he did so in a manner inviting them to live up to expectations. As noted in the previous chapter, he was sensitive to the narrow political self-interest displayed by most of the aristocrats in Parliament. In short, Jebb judged the aristocracy according to their social utility and found them wanting.

---

[7] *Thoughts on ... Prisons*, Jebb II, p. 567.

[8] 'God no respecter of persons' Acts 10:34, Jebb II, p. 92.

[9] BL Cole mss. 5873:70.

[10] John Disney to J.C. Brooke, 17 August 1782, 'Letters of J.C. Brooke', BL English letters c222.

[11] Martha Zebrowski, 'The Corruption of Politics and the Dignity of Human Nature: the critical and constructive radicalism of James Burgh', *E&D*, 10 (1991), p. 81.

[12] AJ, *Two Penny-worth of Truth* (20 December 1792), p. 13.

[13] Cited in Page Smith, *John Adams* (New York, 1962), p. 714.

Historians disagree as to whether the aristocracy or middle class were more culturally dominant, but it is generally accepted that there was a growing divide between polite and common people in eighteenth-century England. Recent studies have emphasised the significant electoral clout wielded by Dissenters.[14] In light of this, Seed has argued that the leading ministers of Rational Dissent (men such as Price, Priestley, Andrew Kippis and Joseph Towers) were representatives of a large, wealthy and influential section of the political nation. While these men were prominent critics of the political and religious status quo, they supported moral reform and the rationalisation of legal restraints on the poor. It was this combination of religious and political liberalism with a fear of 'the mob' that saw many Rational Dissenters at first embrace the French Revolution and then back away from the threat to property posed by Paineite radicalism. It is important to remember that Rational Dissenters employed servants.[15] While there was, to some degree, a religious and political divide between Rational Dissent and the establishment, there was an even greater social divide between the Rational Dissenters and the lower orders.

The supposedly harsh individualism of Rational Dissenters should not be exaggerated. Even a thinker like Priestley displayed many paternalist and mercantilist values. Like his fellow Rational Dissenters, Priestley was primarily concerned with religion rather than economics and thus viewed all questions of social inequality primarily in light of moral improvement rather than economic efficiency.[16] Thus it is not surprising that when he settled in America Priestley was shocked by the independence and lack of deference of the lower orders, and declared: 'If there were more subordination, it would be better for them all'.[17] Rational Dissenters were committed to moralising and instructing the lower orders. In his *Farewell Address* Lindsey instructed his parishioners in Catterick to be obedient to their superiors, and criticised them for indulging in riotous games, foul language and drunkenness.[18] John Disney advocated the stricter regulation of alehouses.[19] Even the radical London Wilkites distinguished themselves from both plebeian and patrician alike, and revealed the middle-class attitudes of shopkeepers and traders. Their calls for stricter policing of the streets 'indicate a greater sensitivity to the fate of movable property than to the misfortunes of the labouring poor'.[20] Jebb himself sat on the committee of a

---

[14] J. Phillips, *Electoral Behaviour in Unreformed England*; Frank O'Gorman, *Voters, Patrons and Parties: the unreformed electorate of Hanoverian England, 1734-1832* (Oxford, 1989); James E. Bradley, *Religion, Revolution and English Radicalism*; *Popular Politics and the American Revolution: petitions, the crown and public opinion* (Cambridge, 1986).

[15] Seed, 'Rational Dissent and Political Opposition', p. 168.

[16] Margaret Canovan, 'Paternalistic Liberalism: Joseph Priestley on rank and inequality', *E&D*, 2 (1983), pp. 34-35.

[17] Joseph Priestly to Theophilus Lindsey, 12 July 1795, *Works*, I, pt 2, p. 310.

[18] Theophilus Lindsey, *A Farewell Address to the Parishioners of Catterick* (1774), p. 17.

[19] John Disney, *The Duty of Circumspection in Licensing Public Ale-houses* (1776).

[20] John Brewer, 'The Wilkites and the Law 1763-74: a study of radical notions of governance', in John Brewer and J. Styles, *An Ungovernable People* (1980), p. 170.

workhouse in his Suffolk parish, and there are definite paternalist overtones in his medical practice. If Jebb attacked the dominance of landed wealth in the political system, he nevertheless remained respectful of the rights of property and accepting of economic inequality as natural.[21] Ann Jebb insisted that the French and the English reformers were only demanding political equality and that 'poverty be no bar to merit', not something 'so wild as an equal division of property'.[22]

Rational Dissenters did, however, display a distinctive attitude toward the poor. While they often divided people into the stereotypes of 'industrious' and 'undeserving', Ditchfield has argued that they 'did not share the increasingly negative attitude towards the poor near the end of the eighteenth century detected by some historians', but tended to view the poor as 'fellow victims of an oppressive church-state'. Rational Dissenters were also wary, if not hostile toward the growth in charitable organisations because they saw them as forcing particular religious and political doctrines upon the poor. Substantial assistance for the poor and general human improvement, according to Rational Dissenters, could only come from a growing number of independent, religiously inspired enlightened individuals – like themselves.[23]

Aside from internal divisions, the failure of the Association movement owed something to the fact that it remained a gentry and middle-class enterprise. The Association movement would have had a greater impact if it had actively sought to mobilise the masses of discontented artisans.[24] As the very aim of the SCI indicates, Jebb was keen to see people from the lower orders become politically active. At a meeting in Westminster Hall on 2 February 1780 he expressed delight in seeing 'the nobleman, the gentleman, the artisan, the mechanic; in short every description of men, united in opposing the arbitrary measures of an abandoned administration'.[25] Yet despite such idealistic sentiments, the cost of membership placed the SCI out of the reach of working men.

While the eighteenth-century practice of forming coffeehouse clubs contributed significantly to the development of extra-parliamentary politics, it also entrenched the exclusion from political debate of women and the lower orders.[26] Only in the 1790s did Corresponding Societies emerge that were organised by and within the financial reach of workingmen. Indeed, Langford has argued that prior to the French Revolution the lower classes were actually pushed out of politics by the increasingly literate, middle-class domination of

[21] 'The labours of the lowliest of the sons of men are necessary to the well-being of the whole'. Jebb I, p. 22.
[22] AJ, *Two Penny-Worth of Truth for a Penny* (20 December 1792), pp. 6-7.
[23] G.M. Ditchfield, 'English Rational Dissent and Philanthropy, c.1760-c.1810', in Hugh Cunningham and Joanna Innes eds., *Charity, Philanthropy and Reform from the 1690s to 1850* (1998), pp. 193-207, quoted at 198-99.
[24] Bradley, *Religion, Revolution and English Radicalism*, p. 429; Cannon, *Parliamentary Reform*, pp. 68-69.
[25] 'Life of Jebb', p. 147.
[26] Brewer, 'Commercialization of Politics', in McKendrick, *Birth of a Consumer Society*, p. 219.

extra-parliamentary agitation.[27] In the end it is unclear how aware radicals prior to the 1790s were of the social implications of their proposals. Despite their rhetoric, they did not draw lower-class people into the centre of the Association movement. They thought that if the franchise were widened, and they provided the masses with 'constitutional information', the lower orders would naturally elect their social betters – sturdy, independent, well-educated individuals from the middle and upper classes. Indeed, as noted in the previous chapter, Jebb believed that the masses would become more disciplined and industrious if they were given a say in government.

Conservatives and radicals aimed at the same end (an orderly society), but differed as to how it could be achieved. Conservatives tended to emphasise the use of paternalism and punishment. Jebb's moral philosophy, however, led him to believe that education would improve the morality and patriotism of the lower orders. This attitude gave Ann Jebb the confidence to declare that 'I never knew a man make the worse servant for being able to read his duty'.[28] If equal representation were granted, she argued, the British people '(trusting that every other necessary reform would follow of course) would soon astonish the world with their tameness'.[29] In the same vein, she claimed that the soldiers of revolutionary France had shown that 'obedience to their leaders, was not incompatible with a zeal for freedom'.[30]

Political reform was desired so that the state would be governed by an elected meritocracy who would provide fiscally prudent government, a rational legal code, and ensure religious and political liberty.[31] Ultimately the radical rhetoric of Rational Dissent was bound within 'limits established by the property relations of late eighteenth-century English society'.[32] We can, however, see the degree to which Jebb was both bound by and pushed against these limits through an examination of his attitude toward women and slavery, and his interest in legal reform.

Eighteenth-century England was a patriarchal and in some respects misogynist society. The rhetoric of Wilkite patriotism was drenched with references to 'masculine virtue' and 'effeminate depravity'. The Duchess of Devonshire had to endure considerable ridicule when she assisted Charles James Fox on the hustings during the famous 1784 election. And there were constant calls to restrict legal rights and freedoms enjoyed by women. For example, in 1778 the House of Commons barred women from listening to debates, as they had increasingly done since mid-century. Yet the increasing awareness of, and contribution to public life made by women is inescapable.[33] Of particular note

---

[27] Langford, *Polite and Commercial People*, p. 720.
[28] AJ, *Two Penny-worth of Truth* (20 December 1792), p. 14.
[29] AJ, *Two Penny-worth of Truth* (20 December 1792), p. 16.
[30] AJ, *Two Penny-worth More of Truth for a Penny* (26 January 1793), p. 5.
[31] Jebb argued that without parliamentary reform taxes would not be imposed equitably. 'Speech at a general meeting of the electors of Westminster', 17 July 1782, Jebb III, p. 301.
[32] Seed, 'Rational Dissent and Political Opposition', p. 168.
[33] Colley, *Britons*, pp. 238-50.

was the participation of women in London debating societies as both audience and speakers.[34]

Locke had claimed that the development of rationality was connected with an increasing divide between public and private. The public sphere, he argued, should be the province of rational exchanges between men, while indulgence in passion should be confined to the domestic realm. Thus, while Locke argued against patriarchalism in politics, he concluded that the customary subjection of wives to the will of their husbands was natural. As Catherine Hall has written, 'for both Hobbes and Locke the fundamental subject matter of political philosophy was not the adult human individual but the male-headed family.'[35] In both traditional and Enlightenment thought it was assumed that women should be politically represented through their husbands and fathers. John Cartwright argued that women had no right to representation in Parliament because they were 'by nature' unable to perform the legal and militia duties of a citizen.[36]

Both conservative and radical women agreed that their role should be confined to exercising a moral influence on politically active men. In short, the vote for women was not an issue in the eighteenth century. As the radical Harriet Martineau wrote: 'I want to be doing something with the pen, since no other means of action in politics are in a woman's power'.[37] Thus, eighteenth-century 'feminists' concentrated upon arguing that women had the same intellectual abilities and moral worth as men.[38] They applied the language employed in debating the political rights of men to the civil and domestic relationship between men and women. Even the most advanced advocates of women's rights in the 1790s only argued for, in Mary Wollstonecraft's words, a 'revolution in female manners'. This would be achieved by greater domestic equality, and by giving women a political voice through influence on their husband's vote.[39]

Rational Dissent played an important role in promoting greater social equality for women. It has been argued that 'godliness' provided seventeenth-century Puritan women with a means through which they could transcend some of the restrictions imposed by gender, and enabled them to become active agents within their congregations.[40] There seems to have been a similar egalitarian dynamic at work in Rational Dissent. According to Ruth Watts, 'Unitarians

---

[34] Donna T. Andrew, 'Popular Culture and Public Debate: London 1780', *The Historical Journal,* 39 (1996), pp. 405-23.

[35] Catherine Hall, *White, Male and Middle Class: explorations in feminism and history* (Cambridge, 1995), p. 155.

[36] John Cartwright, *An Appeal, Civil and Military, on the Subject of the English Constitution* (1799), p. 17; cited in Dickinson, *Politics of the People*, p. 184.

[37] Cited in Dickinson, *Politics of the People*, p. 156.

[38] Alice Browne, *The Eighteenth-Century Feminist Mind* (Brighton, 1987), p. 139.

[39] Susan E. Brown, 'Rational Creatures and Free Citizens: the language of politics in the eighteenth-century debate on women', *Historical Papers* (Canadian Historical Association, 1988), pp. 41-2.

[40] Diane Willen, 'Godly Women in Early Modern England: Puritanism and gender', *Journal of Ecclesiastical History,* 43 (1992), pp. 561-80.

played a significant role in changing ideas on women's abilities and what they could do. This, in turn, was an important basis from which the balance of power in gender relationships could be changed.'[41]

It is striking how much some of the leading lights relied upon the domestic and intellectual support of their partners. Mary Priestley was 'a very industrious woman, never at rest except when she was asleep', and she held the purse strings, doling out pocket money to her husband whenever he left the house. Joseph always said that he was only a lodger in Mary's house, and when she died he was unable to manage his domestic affairs.[42] Hannah Lindsey seems to have been a formidable woman, whose stern manner contrasted sharply with her husband's kind disposition. She managed the household budget, worked with the servants in house and garden, taught Sunday school, ran an apothecary shop and used her considerable medical knowledge in tending the poor. When Catherine Cappe exclaimed 'how I would exult if I had your knowledge, and could apply it?' Hannah Lindsey replied: 'Exult! You would have no reason; do you not think, that if it were the will of God that these poor persons should recover, he could not easily have employed other means equally effectual without my feeble agency?'[43] The women of Rational Dissent were encouraged to be active, industrious and strong-minded; and they clearly benefited from the egalitarian implication of Acts 10:34: 'God is no respecter of persons, but in every nation he who feareth him, and worketh righteousness, is accepted of him'.[44]

Probably the best testimony to the relatively equal domestic relations of Rational Dissenters is their express opinions regarding women. Priestley declared that 'the minds of women are capable of the same improvement, and the same furniture, as those of men', and praised the Cambridge Rational Dissenter Robert Robinson for providing his daughters with the same education as his sons.[45] Jebb and Robinson were on friendly terms. Jebb wrote in his private notebook: 'women are not dealt with justly by the laws of the land. All laws of inferiority should be repealed. Compact supposes equality.'[46] He was probably referring to a recent publication, which asserted that through marriage women lose their 'legal existence'.[47] Jebb's use of the word 'compact' suggests

---

[41] Ruth Watts, *Gender, Power and the Unitarians in England 1760-1860* (1998), pp. 1-2.
[42] Alan Ruston, 'A Servant's View of Joseph Priestley', *E&D*, 8 (1989), pp. 115-19; H. John McLachlan, 'Mary Priestley: a woman of character', in Schwartz and McEvoy, *Motion Toward Perfection*, pp. 251-64.
[43] Cappe, *Memoir of Mrs Lindsey*, p. 6.
[44] Cappe concludes her *Memoir of Mrs Lindsey* with this text; and Jebb chose it as the starting point for one of his more controversial Cambridge sermons, Jebb II, pp. 87-106.
[45] Joseph Priestley, *A Sermon on the Occasion of the Death of the Rev Robert Robinson* (Birmingham, 1790); Watts, 'Joseph Priestley and Education', pp. 88-89.
[46] Jebb II, p. 180. This comment was squashed into the bottom of the last page of his miscellaneous notes, and would have been written in the mid-1780s.
[47] [?], *The Laws Respecting Women as they Regard their Natural Rights* (1777), cited in Colley, *Britons*, p. 238. The author claimed that 'By marriage the very being or legal existence of a woman is suspended. ... She can't let, set, sell, give away, or alienate any

that he was privately entertaining the idea of women having political rights. David Williams, who shared political views that were similar to Jebb's, was not afraid to suggest that the franchise be extended to single women and widows.[48] In light of such sentiments it is not surprising that Mary Wollstonecraft drew on her contact with Rational Dissenters in formulating her ideas on the rights of women.

Ann Jebb clearly enjoyed an intellectually vigorous relationship with her husband, and was liked and respected by their friends. John Disney wrote: 'Mrs Jebb may be less known to the world at large than our female historian [Catherine Macaulay]: but in the circle of her friends she is respected as well for the soundness of her judgement, and the sincerity of her friendship, as for the eminent integrity and candour of her mind.'[49] In addition to encouraging his wife to write in support of religious liberty to the newspapers, John Jebb was evidently influenced by her opinion on political matters.[50] Ann may also have had some more direct engagement in political activities. The Cambridge High Churchman William Cole observed that Jebb and his wife often went to London to attend meetings of the petitioning clergy. That Ann may have been more than just a passive observer at these meetings is suggested by Henry Taylor, when he hoped to see her 'chairman at the next meeting of the Feathers'.[51] Taylor may have been jesting as was often his want, but we should not underestimate the important role women played in supporting religious and political dissent. Thus one critic of the Feathers Tavern petition was led to exclaim that it was not the Church that needed reform, but rather 'the age, your consciences, your lives, your friends, associates – nay your modish wives'.[52] While Rational Dissent did not challenge male domination of the public sphere, in its intellectual and social composition it promoted greater domestic equality and encouraged women to lead socially and intellectually active lives. As a result women like Ann Jebb found themselves implicitly challenging conventional notions of femininity. Taylor lyrically expressed this: 'you confess yourself to be neither fish nor flesh, but a kind of an otter, between a fine lady and a Philosopher'.[53]

The slave trade attracted moral indignation from Jebb's circle. Francis Blackburne had expressed an abhorrence of slavery at the start of the Seven Year's War, and attributed 'our present dangerous situation' to the 'the cries of these poor wretches against us'.[54] While Jebb himself expressed a disdain for

---

thing without her husbands consent. Her very necessary apparel, by the law, is not her's in property'. p. 65. See Colley, *Britons*, p. 238.

[48] James Dybikowski, 'David Williams and the Eighteenth-Century Distinction between Civil and Political Liberty', *E&D,* 3 (1984), p. 34.

[49] Disney, *Memoirs of Thomas Brand Hollis*, p. 43n. In the late nineteenth century the Unitarian historian Robert Spears wrote that Ann Jebb was 'a woman of extraordinary mental powers'. *A Record of Unitarian Worthies* (1876), p. 282.

[50] Meadley, *Memoir of Ann Jebb*, p. 16.

[51] Henry Taylor to Ann Jebb, 25 January 1773, CUL Taylor papers.

[52] [Anon.], *London Chronicle*, 17 March 1774.

[53] Henry Taylor to AJ, [?], CUL Taylor papers.

[54] Francis Blackburne to Theophilus Lindsey, 19 March 1756, DWL Blackburne-Lindsey correspondence.

'the abominable slave trade' (which he hoped American Independence would bring to an end), he did not involve himself directly in the fledgling abolitionist cause.[55] Nevertheless, he became a familiar acquaintance of Granville Sharp, the pioneering evangelist.[56] In 1776 Jebb thanked Sharp for a copy of his book against slavery. He expressed agreement with Sharp's stance on this 'very serious affair', and wrote: 'I am clear in my opinion and have for many years maintained that no considerations of trade, or any other consideration whatever can be offered in excuse for so horrible a practice.' He commended Sharp for founding his arguments on 'proofs from Scripture', and concluded that 'this practice is as offensive to the Supreme Being, as it is contrary to reason and Humanity. Indeed, a stronger and more wanton violation of Man's Rights cannot possibly be conceived.'[57]

It was easy for reformers to link the issue of slavery to their other concerns. Sharp believed the slave trade 'to be the cause of all our misfortunes in America' because it violated God's laws.[58] Jebb died before the campaign against slavery really gained momentum, but Sharp would have kept him up to date with developments. For example, two days after the African Gustavas Vasa had related 'an account of 130 Negroes being thrown alive into the sea from on Board an English slave ship', Sharp called on Jebb while in the middle of urging a 'prosecution in the Admiralty Court against all Persons concerned'.[59] Such stories led the SCI to support a petition by the Quakers for abolition of the slave trade in August 1783. They also reprinted Thomas Day's *Letter on the Slavery of the Negroes* (1776) because 'the practice of Negro Slavery is still shamefully countenanced and supported in some parts of the British Dominions, although directly contrary to the Spirit of the English Constitution as well as the Dictates of Christianity'.[60] Jebb also appears to have been acquainted with the young William Wilberforce, and John Disney wrote that the abolition of the slave trade 'did not fail greatly to interest the heart of Dr Jebb, on many occasions'.[61] He may have played a more active role in the campaign for abolition had he not died in 1786.

Jebb's attitude toward other social orders, women and slavery testifies his commitment to an expansion of civil rights. Yet it also indicates that he assumed some degree of 'natural' social inequality. Everyone should be treated as equal in the eyes of God and the law, be allowed to voice their opinion, and a broad range of people should be able to exercise a degree of political influence consonant with their social rank. Yet on the other side of the coin, all should

---

[55] JJ to Dr William Chambers, 16 July 1775, 'Life of Jebb', p. 94.

[56] They met and dined together on a number of occasions. GRO Sharp Diary, I, 5 June 1781, 20 December 1781, 25 April 1782, 21 March 1783.

[57] JJ to Sharp, 25 November 1776, GRO Sharp papers; Granville Sharp, *An Essay on Slavery* (Burlington, 1773; reprinted London, 1776).

[58] 17 December 1781, GRO Sharp Diary, I, p. 133.

[59] 19-22 March 1783, GRO Sharp Diary, II, p. 1.

[60] On the Quaker petition: PRO SCI Minutes II, pp. 25-26; and SCI, *Constitutional Tracts*, II, pp. 117-18. On Day's *Letter*: PRO SCI Minutes II, p. 70, 11 June 1784.

[61] Wilberforce related an anecdote regarding Jebb to Cartwright, *Life of Cartwright*, p. 164. Jebb I, p. 228.

resign themselves to fulfilling the duties of that station in which they had been placed by Providence. An examination of Jebb's attitude toward law reform further illuminates the liberal and disciplinarian aspects of his enlightened thought.

CRIME AND PUNISHMENT

According to John Disney, Jebb 'loved the study of the law, rather than the profession of it'. Yet when it became evident that his efforts to be appointed as a doctor in a London hospital would always attract powerful opposition, Jebb thought of changing profession yet again and becoming a lawyer. According to Disney, to this end 'he admitted himself of Lincoln's Inn, the 9th of November 1780'. Yet he gave up the idea and concentrated on building up his private medical practice.[62] No doubt, Jebb was daunted by the prospect of re-training for a third career at the age of forty-four after having invested so much time and effort in medical training. Nevertheless, the passing thought of becoming a lawyer further demonstrates Jebb's frustration with the political climate, and his interest in the law as a bulwark of English liberties. This section will discuss Jebb's interest in the law, his views on criminal law and punishment, and consider the debate over law and civil liberty.

The law underpinned the social and political structure of eighteenth-century Britain.[63] Differing views of jurisprudence were inextricably intertwined with, and illustrative of, social, religious, philosophical and political opinions. The interest many Rational Dissenters took in law reform is certainly understandable. As Wilfrid Prest has observed, Dissent itself 'was at very least defined, and in one sense actually created, by a body of statute law'. Thus, in light of his philosophical, religious and political interests, it is not surprising that Joseph Priestley was 'thinking along the lines of a positivist analysis of the legal and constitutional "machine of government"'.[64] It would seem that Priestley's interest in legal history and reform owed much to his determinist philosophical view.[65] For Priestley,

> the laws of a country are necessarily connected with everything belonging to the people of it; so that a thorough knowledge of them, and of their progress, would inform us of everything that was most useful to be known about them ... from the knowledge of the progress of laws, and changes of constitution, in a state, a politician may derive more useful

[62] 'Life of Jebb', pp. 159-60.

[63] Douglas Hay et. al., *Albion's Fatal Tree: crime and society in eighteenth-century England* (Harmondsworth, 1975).

[64] Wilfrid Prest, 'Law, Lawyers and Rational Dissent', in Haakonssen, *Enlightenment and Religion*, pp. 184-85.

[65] Gatrell sees Locke and Hartley's psychology of association behind many arguments against 'irrational' punishments in favour of 'reformative penal systems'. V.A.C. Gatrell, *The Hanging Tree: execution and the English people, 1770-1868* (1994), p. 328.

information, and a philosopher more rational entertainment, than from any other object he can attend to.[66]

In like manner, Jebb read Montesquieu and Beccaria while at Cambridge, and in 1773 he began to prepare a course of 'political or constitutional lectures' (which he evidently failed to complete).[67] Near the end of his life, when sick and confined to his bed, he 'studied the Saxon language, Anglo-Saxon laws, English history and antiquities, with a view to examine into our criminal code, and particular points of liberty'.[68] Finally, John Disney notes that Jebb 'had much considered the state of the criminal law in this country, and was convinced of the great necessity of a revision of the whole penal code', and encouraged Capel Lofft to publish his 'catalogue of penal statutes'.[69]

The second half of the eighteenth century witnessed increasing debate over the nature of law and punishment, and one historian has observed that 'the really giddy time for law reformers was the 1770s and 1780s'.[70] In England before 1775 the main criminal punishments included hanging, transportation, the pillory and whipping. While it was hoped that minor offenders and those in the early stages of crime could be turned back to moral and socially responsible behaviour by chastisement (such as that offered in houses of correction), it was generally assumed that serious offenders were incorrigible.[71] Yet in the years leading up to the American war there was increasing public debate over the possibility of using imprisonment with hard labour as a substitute for capital punishment in relation to all but the most serious crimes, and also to provide a means of reforming criminals. This suggestion was motivated by two broad concerns. First, the perceived increase in crime suggested that current means of punishment were failing to discourage or prevent crime. Some argued that crime was actually being encouraged by the lack of proportion between offences and punishments at both ends of the spectrum (if you have capital punishment hanging over your head for a theft, why not add murder to your list of crimes?). Second, some argued that offenders could be reformed by a combination of hard labour and imprisonment.[72]

Jebb read with approval the famous essay *On Crimes and Punishments* (1764) by the Italian Cesare Beccaria. A reference in his theological notes shows that he was familiar with Beccaria's book in the early 1770s, and he refers to 'the incomparable Beccaria' in a footnote of his *Address to Middlesex*.[73] *On Crimes and Punishments* was an enormously popular work, and Jeremy Bentham acknowledged it as one of the most stimulating and influential that he

[66] Cited in Prest, 'Law, Lawyers and Rational Dissent', p. 186.
[67] 'Life of Jebb', p. 50.
[68] 'Life of Jebb', p. 216.
[69] Attached to Jebb's *Thoughts on the Construction and Polity of Prisons* (Capel Lofft ed., 1785).
[70] Gatrell, *The Hanging Tree*, p. 326.
[71] J.M. Beattie, *Crime and the Courts in England: 1660-1800* (Princeton, 1986), pp. 422-23; Michael Ignatieff, *A Just Measure of Pain: the penitentiary in the industrial revolution, 1750-1850* (New York, 1978), pp. 24-25.
[72] Beattie, *Crime and the Courts*, p. 554.
[73] Jebb II, pp. 160, 482.

had read.[74] Beccaria judged society by the principle that the greatest number should share the greatest happiness, and it was this attitude that informed his views on the law. He combined Rousseau's sentimentalism (the love of virtue, equality and abhorrence of cruelty) with a strict rational critique of the prevailing administration of the law in European countries. Beccaria argued that the state had no business in punishing crime as both an offence against society and a sin. The Church could rail against sin, but the task of the state should be confined to the secular and utilitarian aim of repairing the damage done to an individual and society by a crime. Beccaria launched an eloquent attack on capital punishment and torture (which he wanted entirely abolished) as both an infringement on natural rights and unjustifiable in terms of utility.[75]

The push for penal reform in Britain came largely from utilitarians, radicals, evangelicals and nonconformists (in particular Quakers). While Jeremy Bentham has received much attention by historians, his influence was confined to small circles and did not become widely publicised until the 1820s. Far more important in the decades on either side of 1800 were practicing lawyers and doctors who urged penal reform, some of whom (like Jebb) were members of the Society for Constitutional Information.[76] Several lawyers supported Lindsey's Essex Street chapel: James Adair, Joshua Grigby and John Lee were MPs. There was also Sir Thomas Bernard who became a barrister in 1780, and Michael Dodson who practiced law, indulged in scripture criticism and was the subject of a 'Memoir' by John Disney.[77] Others who are not recorded as members of the Essex Street congregation, but can be considered as Rational Dissenters, included William Jones, Capel Lofft, Thomas Day, Samuel Heywood, Francis Maseres, Manasseh Dawes and George Tierney (who had been at Peterhouse under Edmund Law).[78]

Perhaps even more significant was the young Samuel Romilly (1757-1818), who was nominated as a member of the SCI by his close friend John Baynes, and seconded by Jebb.[79] In 1782 and 1783 he spent time in France and Switzerland, meeting the ageing Enlightenment sages Diderot and Benjamin Franklin.[80] He was admitted to the English bar in 1783, involved himself in the campaign against slavery and, when elected to Parliament in 1806, vigorously campaigned for reform of the criminal law. In her last years Ann Jebb was pleased to observe the efforts of 'our friend Romilly' to reform the penal code – a subject he had discussed as a young man with her husband.[81] This is attested

---

[74] Franco Venturi, *Utopia and Reform in the Enlightenment* (Cambridge, 1971), p. 101.

[75] David Young, 'Despotism and the Road to Freedom: Cesare Beccaria and Eighteenth-Century Lombardy', *Studies in Eighteenth-Century Culture*, 13 (1984), pp. 271-79.

[76] Gatrell, *Hanging Tree*, pp. 328-29.

[77] John Disney, *A Short Memoir of Michael Dodson* (1800).

[78] Prest, 'Law, Lawyers and Rational Dissent', p. 179.

[79] 7 November 1783, SCI Minute Book, II, p. 36.

[80] Diderot was 'all of warmth and eagerness, and talked to me with as little reserve as if I had been long and intimately acquainted with him. Rousseau, politics and religion were the principal topics of conversation and he inveighed with great warmth against the tyranny of the French government'. Cited in Patrick Medd, *Romilly* (1968), p. 40.

[81] Meadley, *Memoir of Ann Jebb*, pp. 45-46.

by Romilly himself when he refers to his anonymous *Observations on a late Publication, entitled, 'Thoughts on Executive Justice'* (1785) being 'highly approved' by 'a few of my friends' including Dr Jebb.[82] Romilly's target was a tract by Martin Madan, a Surrey magistrate, who had argued that a strict and severe application of the capital laws was the only way to deter criminals and decrease the number of executions in the long run.[83] Jebb thought the enormous popularity of Madan's tract in England 'a reproach to our wisdom and virtue', and may have encouraged Romilly to write his reply.[84] The latter argued that an increase in the frequency of execution would prove no greater deterrent to crime. Only one hundred copies of Romilly's tract were sold.[85] The important point for us is that Jebb was among the minority who believed that capital punishment should at least be greatly restricted, in comparison to the vast majority of educated men who continued to support public execution.

It has been claimed that the rational reformers were primarily concerned with 'the capital code's ineffectiveness, not its cruelty'.[86] Though this may be a little harsh, it is true that while Beccaria had argued for the complete abolition of capital punishment, this was not the aim of most English reformers.[87] What they could unite around (and would struggle to achieve) was reform of the seemingly wide, disproportionate, indiscriminate and frequent use of execution. Manasseh Dawes thought (in 1782, prior to the mid-1780s increase) that a decrease in public executions since the sixteenth century had been caused by the progress of 'philosophy, knowledge, and liberty', and to complete the triumph there should be an 'extinction of death as a punishment for human offences'. Yet while Dawes attacked capital punishment as homicide by society, he allowed the death penalty for murder as 'justified by holy writ and human prudence'.[88] Romilly condemned the indiscriminate use of the death penalty, but wrote: 'I confess, however, that to myself it seems absolutely impossible, even if it were to be wished (of which I am not quite sure) to omit death in the catalogue of human punishments'.[89]

In general, total abolition was not an issue. Nevertheless, among Jebb's circle capital punishment was seen, at the very best, as a necessary evil that should be employed with great care and reluctance. Cartwright dismissed a long-

---

[82] 'A few of my friends, – Baynes, Vaughan, Lord Lansdowne, Dr Jebb, Wilberforce, and Sir Gilbert Elliot, knew that the work was mine, and highly approved it'. Romilly, *Life,* I, pp. 6.

[83] Martin Madan, *Thoughts on Executive Justice* (1785).

[84] 'Life of Jebb', p. 216n.

[85] Romilly, *Life*, pp. 65-66.

[86] Gatrell, *The Hanging Tree*, p. 328.

[87] William Eden, *Principles of Penal Punishment* (1771), was a popular tract that argued that capital punishment would act as a deterrent only if employed for the most serious offences. While there is no direct evidence, Samuel Romilly (and Jebb) would almost certainly have read this work. Medd, *Romilly*, p. 210

[88] Manasseh Dawes, *An Essay on Crimes and Punishments; with a view to a commentary upon Beccaria, Rousseau, Voltaire, Montesquieu, Fielding, and Blackstone* (1782), pp. xxi, 74, 84.

[89] Samuel Romilly to Jean Roget, [?] 1784, cited in Mead, *Romilly*, p. 50.

standing servant because he attended an execution after being expressly forbidden.[90] Lofft railed against the 'vindictive jealousy' of penal laws which were calculated to protect the 'amusements of the great and wealthy' as though they were 'the very existence of society'. He condemned the uneven, inconsistent, and irrational nature of laws that were too often applied to innocent and helpless sufferers, or those who had committed trifling crimes. 'The laws as they are', declared Lofft, 'will not be executed with that constancy which is indispensable to ensure their observance. Indeed, certainty of punishment does appear essential to sound policy: but reasonableness in the kind and degree of punishment allotted to offences must first be established, and the community satisfied that it is, before that certainty can produce the proper effect, or be reconciled to justice and humanity.'[91] In 1800 Lofft was removed from the magistracy for 'improper interference' in the case of a young servant girl condemned to death for petty theft.[92]

Jebb joined with his lawyer friends in desiring that the penal code be reformed, and told a friend that 'I carry my ideas further than many men on these subjects. The sufferings of Human creatures are made too familiar by the practice of most legislatures.'[93] Ann Jebb became completely opposed to capital punishment. In 1792 she expressed the belief that the death penalty was 'a punishment so contrary to the principles and the feelings of many in this age, that I trust that the time will soon arrive, when it will be totally abolished from our courts of justice'.[94]

A desire for greater use of imprisonment accompanied arguments for reform of the penal code, and this in turn led to calls for prison reform. Minds were concentrated on the issue of prison reform by two things: the American Revolution abruptly terminated the major outlet for transported convicts, and there was increasing concern about the dangers of 'gaol fever' spreading to the wider community.[95] One of the most important figures who helped justify, explain, increase and improve the practice of imprisonment was the nonconformist philanthropist, John Howard. During the mid-1770s he visited every prison and house of correction in England, many on the Continent, and often at great danger to his health. The result was a detailed description of the appalling and inhumane conditions within English prisons. Howard presented abundant evidence that the entire system needed an overhaul: prisons must be cleaned up, their social structures reorganised and provided with medical and religious attention. Most important, the prisons and their administrators should be subjected to regular and independent inspection to ensure the maintenance of standards. He wanted nothing less than a lasting 'reformation' of the prison

---

[90] *Life of Cartwright*, pp. 162-63

[91] John Jebb, *Thoughts on the Construction and Polity of Prisons* (Capel Lofft ed., 1786), pp. vi, x, 34-5, 95, cited in Gatrell, *Hanging Tree*, pp. 343-44.

[92] Gatrell, *Hanging Tree*, pp. 340-53.

[93] 'Life of Jebb', p. 213; JJ to Francis Dobbs, 5 October 1783, NLI Dobbs papers.

[94] AJ, *Two Penny-worth More of Truth for a Penny* (26 January 1793), p. 14.

[95] Robin Evans, *The Fabrication of Virtue: English prison architecture, 1750-1840* (Cambridge, 1982), pp. 94-117.

system.[96] Along with Jonas Hanway, Howard made believable the idea that prisons were a feasible alternative form of punishment, capable of reforming criminals. Their writings were influential because they outlined how cruel, filthy, disease-ridden institutions could be cleaned up and regulated, and emphasised the possibility of reforming criminals by teaching them basic Christian principles. The unregulated filth and brutality of prisons could be done away with, the reformers argued, and in a disciplined and healthy environment moral fetters could be applied to the mind.[97]

Traditionally historians have used Howard's writings as an accurate description of the eighteenth-century prison: that reform begun in the 1770s brought improvement to squalid institutions essentially unchanged from medieval times. Yet the history of prisons has attracted considerable interest from radical historians in recent decades. Many have argued that rational reform of prisons was not really an improvement for those incarcerated, as it was part of a plot by the increasingly powerful middle class to mould, control, and confine the lower orders of society.[98] Others have questioned the traditional picture of the eighteenth-century prison, pointing out that many prisons functioned well in an eighteenth-century context and that there was often improvement made at a local level before the era of reform.[99] Whatever the outcome of such debates, it is sufficient for present purposes to say that Jebb's views were expressed in the context of a generally increasing interest in reforming the prison system as a means of both punishing and reforming prisoners.

Howard's work has been described as a 'landmark in the history of social welfare', and was recognised as such by his contemporaries.[100] The young Samuel Romilly praised Howard's book as one of those that 'have been rare in all ages of the world – being written with a view only to the good of mankind'.[101] And Jebb's friend and former student, John Baynes, recommended *On the State of the Prisons* to Benjamin Franklin as 'one of our best printed books'.[102]

In 1785 Capel Lofft published Jebb's *Thoughts on the Construction and Polity of Prisons*, which had been inspired by Howard's 'immortal work' – a book Jebb thought 'at once the strongest exhibition of philanthropy since the

---

[96] John Howard, *The State of the Prisons in England and Wales, with preliminary observations, and an account of some foreign prisons and hospitals* (1929 [1777-80]), p. xxi.

[97] Beattie, *Crime and the Courts*, pp. 568-69.

[98] The most influential exponent of this view was Michel Foucault, particularly his *Discipline and Punish* (1977 [French edn. 1975]). See also, Ignatieff, *A Just Measure of Pain*.

[99] Margaret DeLacy, *Prison Reform in Lancashire, 1750-1850: a study in local administration* (Manchester, 1986).

[100] Langford, *A Polite and Commercial People*, p. 487.

[101] W. Peter, *The Speeches of Sir Samuel Romilly in the House of Commons* (1820), vol. I., p. 29.

[102] John Baynes, 'Journal', in Romilly, *Life*, p. 457.

foundation of our religion, and the severest satire on the species'.[103] Jebb felt that he could make some practical suggestions regarding the layout of prisons 'suggested principally by observations' made in the course of his medical practice.[104] Jebb agreed that regular inspection was needed to relieve prisoners from 'the tyranny of their keepers, and other severities' associated with their condition – indeed, like Howard, he thought the 'grand obstacle' to the improvement of prisons was 'the infrequency of their inspection'.[105] As a doctor, Jebb was concerned that 'the health of persons confined cannot be consulted in any tolerable measure'. As noted in chapter 7, there was a growing interest in the relationship between environment and disease, and prisons were considered one of the most prominent examples of the connection between dirty, cramped conditions and the generation and spread of 'fevers'.[106] The 'lofty walls and iron doors', Jebb wrote, 'enclose disease, as well as misery of other kinds, which prevents the compassionate' from inspecting the prisons or helping 'lessen the calamities of confinement'. He wanted to see prisons transformed from places where criminals were locked away, ignored, and left to rot by society, into places were the necessary period of confinement would not be unendurable, and could even contribute to reforming the character of the inmates.

Jebb made a number of practical recommendations to improve the construction of prisons around the theme of preventing the spread of disease caused by miasma and contagion. Prisons should be 'ventilated frequently, by currents of fresh air moving freely in a horizontal direction' in order to 'remove the bad effects of that stagnation of air and accumulation of putrid effluvia from living bodies'. He thought Howard's suggestion of positioning prisons at a distance from other buildings, on elevated ground and with a stream of running water was 'certainly preferable to the present practice of erecting them in the closest part of towns'. Yet this would be to little avail if the prison were still constructed with four high walls that would trap the putrid air within. Jebb's solution to this problem was to surround the prison with a 'dry moat, with shelving sides, covered with grass' approximately thirty feet deep, with a wall rising from the bottom of the moat to level with the surface. 'Thus would the security at present aimed at by the high walls, be still enjoyed, without their numerous inconveniences'. Jebb agreed with Howard's suggestion that the

[103] Howard, *The State of the Prisons*; Jebb II, p. 558. John Disney wrote in his diary: 'Received Mr Howard's third edition of his State of the Prisons, a present from the author'. John Disney, 'Diary', 30 April 1784.

[104] Jebb II, pp. 558-59.

[105] For this and the following see *Thoughts on the Construction and Polity of Prisons*, Jebb II, pp. 557-68.

[106] Howard does not seem to have been concerned with contagion to any real degree. He thought that the putrid and malignant air was unhealthy for the convicts, but he had noticed some foreign prisons that were just as dirty and cramped as those in England, where 'gaol-fever' was unknown. He thought that gaol-fever was caused more by 'the sudden change in diet and lodging [which] so affects the spirits of new convicts, that the general causes of putrid fevers exert an immediate effect upon them'. It was the treatment of prisoners in England (being clamped in irons, deprived of food and clothing, and kept in idleness) that made them sickly. Howard, *State of the Prisons*, pp. 4, 258-59.

compound itself should consist of separate buildings two stories high and not more than 'six or eight apartments' each. With respect of the issue of security, Jebb felt that too much emphasis had been placed on the construction of stone prisons with 'mechanical expedients to guard against escape'. He felt that a better and less costly approach would be to construct separate, more spacious brick buildings 'into whose recesses the eye of vigilance can penetrate with greater ease'. The emphasis should be on 'a judicious mode of conducting their internal polity'. Good lighting, regular patrols and a system of alarms would 'afford more real security, with less expense, and less injury to the feelings of humanity' than the prevalent prison structure. 'Let us imitate nature', Jebb urged, 'she effects her purposes by the simplest means'.[107]

Jebb was wary of the danger of oppressive and authoritarian practices being instituted by prison warders. Following Howard, he argued that 'the utmost care should be taken, that the restraint of liberty, even in the case of the most atrocious crimes, should be as mild as circumstances will admit: that the establishment of the proper rules and orders, and the mode of carrying them into execution, should be entirely under the control of the magistrates and the gentlemen of the district.'[108] There should be no involvement of the army, and the 'tyranny or over-bearing influence of any man, or set of men, who hold their appointment from the crown' should be guarded against. Any introduction of the French system of police should be avoided at all costs as it would lead to a situation where 'liberty, the choicest gift of heaven to man, without which no other blessing can convey real enjoyment to the rational mind, should be impaired, perhaps, totally destroyed'. To guard against any abuse of power by prison officials, Jebb suggested a model taken from his experience as a supervisor of a workhouse in rural Suffolk. Each prison should have a spacious committee room, available for weekly meetings involving a rotating selection of 'the principal gentry, clergy, and tenantry, in the county', who would supervise conditions. Jebb assured his readers that no one would complain 'of the fatigue of attendance' as they would take 'pleasure in the discharge of so useful an employment'. By this means, the functioning prison would be under constant and independent scrutiny.

Jebb hoped that improving the structure and governance of prisons in this way would ensure that 'the feelings of humanity, at present wounded by every reflection upon the complicated sufferings endured in these melancholy mansions, be effectually consulted, without offering the minutest injury to substantial justice'. The tract on prison reform was written during one of the frequent bouts of ill health that plagued Jebb prior to his death. It was published and distributed by Capel Lofft in the county of Suffolk in 1785, as part of a successful campaign to have an antiquated gaol demolished and replaced with a

---

[107] Howard, *State of the Prisons*, pp. 19-45. As always Jebb professed a modest and empiricist stance: 'With respect to the specific regulations of internal polity, I do not presume to give a formal opinion: being conscious that much must depend upon experiment, and that my habits of life do not enable me to point out the form that would be most expedient'. *Thoughts on ... Prisons*, Jebb II, p. 564.

[108] *Thoughts on ... Prisons*, Jebb II, p. 564.

larger and cleaner prison.[109] The idea of a dry moat was not adopted for any prison, but was used in a lunatic asylum at Wakefield.[110] Lofft printed posthumously a second edition with Jebb's revisions for a wider audience in 1786.[111] While of minor significance in terms of its impact, this tract provides a valuable insight into the character and limitations of radical thought in the early 1780s. Such views on penal reform were inseparable from the wider agenda of political reform, as indicated by Capel Lofft when he declared that 'the people of this country will remember, that unequal severity in the laws is always either consequent or preparatory to despotism in the constitution.'[112] In short, Jebb's views on crime and punishment reflect his social, religious and political attitudes.

JURIES AND LIBEL

There was one legal debate that bore an immediate relation to the preservation of liberty, and that was the rights and duties of juries in regard to trials for libel. In 1783 the SCI involved itself in a celebrated court case that revolved around the issue of freedom of speech and the rights of juries. William Shipley, the Dean of St Asaph, published a Welsh edition of *A Dialogue between a Scholar and a Peasant* by William Jones – a brief appeal for universal manhood suffrage. In response, Welsh conservatives tried to persuade the government to prosecute for seditious libel. When the administration refused, another William Jones, a solicitor from Ruthin, Denbighshire, undertook a private prosecution for seditious libel in April 1783.[113] The SCI responded by devoting most of its attention to the case; it resolved to print another 3,000 copies of the *Dialogue*, sought legal endorsement for their publications from sympathetic MPs and raised a fund of 270 pounds to publicise the case.[114] Richard Brocklesby and Thomas Oldfield were sent into Denbighshire to distribute SCI publications to vindicate Shipley and, if possible, divert the prosecution onto itself as the original publisher, for which a trial would be held in London. Among the publications distributed were extracts from Joseph Towers' *British Biography* on John Lilburne and Judge Jefferies, which argued that juries should be judges of law as well as fact. The Society devoted much attention to this prosecution which dragged on for one and a half years; and rightly so, as this was, according to Thomas Green, 'unquestionably ... the most important seditious libel prosecution since the *Seven Bishops' Case*'.[115]

---

[109] Richard H. Condon, 'Capel Lofft', *BDMBR* I, p. 298.
[110] Evans, *Fabrication of Virtue*, p. 113; Charles Watson and James P. Pritchett, *Plans etc. and Description of the Pauper Lunatic Asylum* (York, 1819).
[111] 'Life of Jebb', pp. 217-18.
[112] Capel Lofft, Appendix to Jebb, *Thoughts on ... Prisons*, pp. 36-7
[113] Black, *Association*, pp. 197-98.
[114] PRO SCI Minutes II/961, pp. 7-8.
[115] Thomas Green, *Verdict According to Conscience: perspectives on the English criminal trial jury, 1200-1800* (Chicago, 1985), p. 328.

At the opening of the trial the prosecution argued that no unprejudiced jury could be selected in Denbighshire because of the Society's campaign. The judge responded by shifting the case to the Shrewsbury Assizes, where it was finally tried before Francis Buller of the Court of King's Bench on 6 August 1784. The eloquent trial lawyer Thomas Erskine had lent Shipley his services and turned in one of his best performances, but Buller summed up strongly against Shipley, declaring that the tract was a libel. The jury, however, having been won over by Erskine, brought in a verdict of 'guilty of publishing only'. Lord Mansfield, who upheld Buller's decision as conforming to judicial practice since the Revolution, rejected an appeal for a new trial. Shipley was eventually granted an 'arrest of judgement' based on the insufficiency of the indictment and the findings.

The case re-ignited a debate occasioned by the prosecution of John Wilkes for publishing the *North Briton*. Jebb's opinions on libel are expressed in an anonymous public letter 'To Mr Justice Buller' dated 8 September 1784. According to Jebb, the position of the bench 'that the truth of a libel is an aggravation of the guilt incurred by its publication, rests upon the idea, that this composition derives its criminality from its tendency to produce a breach of the peace; an idea, originating in feudal principles, and altogether foreign to the just object and end of punishment in this instance.' Jebb stated his position clearly: 'the freedom of the press, which is the bulwark of English liberties, cannot be duly exercised, unless every individual be allowed to freely canvass the public actions of public men'. In light of this he felt that Buller's 'doctrine' should be condemned. To illustrate the issue, Jebb explained that if he misrepresented the 'fact' of Buller's conduct at the trial, he would be guilty of injustice and 'liable to the proper censure'. If, however, 'I justly state the fact, but err in my inferences, my judgement may be called in question, but my person ought to be secure from prosecution'. And if he both accurately reported and assessed the situation, then he would earn the approbation of his 'fellow-citizens', and 'an impartial and duly informed jury of my countrymen' would protect him from any prosecution 'openly or secretly encouraged by the friends of despotism'.[116]

That the system did not work this way was evidenced by Buller's conduct in the Shipley case.[117] Jebb asked Buller why he repeatedly refused to record the jury's verdict of 'guilty of publishing *only*', and insisted upon recording it as 'guilty of publishing this libel'. 'Surely', Jebb asked, 'as they neither found that the pamphlet was a libel, nor any criminal intention in the publisher, it was fair for you to conclude, that it was their intention to acquit the defendant.' Jebb admitted that the jury did not appeal to the discretion of the court according to 'the 13th of E.1.c.30, whereby the jury, doubting of the complexion of the fact, are permitted, in a particular instance, to find a special verdict, more properly styled a "verdict, at large"'. But that they expressly insisted on the inclusion of the word 'only' means they definitely rejected 'every idea of guilt'. Buller could have either honestly interpreted the jury's decision,

[116] Jebb III, pp. 368-76.

[117] For a narrative of the trial, see James Oldham, *The Mansfield Manuscripts* (Chapel Hill, N.C., 1992), pp. 794-800.

or allowed them to leave the court to reconsider their verdict (presumably with access to legal advice). Then the outcome may have been similar to the trial of William Penn in 1670 for preaching to an unlawful assembly. In this case the jury confined itself to finding Penn guilty of 'preaching to an assembly'. When the judge refused to accept this they changed their verdict to 'not guilty' and the case was concluded.[118]

The Shipley case testifies to the perceived importance of trial by jury as a bulwark of civil liberty. In August 1783 Jebb chaired a meeting of the SCI that resolved that in order to preserve liberty of the press, 'British Juries should be well acquainted with the powers with which the Constitution has invested them, especially in prosecutions for libels'.[119] Jebb had 'some apprehensions' regarding the Foxite suggestion of a declaratory law respecting juries: this stemmed from his fear that defining and setting rights down in legislation would also limit them. Rather, he hoped that Parliament would legislate to require 'that in all criminal cases, the jury be obliged, not barely permitted, to find a general verdict'. Again Jebb expressed his concern with the duties of citizenship: the jury 'should never be permitted to find the truth of indifferent facts, and leave the legal complexion of those facts to the justices; for by such conduct they, in fact, desert their charge, and deliver up their fellow-citizen, who has put himself upon their judgement for good and evil, to the professional prejudices of men, who, not being sworn to the specific case, cannot have their feelings much alive.'[120] Jebb also thought that libel should be considered a civil case, and payment of damages the only penalty.[121]

The Shipley case provoked a flurry of pamphlets. The main contribution by the SCI was a tract by Joseph Towers, which set forth in greater detail the same arguments that Jebb had urged against Justice Buller.[122] This debate culminated in Fox's Libel Act of 1792, which finally granted to the jury the right to find the fact of libel as well as the fact of publication. Thus a reform was accomplished by legislation that Lord Mansfield could have made by granting a re-trial and directing the jury to consider the 'whole matter'. Calls for reform were neither unreasonable nor unrealistic. While Mansfield was known for modernising the law in his commercial decisions, he did not carry this spirit over into the realm of politics. Mansfield was a conservative who considered the tracts published by the SCI to be seditious. As James Oldham has observed, 'the position taken by Fox, Camden, Erskine – the position that ultimately prevailed

[118] Jebb drew this from a tract he wished the Shipley jury had read: Sir John Hawles, *The Englishman's Right, a dialogue between a Barrister at Law and a Jury-man* (1752 [1680]).

[119] PRO SCI Minutes II, p. 22.

[120] 'Life of Jebb', p. 212.

[121] 'Life of Jebb', p. 213.

[122] Joseph Towers, *Observations on the Rights and Duty of Juries in trials for libels* (1784). This tract was presented to the SCI 3 Dec. 1884. SCI Minute Book, II, p. 89; F.K. Donnelly, 'Joseph Towers and the Collapse of Rational Dissent', *E&D*, 6 (1987), p. 33.

– was not merely a differing view of the jury function; it was a differing vision of government'.[123]

Though his contribution in terms of publications was small, Jebb took an active interest in law reform and encouraged young friends like Lofft and Romilly in their work. His attitude to the law and its administration further reveals the compassionate aspect of his rational piety, and his habit of combining natural rights and utilitarian arguments in the cause of both rational reform and the defence of perceived ancient English liberties. It also reflects his position as a self-conscious representative of the middle classes.

[123] Oldham, *Mansfield Manuscripts*, II, p. 808.

11

Democratic Agents

> We are agents for the democratical part of the constitution, and … it is not reasonable to expect that we shall be strenuously supported by the nobility, unless when the common danger shall become extreme.[1]

The first half of the 1780s witnessed one of the most turbulent periods in the history of the English Parliament. After the initial flurry of agitation in 1780, the various out-of-doors organisations struggled to revive interest in parliamentary reform. Indeed, Jebb and his fellow radicals might have fallen silent had it not been for a series of political crises. These centred on the problem of finding a prime minister who had both the support of George III and a working majority in the Commons. In the course of these high political tussles, Rockingham, Charles James Fox and William Pitt the Younger at various times courted the support of the reformers.

The reformers, however, were fatally divided between the moderate platform of Christopher Wyvill's Yorkshire Association, and the more radical but less broadly appealing proposals doggedly espoused by Jebb's metropolitan radicals. While historians have long recognised his prominent role in the extra-parliamentary reform movement, Jebb has been characterised as an inflexible extremist.[2] Jebb himself explained that 'I am supposed by many, too pertinacious in my sentiments, and have by some, of what are called moderate men, been called *impractical*; but I do not repent. I labour in the first place to explore political truth; when found, I avow it, support it, diffuse it, act upon it, and never renounce it.'[3] Rather than dismiss his conduct as naïve, Jebb's political activities need to be seen as deeply rooted in his radical Enlightenment convictions.

---

[1] *Letter to Sir Robert Bernard*, Jebb II, p. 512.
[2] Christie, *Wilkes, Wyvill and Reform*, pp. 115, 199.
[3] JJ to Archibald Hamilton Rowan, 29 September 1785, *Autobiography of Archibald Hamilton Rowan*, p. 130.

POLITICAL INSTABILITY, 1780-84

Despite the best efforts of the opposition, Lord North preserved his ministry through skilful parliamentary management in 1780 (see chapter 8). Jebb was not surprised at the parliamentary defeat of Burke's 'economical reform'. Buoyed by the establishment of the Society for Constitutional Information, he remained confident that substantial reform would eventuate. In mid-May he told Wyvill:

> the friends of Mr Burke cry out the affair is over, nothing but despondency reigns among them, and they dispirit the troops amazingly. I own I think everything looks well. You and I were from the beginning persuaded that the Influence of the Crown would not be diminished by the instrumentality of that Body which was the very object of that influence.[4]

The mood of the nation remained one of disaffection. The staunch Whig Samuel Kenrick informed his friend in Scotland that 'all the world I see seem greatly dissatisfied with our now governors and their measures: and seem all to apprehend some dreadful resolution, if not impending ruin of the country'.[5]

At the start of summer some of this dissatisfaction found a dramatic outlet in the form of crowd violence. On a warm Friday 2 June, thousands of members of the Protestant Association marched on the House of Commons to present a petition against the Catholic Relief Act. The four columns swelled as they converged on the Parliament, where the crowd began to jostle and assault the arriving MPs. For the next week London witnessed widespread rioting in which houses were burned and looted, prisoners liberated and distilleries raided. In particular, prominent Catholics and supporters of religious toleration like Sir George Savile were singled out, and the Essex Street chapel was lucky to be spared.[6] Enlightened sensibilities were given a rude shock, with Edward Gibbon exclaiming that 'forty thousand Puritans, as they might have been in the time of Cromwell, have started out of their graves'.[7] 'No Popery' demonstrations and civil disturbances flared in several provincial towns.[8]

For those advocating universal suffrage it was a public-relations disaster. Twenty years on, Capel Lofft blamed the failure of reform in 1780 on

---

[4] 'I hold to my old doctrine', he continued, 'and what others lament, viz. the weakness of our Power in the House of Commons, gives me wonderful content. The eyes of all must open in due time, they must see that nothing but Annual Parliaments &c will effect our great work'. JJ to Christopher Wyvill, 13 May 1780, NYRO Wyvill mss.

[5] Samuel Kenrick to James Wodrow, 12 May 1780, DWL Wodrow-Kenrick correspondence.

[6] Theophilus Lindsey to William Tayleur, 10 June 1780, in H. McLachlan, 'More Letters of Theophilus Lindsey', *Transactions of the Unitarian Historical Society,* 3 (1923-26), p. 365; John Stevenson, *Popular Disturbances in England 1700-1870* (1979), pp. 76-90; Haydon, *Anti-Catholicism*, pp. 204-44. For an entertaining account of the riots see Christopher Hibbert, *King Mob* (1959).

[7] Cited in Roy Porter, *Gibbon: making history* (1988), p. 133.

[8] Colin Haydon, 'The Gordon Riots in the English Provinces', *Historical Research,* 63 (1990), pp. 354-59.

the 'savage outcry against Popery'.[9] With thousands surrounding the Houses of Parliament on the first day, abusing and assaulting peers as they arrived, the Duke of Richmond persisted with a speech in favour of annual parliaments, and tried depict the riots as a response to the Quebec Act, rather than as a protest against toleration of Catholics within Britain.[10] But, in the words of Lecky, 'no serious discussion was possible. Pale, bruised and agitated, with their wigs torn off, their hair dishevelled, their clothes torn and bespattered with mud, the peers of England sat listening to the frantic yells of the multitude who already thronged the lobbies'.[11]

The general response of the reformers was to attribute this wild outburst of plebeian anger to the ignorance and corruption they were trying to combat. As the crowd began to thin in the evening, Jebb, Brand Hollis and five other members of the SCI met at a tavern in the Strand and decided to print five hundred subscription sheets and two thousand ballot papers. The following week, with the rioting in full swing, they resolved to print four thousand copies of Cartwright's *Declaration of Those Rights of the Commonality of Great Britain without Which They Cannot Be Free* – a vivid illustration of how they perceived themselves as middle-class thinkers who were duty bound to enlighten the ignorant and deluded masses.[12] The Society tried to ignore the riots as much as possible, and eighteen months later printed *On the Legal Mode of Suppressing Riots* (1781) by William Jones. He argued that citizen militias were the only way of reconciling political liberty and the need to preserve law and order. Indeed, for committed Whigs the worst consequence of the riots was the excuse they gave for the use of a standing army.[13]

Lord North took advantage of the conservative mood that swept the country following the riots, and called an election for September 1780. The campaign was hard fought, with 'party' contests in half of the electorates. The North ministry was returned with a slightly reduced majority, but still reliant upon the support of independents. As E.C. Black has pointed out, 'the same House would support North, then Rockingham, Shelburne, Fox and North, and the younger Pitt'. The Associations campaigned hard and won Yorkshire, Westminster, Kent, Middlesex, Surrey and Gloucester.[14] During the campaign Jebb tried to keep the issue of parliamentary reform alive with an address 'To the People of England' under the pseudonym 'Alfred'. 'Full of anxious apprehensions for my country', he pleaded with the people to use the dissolution of parliament as an opportunity to pursue 'any plan which shall be proposed for

---

[9] Capel Lofft, *On the Revival of the Cause of Reform in the Representation of the Commons House of Parliament* (1809), p. 9.

[10] Hibbert, *King Mob*, pp. 51-52, 64.

[11] W.E.H. Lecky, *History of England in the Eighteenth Century* (1892), IV, p. 311.

[12] On 9 June they decided to print four thousand copies of the *Declaration of Rights*. PRO SCI Minutes, I, pp. 12-14.

[13] Ian McCalman, 'Mad Lord George and Madame La Motte: riot and sexuality in the genesis of Burke's *Reflections on the Revolution in France*', *Journal of British Studies*, 35 (1996), p. 356.

[14] Black, *Association*, pp. 73-74.

your deliverance', and warned that the cause of reform would be greatly hurt if a new septennial parliament were elected.[15] The SCI distributed two thousand copies of the *Report of the Westminster Subcommittee*, but lapsed into a period of malaise following North's victory.

The Associations had played an important and moderately successful role in preventing the government from obtaining a comfortable majority. Yet the result fell far short of Jebb's unrealistic expectations. 'The present Parliament will, in all probability, on the first day of its meeting give us a foretaste of what we are to expect the ensuing seven years', Jebb wrote, 'or, in other words, it will be as venal as the last.'[16] All England looks to Yorkshire at this moment', Jebb wrote challengingly to Wyvill after the election.[17] The latter, however, was becoming a political realist and cautioned against 'engaging with any new matter' until success was more probable.[18] Through the independent Whigs George Savile and Lord Mahon, Wyvill was quietly trying to court Rockingham's support for economical reform and the introduction of one hundred county members, while leaving the duration of parliaments untouched. Sensitive to the direction in which Wyvill was leaning, Jebb warned him that Burke's economical reform bill 'does not suit my idea. Moving the People of England to carry so small a reform, would be tempesting the ocean to drown a fly'.[19]

While courting the Rockingham Whigs, Wyvill was also trying to unite the extra-parliamentary reformers behind his plan for an additional one hundred county representatives and triennial parliaments.[20] But Jebb was also actively promoting his own cause. The ever-watchful William Cole observed: 'At this time Jan: 1781 [Jebb is] an active man with Sir Robert Bernard and the Huntingdonshire Patriots and Associators, corresponding with the committees of Westminster in favour of Rebellion and Confusion, the harvest of such Patriots.'[21]

A second convention of Association delegates was held at Guildhall in early March, but agreement on a specific program proved impossible. Jebb unsuccessfully moved that if one hundred county members were to be added to the Commons, then the same number of borough seats should be abolished. He followed this with equally unsuccessful motions for annual parliaments and universal manhood suffrage. Eventually a generally worded petition calling for economical and parliamentary reform was adopted and subsequently rejected by the House of Commons. In light of his earlier criticism of petitions as ineffectual, Jebb felt compelled to publish a tract explaining that he had endorsed the petition in the hope that if it were rejected popular interest in an

---

[15] 'Alfred' [JJ], 'To the People of England', Jebb III, pp. 285-89.
[16] JJ to Christopher Wyvill, 14 October 1780, *Wyvill Papers,* IV, p. 495.
[17] JJ to Christopher Wyvill, 14 October 1780, *Wyvill Papers,* IV, p. 495.
[18] Christopher Wyvill to JJ, 18 November 1780, *Wyvill Papers,* IV, p. 498.
[19] JJ to Christopher Wyvill, 19 December 1780, *Wyvill Papers,* IV, p. 500.
[20] Christopher Wyvill, *Address to the Electors of Great Britain* (January 1781). This was published on behalf of the Yorkshire Association.
[21] BL Cole papers 5873:71.

extensive reform of Parliament would be revived.[22] Yet public interest in reform remained at low ebb. For most of 1781 poorly attended Westminster Committee meetings were only held monthly.

When Jebb was invited to give advice to the Irish reformers in 1783, he was adamant that petitioning Parliament would be to no avail.[23] In the meantime the argument against petitions had been advanced in an important work of political philosophy by the deist David Williams.[24] A reviewer was led to declare: 'It is ... our duty to observe that Dr Jebb has done him [Williams] the honour to adopt some of his opinions; but without any proper acknowledgement'. Some years later Williams himself observed that the advice given to the Irish revealed that some English reformers had converted to his view.[25] This, however, was unfair. Jebb had been sceptical about petitions since the failure of the Feathers Tavern, and he had sought to justify his signing of the 1781 petition in his *Letter to Sir Robert Bernard.* Williams was not afraid of making enemies if it would promote the appearance of his being independent. He had addressed his *Letters* to James Martin, a reform-minded member of parliament who had recently been elected as president of the SCI. Williams indicated that Martin had doubts about the prospects of the reform movement. Not surprisingly, while Martin presented the SCI with a copy of the *Letters*, it did not distribute any of Williams's writings.[26] Though this may also be attributed, no doubt, to his express opinion that the constitution that had so impressed Montesquieu was 'one of the most awkward and unmanageable fabrics which has ever been produced by human folly'.[27]

Wyvill continued to lobby Jebb in the hope that he would eventually work with political reality, but their fundamental differences only became more apparent. Because of the 'present despondence of the People', Wyvill suggested that the next move would 'depend upon circumstances; and amongst others chiefly on the appearance of a better and more general support next winter'. But, he reminded Jebb, they were opposed by 'a large body of persons who are from interests or prejudices of various kinds averse to a Parliamentary Reform, however much they may complain of a Corruption of Parliament'. And he warned that if the radicals did not support his moderate plan the county Associations would 'grow tired of a contest so evidently unavailing, and dissolve themselves'.[28]

A strongly worded reply from Jebb reveals the deep division between the London and Yorkshire reformers. He urged Wyvill to stop looking forward to support from the Rockingham Whigs in the winter session. 'Strange', he

---

[22] *A Letter to Sir Robert Bernard, Chairman of the Huntingdonshire Committee* (1781), Jebb II, pp. 493-516. Written 13 May 1781.

[23] *Address to the Volunteers of Ireland*, Jebb II, p. 525.

[24] David Williams, *Letters on Political Liberty* (3rd ed., 1789 [1782]).

[25] Review cited in Dybikowski, *On Burning Ground*, p. 309; Williams, *Letters on Political Liberty*, pp. 114-15.

[26] SCI Minutes I, 19 April 1782; Dybikowski, *On Burning Ground*, pp. 160-61.

[27] Cited in Dybikowski, 'David Williams and Civil and Political Liberty', p. 25.

[28] Christopher Wyvill to JJ, 5 June 1781, *Wyvill Papers*, IV, pp. 149-52.

reflected, 'that it shall be allowed to the Representative to make every innovation in the constitution that selfishness and treason can suggest, at the same time that we hesitate whether the Constituent has a right to reform what the villainy of the Servant hath deranged.' He was dissatisfied with the Yorkshire plan for an addition of one hundred county members, and observed that Burke had been able to ridicule the proposal as a declaration that 'the House of Commons is not sufficiently numerous'. 'I must cordially confess', Jebb wrote, 'that I for one would never have subjected myself to the losses, odium, and anxiety I have suffered, if I had imagined that the Friends of Reformation could have been satisfied with so defective a plan.' He had compromised his position enough already by endorsing the Association petition: 'through a desire of promoting uniformity, not very handsomely requited, I have assented to partial measures, and have been content to use the language of servility to a Tribunal which at the moment I esteemed corrupt'. Jebb was now firmly convinced that 'the spirit of accommodation will ruin all' and that the constitution could 'never be restored gradatium'. Negotiations with the aristocratic opposition were useless because they would never agree to a 'reasonable compensation' for the loss of their 'Borough Interest, until compelled thereto by the Power of the People'.[29]

In response Wyvill restated his belief that without support from the parliamentary opposition, reform was impossible – or at least impossible 'without the hazards of a Civil War'. Their disagreement was fundamental and he suggested that 'it were to no purpose to press any farther consideration of the subject'.[30] But Jebb was not to be put off so easily. Glad that 'we may differ, and yet preserve the utmost mutual regard', he assured Wyvill that Lord Mahon's efforts to strike a compromise between the Yorkshire Association and the Rockingham Whigs would fail, and added that the 'Friends of Liberty in London' placed 'shortened Parliaments ... in the front rank of Reformation measures'.[31] In a subsequent letter Jebb again criticised the aristocracy, declaring that 'family prejudices such as those in Devonshire, &c. do mischief'. John Dunning (a supporter of Lord Shelburne) and Brand Hollis had led Devonshire into the Association movement in 1780, but Dunning and his supporters had backed away when Brand Hollis began to circulate radical SCI pamphlets in the county.[32]

Lord North's government was in trouble following news of the defeat at Yorktown in October 1781. While George III was forcing his prime minister to continue the war, petitions were being drawn up calling for peace. Jebb was delighted, and observed that 'other measures are scheming if remonstrance fails

[29] JJ to Christopher Wyvill, 7 August 1781, *Wyvill Papers*, IV, pp. 501-07.
[30] Christopher Wyvill to JJ, 27 August 1781, *Wyvill Papers*, IV, pp. 508-09.
[31] It is interesting to note that in reminding Wyvill that the 'friends of Liberty in London' place 'shortened parliaments ... in the front rank of reformation measures', he originally wrote 'annual' but crossed it out and wrote 'shortened'. JJ to Christopher Wyvill, 27 September 1781, NYRO Wyvill mss.
[32] JJ to Christopher Wyvill, 27 November 1781, *Wyvill Papers*, IV, pp. 512-14.

– all within the line of peaceable opposition'.[33] On 10 December the republican Sylas Neville attended 'a meeting of Westminster voters in the Hall to agree to a petition & remonstrance. Fox & my friend Jebb harangued the multitude, but there was so much noise & moving about that I could not hear what they said, but we shall have it all in the *Courant* tomorrow. The present powers have certainly brought us into a fine situation. How we are to get out, Heaven knows'.[34] Later in the month Jebb suggested that should the county militia be called upon to expand, the SCI should emphasise a link between bearing arms and the right to vote – 'distress will force the doctrine we think just upon the public ear.' A popularly elected national convention could force the King and House of Lords to agree to parliamentary reform by refusing to pay their taxes.[35] At this time Jebb was busy organising the Quintuple Alliance, a confederation of the London, Westminster, Southwark, Middlesex and Surrey Associations. This was intended to provide the metropolitan radicals with an extra-parliamentary body that could upstage Wyvill's Yorkshire Association.[36]

When Wyvill published his *Political Papers* in 1794 he added a substantial note explaining his relationship with Jebb. While they had remained friends, their 'correspondence was too frequently controversial'. In hindsight Wyvill regretted that he had initially encouraged a suspicious disposition toward the parliamentary opposition, and lamented the inflexibility of the radicals. He had struggled to inspire county support for moderate reform, 'yet the popular Agents in London still protracted discussion, still pressed Yorkshire to advance to more extended changes; not perceiving that these dissentions weakened Yorkshire, without adding to their strength'. The root cause of his disagreements with Jebb, he confessed, was that he had always opposed the idea of electing a national convention to force reform upon the House of Commons. It was 'a proposition totally incompatible with any plan of moderate Reform, and pregnant with hazards to which his too-speculative Friend had not sufficiently adverted'.[37]

The contest in the Commons in early 1782 has been described as one of the 'high points in parliamentary history'.[38] George III refused to enter into peace negotiations with the Americans and Lord North was put in the impossible position of defending an unpopular policy with which he also disagreed. His majority was gradually whittled away until it disappeared and he presented an angry king with his resignation on 20 March. George III was forced to accept an administration headed by Rockingham, with Shelburne and Fox as the principal secretaries of state.[39]

Jebb always distrusted the Rockingham Whigs for their natural opposition to any substantial electoral reform. In mid-1780 he observed that 'the

[33] JJ to Christopher Wyvill, 11 December 1781, *Wyvill Papers*, IV, pp. 514-15.
[34] Monday 10 December 1781, *Diary of Sylas Neville*, p. 283.
[35] JJ to Capel Lofft, 23 December 1781, 'Life of Jebb', pp. 171-72.
[36] Black, *Association*, p. 85.
[37] *Wyvill Papers*, IV, pp. 520-22n.
[38] P.D.G. Thomas, *Lord North* (1976), p. 130.
[39] Ian Christie, *The End of North's Ministry, 1780-1782* (1958), pp. 340-69.

Party of Rockingham ... really are more aristocratic than I could have conceived', and complained of 'determined and uniform opposition' to radical reform within the Westminster Committee.[40] In January 1782 he wrote that 'Richmond is our great support, though Mr Fox and Lord Shelburne are also friendly. With respect to Mr Fox I speak from my own knowledge when I say his mind is truly great and liberal, and I hope everything from his abilities and spirit'.[41] In April 1782 Jebb enthusiastically wrote that 'a large party are strenuous in their exertions to effect reform in England'.[42] 'I look to events with an anxious eye', he wrote to John Forbes in Dublin,

> If adhering to the principles of Virtue and Honour which render men respectable in private life, [the new ministry] shall labour to effect (what I am satisfied is practicable) a *general* peace. If without delay they will grant to Ireland her past demands as stated in the resolutions of her Volunteers. If America they shall acknowledge independent. If they shall look with a [friendly] eye on the efforts in both Countries to reform the representation, which mocks the people of both with the shadow of Liberty, the substance being long since gone. If they will evidence themselves friends of Toleration in its most extreme form – they will then in fact deserve the name Patriots, and late posterity will bless them. My hope is they will do these things, and my affection to many of them causes me to wish it for their sakes as well as for the sake of the Public.[43]

Such hopes were not ill founded. In May the young William Pitt introduced a carefully worded motion calling for the establishment of a committee to examine the state of representation. Yet without support from Rockingham, this was defeated. The Duke of Richmond was outraged, and threatened to cause a cabinet crisis if the government did not throw its weight behind Pitt's proposal. Any such confrontation was averted by Rockingham's death in early July.[44]

Shelburne became the leader of the government and Fox and his closest supporters resigned and returned to the opposition benches. In accordance with the Association convention resolutions of 18 May, another petition calling for reform in general terms was adopted and later presented to Parliament by Fox and Cecil Wray. Jebb spoke at the meeting in Westminster Hall on 27 July and stressed that the petition should have as many signatures as possible, declaring

---

[40] JJ to Christopher Wyvill, 13 May 1780, NYRO Wyvill mss; JJ to [?], 1 May 1782, HUL Jebb letters.

[41] JJ to Francis Dobbs, 25 January 1782, NLI Dobbs papers.

[42] JJ to John Forbes, 13 April 1782, NLI F.S. Bourke collection.

[43] JJ to John Forbes, 20 April 1782, NLI F.S. Bourke collection. According to John Disney, at this time it was suggested to Jebb 'from a very respectable quarter' that a London 'alderman's gown only waited his acceptance'. But Jebb declined the office because his medical practice would not permit time to fulfil his duties. 'Life of Jebb', p. 174.

[44] Black, *Association*, p. 87.

that 'an unarmed people' can affect constitutional reform through 'perseverance and manly firmness'. He urged relentless public censure of parliamentarians who opposed reform, and asserted that even the most arrogant peer would be made uneasy by public criticism. Jebb claimed that parliamentary reform was the only way to ensure that the tax burden occasioned by the war was spread evenly. He explained that the petition was expressed in general terms in order that those like himself, Cartwright and the Duke of Richmond who were committed to radical reform could support it. With Shelburne, Richmond and the younger Pitt in power, Jebb declared that the times were 'singularly favourable' for the introduction of 'equal, annual and universal representation'. The 'ancient constitutional connection between the House of Commons and the people' had been destroyed, and the majority of the lower house was now either 'the dependants of nobles, or the creatures of the crown'.[45] Christopher Wyvill was delighted with Shelburne's assurance that he would 'act nobly' toward the Association movement.[46] Yet privately the Jebbs were not so confident; Ann thought Shelburne was 'the King's own minister, and ... if he cannot govern the King – the King will govern him. But while the Duke of Richmond continues in the People will have great hopes'.[47]

Jebb's private reservations regarding Shelburne's disposition were strengthened by the proposed revival of ship money in Suffolk. He rejected as unconstitutional the idea of granting money to the executive independently of Parliament, and thought that the English counties would do better to follow the Irish example and spend their time and money forming volunteer militias.[48] 'Unconstitutional, illegal, invidious, oppressive, and abominable', Jebb believed that ship money was to be revived with the intention of destroying the commerce of the American states.[49] 'O America! Liberated, triumphant, independent, nurse of heroes, asylum sacred to suffering humanity!' Jebb cried out, while condemning Shelburne's reluctance to recognise American independence.[50] He concluded that Shelburne had determined 'this island, once the seat and patroness of freedom, should ... continue to riot in fraternal

---

[45] 'Speech at a General Meeting of the Electors of Westminster', 27 July 1782, Jebb III, pp. 298-307.

[46] John Cannon, *The Fox-North Coalition: crisis of the constitution, 1782-84* (Cambridge, 1969), p. 31.

[47] AJ to John Forbes, 11 July 1782, NLI F.S. Bourke collection; In 1780 Jebb had been deputised along with Brand Hollis and Sir Cecil Wray to thank Shelburne for 'the manly support his Lordship has constantly and uniformly given to the cause of the People'. BL Minutes of the Westminster Committee, 25 March 1780.

[48] 'Alfred' [JJ], 9 August 1782, Jebb III, pp. 308-11. This letter later inserted in the *Bury Post* by Capel Lofft, and it sparked an exchange on the subject in that paper which was later published as *An Inquiry into the Legality and Expediency of increasing the Royal Navy by Subscription for building County Ships. Being the correspondence on the subject between Arthur Young and Capel Lofft* (1783).

[49] 'Hampden' [JJ], 'To the Inhabitants of London and Westminster', 10 August 1782, Jebb III, pp. 312-14.

[50] 'Hampden' [JJ], 'To the Inhabitants of London and Westminster', 14 August 1782, Jebb III, pp. 314-21; 'Hampden' [JJ], 23 August 1782, Jebb III, p. 329.

blood'.[51] Such despondent thoughts were no doubt encouraged by ill health, as at the end of November Jebb was confined to his bed for six weeks by a 'putrid fever' contracted from some patients.[52]

According to Langford, 'by 1783 Wyvill and the Associators represented only themselves'.[53] Yet the persistence of the reformers remained a constant annoyance to conservatives. Elizabeth Montagu dryly commented that 'modern Patriots treat the constitution of England as apothecaries do their patients; they endeavour to give a motion every day and fancy that they will carry off all distempers.'[54] In late January 1783 Jebb discussed the forthcoming Quintuple meeting with the Duke of Richmond. While Pitt was going to support Wyvill's plan, Richmond agreed to push for the establishment of a parliamentary committee to draw up reform proposals.[55] Not surprisingly, Jebb thought Richmond above praise as 'one of the truest friends of the Constitution and of Human Nature the Country has yet seen'.[56]

While Shelburne managed to get peace negotiations under way, he could not maintain a working majority in the Parliament in the face of a formidable and unexpected alliance between Fox and North. He resigned in February 1783 and for five weeks the country was without a prime minister. Eventually, having contemplated abdication, George III was forced to accept a coalition government between the man whom he considered to have deserted him, and a man whose anti-monarchical stance he detested.[57] Jebb wrote to Fox pleading against a coalition. At the Shakespeare Tavern in Covent Garden on 6 March, Jebb condemned the rumoured coalition in a long speech to the electors of Westminster. He could not believe that Fox would contemplate entering into government with those who had conducted the war against America, and who sought to render George III 'as despotic as his most arbitrary neighbours'. Jebb warned that there would come a point when Fox could no longer continue to work within the coalition and he would have to return 'to the people dishonoured and disgraced'.[58] According to Jebb, he delivered this speech 'with all the vehemence which the action called for, to the great offence of Mr Fox's friends', though Fox himself 'behaved with great candour and politeness'.[59] In the course of their political alliance Jebb had always endeavored to 'impress [Fox's] mind with the persuasion, that by employing his splendid talents in the support of constitutional liberty ... he would attain the utmost height of power, to which an honest ambition could aspire'. But such encouragement was to no

51 'Laelius' [JJ], [October?] 1782, Jebb III, p. 360.
52 'Life of Jebb', p. 180.
53 Langford, *Polite and Commercial People*, p. 564.
54 Cited in Derek Jarrett, *The Begetters of Revolution* (1973), p. 163.
55 JJ to John Cartwright, 27 January 1783, 'Life of Jebb', p. 180. John Disney accompanied Andrew Kippis to the Club of Honest Whigs at the London Coffee House on 6 February and found the meeting 'large and agreeable'. Disney, 'Diary', 6 February 1783.
56 JJ to John Forbes, 20 April 1782, F.S. NLI Bourke collection.
57 Cannon, *Fox-North Coalition*, pp. 65-82.
58 'Life of Jebb', pp. 183-84. See also *The Remembrancer* 15 (1783), p. 205.
59 'Life of Jebb', p. 185.

avail. Fox entered into a coalition with North and became, in the eyes of Jebb, the 'associate and advocate of men, in principle and practice most despotic'. In a private letter, Jebb lamented 'the influence his party has upon him' and reflected in Hartlean tones that 'his intimacies, his connections, ... and the habits of his life have gotten too much hold of him, and ambition is his ruling passion'.[60]

The coalition confirmed Jebb in the belief that reform would only be forced by those 'outside of parliament'.[61] Since the heady days of 1780 Fox had attempted to distance himself from the radicals without losing their support. Something of the state of the relationship is indicated by a letter to Jebb on 30 June 1782, in which Fox asked that his name not appear on an advertisement for a meeting of the Westminster Committee. While Fox promised to visit Jebb's house at 3 pm the following day, Jebb noted on the letter that 'Mr Fox did not come, the Marquise of Rockingham dying about 12 o'clock that morning'.[62] With the formation of the coalition government Fox was able to turn his back on the radicals, declaring to Jebb at a dinner that he had 'never disguised ... his decided aversion to their schemes of parliamentary reform'.[63] Trying to look on the positive side, Cartwright hoped that the Coalition had 'taught the people to depend upon *themselves*'.[64]

During the summer of 1783 Jebb had 'various fluctuations in his health and spirits' and went to Brighton to recover.[65] He lost all confidence in politicians, especially as he observed the Coalition doing their level best to 'damp the rising spirit' of liberty in Ireland.[66] He thought that 'the North part' dominated the administration, and that 'the other part are too much crippled'.[67] 'Our newspapers', he complained, 'are entirely under the influence of the Coalition, both divisions of which are the decided Enemies of all Reform'.[68]

At this time political and intellectual division also troubled the Royal Society. The thirty-five-year-old Joseph Banks became president of the Royal Society only three months before Jebb was elected. While the previous president, Sir John Pringle, had been politically opposed to George III, Banks was on good terms with the King. He was keen to rejuvenate the Royal Society and develop it as a scientific institution in service of the state. As a botanist, Banks also wanted the Society to focus upon the biological as opposed to the physical sciences. Yet he attracted opposition through the high-handed manner with which he set about reforming the internal administration of the Society.

---

[60] Jebb II, p. 552n; 'Life of Jebb', p. 199.

[61] JJ to John Cartwright, 12 April 1783, *Life of Cartwright*, p. 155.

[62] Charles James Fox to JJ, 30 June 1782, BL Fox papers, reel 4.

[63] Cited in Mitchell, *Charles James Fox,* p. 253.

[64] John Cartwright to JJ, 14 May 1783, *Life of Cartwright*, p. 154.

[65] 'Life of Jebb', p. 185; JJ to Francis Dobbs, 15 August 1783, NLI Dobbs papers. Jebb returned to London at the start of September with his health little improved, though 'he left Dr Price there much better' and Andrew Kippis. Theophilus Lindsey to William Tayleur, 1 September 1783, JRL Lindesy – Tayleur correspondence.

[66] JJ to John Cartwright, 13 December 1783, *Life of Cartwright*, p. 160.

[67] JJ to John Forbes, 15 August 1783, NLI F.S. Bourke collection.

[68] JJ to Henry Joy, 8 October [1783], LHL Joy papers.

Despite the rhetoric condemning the President's 'despotism',[69] this conflict cannot be characterised as a political clash between radicals and conservatives within the scientific community. The conservative cleric and mathematician Samuel Horsley, who accused the President of making himself 'the Monarch of the Society', led the opposition to Banks. Horsley may have had his eye on the presidency, and he probably helped Banks by what Andrew Kippis called a 'high tone ... [which] went beyond the usual custom of public debates'. Claiming to be neutral in the contest, Kippis himself approved of the 'numerous introduction' of 'the nobility, and gentlemen of rank and fortune' encouraged by Banks. And, in a characteristic display of independence, the President was supported by none other than the 'republican bishop' Richard Watson. In the end, a motion of confidence in Banks was passed in January 1784, which he won 199 votes to 42.[70]

This incident further illustrates how political alignments during the period could alter according to time, place and issue, and the absence of a unified 'reform movement'. Yet while the controversy over the administration of the Royal Society reflected subject and personality differences, it is not surprising that some saw it in terms of the wider debate over representation. One of the most prominent opponents of Banks was Paul Henry Maty. Assistant librarian of the British Museum, Maty was a Secretary of the Royal Society and a close friend of Jebb. He publicly criticised Banks for opposing twelve candidates for the Society in four years (the signature of John Jebb appeared on the nomination certificate for two of these candidates).[71] Maty argued that any well-supported candidate should be elected unopposed. 'We are not an Academy of Sciences, ie. a receptacle for the Great in Science', he declared, 'but a Society of Gentlemen, of all ranks and professions, all opinions, and, we must add, all kinds of learning (or no learning), paying 52 shillings a year for the encouragement of literature.'[72] Personalities and vested interests aside, in this clash within the Royal Society we can hear the echo of enlightened civic humanism versus state-driven specialisation.

In December 1783 George III engineered the defeat of Fox's East India bill in the House of Lords and then demanded the resignation of the Coalition ministry. In their place he made the young William Pitt prime minister. Ann Jebb thought there had never 'been such confusion or such conduct, since Charles's time'.[73] While Pitt could depend upon a majority in the Lords, the opposition factions in the Commons outnumbered him, and Fox boasted of the ease with which he would defeat the 'mince-pie administration' when Parliament resumed in January. The stage was set for what Christopher

---

[69] Paul Henry Maty, *An History of the Instances of Exclusion from the Royal Society* (1784), p. 3.

[70] Gascoigne, *Joseph Banks and the English Enlightenment*, pp. 10-13; Mather, *High Church Prophet*, pp. 49-52.

[71] Maty, *An History*, pp. 8, 12. The candidates were Dr Hallifax, a classical scholar, and Dr Beerenbrock who was supported by, among others, John Jebb and Beccaria.

[72] Maty, *An History*, p. 10.

[73] AJ to John Cartwright, 21 December 1783, *Memoir of Ann Jebb*, p. 17.

Hobhouse has described as 'three of the most exciting months in the history of parliament'.[74]

Fox's confidence evaporated as addresses of support for the King and Pitt poured in from the counties. The provisions of the failed East India bill were widely condemned. Radicals feared that appointing a commission of Fox's friends to supervise the Company would further corrupt the parliament by placing a vast amount of patronage in Fox's hands. Tories were outraged at the infringement on royal prerogative.[75] Lindsey reported that 'we see at present no end to our public confusions'.[76] Ann Jebb complained of the 'sound sleep' of the counties with respect to the issue of parliamentary reform. 'If a particle of despair was in my nature', she told Cartwright,

> it would not fail to show itself at such a time as this. The whole attention of the public is taken up with the wranglings of the two parties, the doubts of a dissolution, and now also with the idea of a general coalition. But what can we expect for a grand coalition of all the abilities of the kingdom, meaning you know the abilities of the two Houses, but that, when they feel their own strength, they will plunder the East, and enslave this nation at their leisure?

Nevertheless, she hoped that if Fox refused a coalition (which he did) then Pitt would be forced to court popular support by promising parliamentary reform.[77] But this was unrealistic, and she was forced to admit that her husband's attempts to mobilise support for radical parliamentary reform revealed that 'our party are a rope of sand, and we do not know where to find them, or whether anyone would support us: and if it failed, many would throw all the blame upon the Doctor, for their conduct gives us no reason to expect a favour'.[78]

The election of 1784 was particularly bitter and hard fought – and nowhere more so than in Westminster. At Westminster Hall on 14 February a squabble broke out between the supporters of the two Members of Parliament for Westminster, Fox and Cecil Wray, as to who should chair the meeting of the electors. A bag of muck was thrown at Fox, and Wray's supporters left to hold a separate meeting outside. Jebb moved resolutions that supported the candidature of Cecil Wray and condemned the Coalition – a 'hateful union' whose aim was 'power, not the good of the country'. He criticised the 'odious and unnecessary restrictions' placed on relations with America, the opposition to parliamentary reform in Ireland and an East India bill that would have imposed a form of government 'more oppressive to the natives than the unjust and unwarrantable domination it proposed to remedy'. Jebb then urged the necessity of 'a substantial and radical reform in the representation', pointed to the encouraging

---

74 Christopher Hobhouse, *Fox* (1934), p. 150.

75 M.D. George, 'Fox's Martyrs: the General election of 1784', *Transactions of the Royal Historical Society,* 21 (1939), pp. 133-68.

76 Theophilus Lindsey to William Tayleur, 27 January 1784, JRL Lindsey – Tayleur correspondence.

77 AJ to John Cartwright, 22 January 1784, *Memoir of Ann Jebb*, pp. 19-20.

78 AJ to John Cartwright, 26 January 1784, *Memoir of Ann Jebb*, p. 20.

signs of extra-parliamentary agitation in Ireland and Scotland, and predicted that commercial prosperity would follow political reform.[79]

The election for the two representatives of Westminster turned into a heated and costly three-way contest between Fox, Wray and the popular war hero and Pittite candidate, Admiral Hood. Unfortunately for the reformers, Wray proved a lacklustre candidate who was unwilling to spend any of his own money in a contest influenced by propaganda and bribery. The Foxites included in their ranks the stunning and charismatic Georgiana, Duchess of Devonshire, who became central to their campaign. She counselled Fox on political tactics and devoted an enormous amount of energy and money to the cause. Freely mingling among the crowds and canvassing through the streets on foot, she became the focus of vitriolic anti-Fox propaganda – much of it sponsored by the government and making liberal use of sexual innuendo and titillation. She was, however, only the most prominent of a number of women who actively participated on all sides of the election contest – one of whom was Ann Jebb. This stimulated a formal debate at Coachmakers Hall on the topic: 'Is it consistent for the FEMALE SEX to interfere at elections?'[80]

In the midst of this three-way contest, the members of both the SCI and the Westminster Committee were divided in their allegiances. Jebb told Wyvill that 'the conduct of the coalitionists is so fundamentally wrong, that ... I most cordially wish entire rout to the party of Fox, Burke, and North'.[81] In return, Fox's supporters ridiculed Jebb in satirical publications. Listed in the 'Enemy's Squadron', the ship 'Inconstant' under 'Captain Jebb' was styled 'a very good ship, but badly manned'. A poem linked his profession and politics:

WHAT diseases (cries Jebb) in the Commons prevail?
They're the vitals of England; and if they should fail,
Let the foul *Primae Vitae* be scour'd; circulation
Will then go on to the health of the nation.
But, if we may judge from some late resolutions,
As you treat your poor patients of bad constitutions,
When you vomit and bleed, bolus, potion, and pill 'em,
Undertaking to *cure* 'em, dear Doctor, you'll *kill* 'em.[82]

It is not surprising that the Westminster Committee adjourned in April 1783 and did not meet again for eight months. When it resumed its sessions in early 1784 under the leadership of Fox's lieutenants, Richard Fitzpatrick and Richard Brinsley Sheridan, it was 'more openly than before the tool of the Fox party'.[83]

Voting was conducted over six weeks in April and May. Standing on the hustings in Covent Garden on the opening day, Wray pledged to follow the

---

[79] Speech at Westminster Hall, 14 February 1784, 'Life of Jebb', pp. 192-94.
[80] *History of the Westminster Election*, p. 352. See also Amanda Foreman, *Georgiana, Dutchess of Devonshire* (Hammersmith, 1998), pp. 136-59.
[81] JJ to Christopher Wyvill, 23 March 1784, *Wyvill Papers*, IV, p. 362.
[82] [J. Hartley], *History of the Westminster Election* (2nd ed., 1785), pp. 69, 459. I was alerted to these attacks on Jebb by Kenneth Pearl, 'John Jebb, a British Radical in the Age of the American Revolution', pp. 187-92.
[83] Christie, *Wilkes, Wyvill and Reform*, p. 198.

instructions of his electors. At his side, Jebb warned that if the Foxites were allowed to 'regain the support and good opinion of the people', other politicians would also 'delude with false shows of patriotism, and afterwards, at their pleasure, insult the honest feelings of their countrymen'.[84] Despite proving a poor candidate, with energetic support from the likes of Jebb it initially looked as though Wray would be returned along with Admiral Hood. But, with the Dutchess of Devonshire in the lead, the Foxites doggedly scoured the city for extra votes and when polling was finally closed in mid-May the result was: Hood 6694; Fox 6234; Wray 5998. Wray's supporters appealed to have the votes scrutinised, and Prime Minister Pitt eagerly agreed. This did not change the result, which was formally announced in March 1785. In the meantime, Fox engineered entry into Parliament via a Scottish seat and claimed the moral high ground with a speech on the rights of elected members in disputed contests.[85] Jebb never forgave the behaviour of his former ally, and in return Fox denounced the radicals as bent on subverting the constitution.[86]

Overall, however, the reformers had contributed greatly to the rout of the Coalition, especially in the eastern counties. Eighty-nine Whig members, nicknamed 'Fox's Martyrs', had lost their seats and Pitt had a comfortable majority. In dramatic circumstances, the 1784 election revealed that the 'Voice of the People' had become an important political fact. The very nature of the contest between Pitt and Fox made it impossible for candidates in the open constituencies to go 'unshackled' to Parliament – they had to commit to one side or the other on the hustings. Irrespective of Pitt's subsequent stance on parliamentary reform, he and the King had 'brought to the fore the new radical principle that the final word in political disputes lay with the people'.[87]

Jebb had initially hoped that Pitt would advance the cause of reform. In July 1782 he praised the 'illustrious son of that illustrious statesman' for proposing a parliamentary committee to examine reform.[88] By April 1783 Jebb was expressing uneasiness, observing that in a letter to the Suffolk Committee Pitt had declared himself 'no well-wisher to reform on the speculative principles of some that have given alarm'.[89] During the election of 1784 Jebb bestowed a qualified approval upon Pitt.[90] Price and Lindsey were hopeful that the sizeable majority Pitt won in the election would enable him to promote reform 'if the attempt be not long delayed'.[91] However, General Robert Cunningham had assured the Irish House of Commons that Pitt's ministry would prove unfriendly to parliamentary reform. Jebb transcribed the speech from the *Dublin Evening*

[84] Speech to the electors of Westminster, 1 April 1784, 'Life of Jebb', pp. 195-98.
[85] Pearl, 'John Jebb, a British Radical in the Age of the American Revolution', pp. 191-92.
[86] Black, *Association*, p. 115.
[87] Paul Kelly, 'Radicalism and Public Opinion in the General Election of 1784', *Bulletin of the Institute for Historical Research,* 45 (1972), pp. 73-88, at 88.
[88] Jebb III, p. 305.
[89] JJ to John Cartwright, 12 April 1783, *Life of Cartwright*, p. 155.
[90] Meadley, *Memoir of Ann Jebb*, p. 16.
[91] Theophilus Lindey to William Turner, 15 April 1784, DWL Lindesy-Turner correspondence.

Post and sent it to Pitt, informing him that many would be indifferent as to who was prime minister if substantial reform was not enacted.[92] By May Jebb was observing that 'I find myself receding very fast from Mr Pitt, without approaching to Mr Fox'.[93]

IRELAND

While the fortunes of the London radicals varied, Jebb kept a sharp eye on developments in Ireland. Having won free-trade concessions from Lord North, and inspired by the Americans, Henry Grattan (1746-1820) and the Irish 'Patriots' went on to demand independence for the Irish Parliament. Such demands had widespread support in Ireland, particularly among the volunteer militias that had sprung up to meet the threat of French invasion. After years of supporting Irish rights on the opposition benches, the Rockingham Whigs had no choice but to grant independence when they found themselves in office in early 1782.[94] Historians have only recently arrived at something like a satisfactory understanding of popular and parliamentary politics in late eighteenth-century Ireland.[95] In the euphoria following Grattan's victory, appeals to natural rights became more frequent. This led some of the leading parliamentary patriots to sound a note of caution. Grattan himself suggested that 'the populace differ much and should be clearly distinguished from the people'.[96] But while the government resisted any extension of the franchise, the radical reformers became more critical of the Irish aristocracy, the Church and British ministers.[97]

Ditchfield thinks it striking that Rational Dissenters displayed 'practically no interest whatever in the affairs of Ireland' aside from the changing legal status of Catholicism.[98] Jebb is a clear exception, as he had family ties in Ireland and had undertaken some of his early education within the Pale. Abigail Adams was led to describe Jebb as 'an Irishman', and found herself dining at the Jebb household with two Irish visitors.[99] In the early 1780s Jebb had several Irish correspondents. Among these was the young Dublin wit, poet, barrister and radical MP Francis Dobbs (1750-1811), who became known

---

92 AJ to John Cartwright, 6 March 1784, *Memoir of Ann Jebb*, p. 21; Jebb's letter is not preserved in Pitt's correspondence.

93 'Life of Jebb', p. 199.

94 Jebb was pleased to see that the Rockingham ministry's stance toward Ireland was 'liberal'. JJ to John Forbes, 13 April 1782, NLI F.S. Bourke collection.

95 S.J. Connolly, 'Late Eighteenth-Century Irish Politics', *Parliamentary History,* 13 (1994), p. 227. On late-eighteenth-century Irish politics, see Foster, *Modern Ireland,* pp. 167-289; R.B. McDowell, *Ireland in the Age of Imperialism and Revolution, 1760-1801* (Oxford, 1979).

96 Cited in Lecky, *History of Ireland*, p. 207.

97 Jacqueline Hill, *From Patriots to Unionists: Dublin civic politics and Irish Protestant patriotism, 1660-1840* (Oxford, 1997), p. 166.

98 G.M. Ditchfield, 'Some Aspects of Unitarianism and Radicalism 1760-1810' (Unpublished Cambridge PhD. thesis, 1968), p. 14.

99 Abigail Adams jr to John Quincy Adams, 13 September 1785, MHS Adams papers.

for his patriot writings.[100] John Forbes MP was a supporter of Henry Grattan in the Irish House of Commons, and a member of the Monks of St Patrick, a fraternal society founded in 1779 in which members mocked Catholic ways and discussed independence.[101] Jebb also kept abreast of developments in Ulster through Henry Joy, a keen reformer and editor of the *Belfast Newsletter*.

With contacts such as these it is not surprising that Jebb also met with Irish Patriots who visited London.[102] In early 1781 Jebb moved a motion in support of Irish free trade and self-government in the Westminster Committee. He was supported by Cartwright and Lofft but 'opposed and defeated by the Rockingham Party in the Committee, and betrayed by some of our own People who think with us but have not the heart to say so'.[103] In January 1783 Jebb warned Dobbs that 'unless you reform the House of Commons you do nothing'.[104] Later that year he was given the opportunity to address the Irish publicly when the Ulster Volunteers wrote to the Earl of Effingham, Richard Price, Cartwright, Wyvill and Jebb requesting advice on parliamentary reform before their next meeting at Dungannon in September.[105] Jebb told the Volunteers that 'the power of delegation appears to me to be as extensive as the obligation of bearing arms for the common defence'.[106] He reiterated his general objection to an increase in the number of county representatives: 'in Lord North's opinion, such a measure would have nothing in it formidable to an administration determined to govern by court influence.' It would make the Irish House of Commons too numerous and increase the cost of elections. County seats were under the control of landholders, Jebb warned, and thus the representative voice of freeholders would decrease. He argued that petitioning was useless and that the Volunteers should draw up a reform plan 'the most extensive and liberal that the times will bear', and then adjourn to give the parliament time to act (or not act) before making their next move.[107]

Such advice contrasted sharply with that of Lord Claremont, leader of the Volunteers, who suggested that a general petition would be most appropriate, leaving the details of reform to the wisdom of parliament. Jebb

---

[100] See *DNB*; J. Hill, *Patriots to Unionists*, p. 169; R.B. McDowell, *Irish Public Opinion 1750-1800* (1944), p. 91.

[101] Neil Longley York, *Neither Kingdom nor Nation: the Irish quest for constitutional rights, 1698-1800* (Washington, D.C., 1994), pp. 120-21.

[102] JJ to Francis Dobbs, 25 January 1782; and 7 April 1782, NLI Dobbs papers; JJ to John Forbes, 8 January 1785, NLI F.S. Bourke collection.

[103] JJ to Francis Dobbs, 23 February 1781, NLI Dobbs papers.

[104] JJ to Francis Dobbs, 27 January 1783, NLI Dobbs papers.

[105] A selection of the replies were later published as *A Collection of Letters which have been Addressed to the Volunteers of Ireland, on the subject of Parliamentary Reform by the Earl of Effingham &c.* (1783). Both Wyvill and Jebb also published their own letters separately: *Letters Addressed the Committee of Belfast on the proposed reformation of the Parliament of Ireland, by the Rev. Christopher Wyvill* (1783); John Jebb, *Letters Addressed to the Volunteers of Ireland, on the subject of Parliamentary Reform* (1783), Jebb II, pp. 517-54.

[106] JJ, 13 August 1783, reprinted in *Address to the Volunteers of Ireland*, Jebb II, p. 520.

[107] *Address to the Volunteers of Ireland*, Jebb II, pp. 521-26.

anxiously awaited the outcome of the Dungannon meeting, and believed that the fate of reform in England and Scotland was dependent upon events in Ireland. He observed that the British government was 'alarmed at the addresses which have lately been made to the Volunteers of Ulster'.[108]

The question of Catholic political rights was the thorniest issue. In the words of R.F. Foster, the 'patriotism' of the Volunteer movement was a form of 'gentry nationalism' that had 'strong affinities with *colonial* nationalism'. The patriots were able to 'take a high line with England *because* they were exclusive in Ireland: had 'patriotism' represented the excluded three-quarters of the Irish nation, they could not have afforded to press so radically for constitutional "liberty"'.[109] John Cannon has observed that Wyvill and Price were hesitant in suggesting that Catholics be given the vote, and that 'Jebb and Effingham took refuge in the observation that only the Irish themselves could have the necessary information for a correct judgement of the problem'.[110] This is true, but Cannon ignores the fact that Jebb then proceeded to argue for full citizenship for Catholics. He acknowledged that most Irish Protestants would object to Catholics being allowed to elect Catholic MPs, and that many would not even allow them to vote for Protestants. 'Local difficulties must be best known to those on the spot', he concluded in his first letter, 'I can only reason from general principles' – from which he proceeded to assert that all should have the vote (while passing over the issue of Catholic politicians).[111] Yet in his next letter he reflected that 'admitting the Roman Catholics to the entire rights of citizenship may appear scarcely worthy of a moment's consideration at no very distant period'.[112] Jebb later assured a sceptical Irish friend that a reformed Parliament would diminish clerical benefices, exclude bishops from the House of Lords and substitute '*a proper payment of the parochial clergy, in lieu of that bane of all improvement, tithes*'. This would 'put an end to priestly avarice and intolerance', and 'the Roman Catholic religion, or at least the worst part of it, would decay. Persecution being removed, light, and learning, and industry would effect the rest'.[113]

In an attempt to halt declining numbers, some Volunteer corps had begun to enlist Catholics, and advanced radicals began to speculate about extending the franchise to include Catholics, if only on a restricted basis. Five hundred representatives from 278 Ulster Volunteer corps attended the Dungannon meeting on 7 September. They called for wide-ranging parliamentary reform, and invited the other provinces to send delegates to a national convention, which would deliberate upon 'what class or description' of Catholics should be granted the vote. The political elites on both sides of the Irish Sea were alarmed at what Charles James Fox thought a '*critical* in the

[108] JJ to Francis Dobbs, 15 August 1783, NLI Dobbs papers.
[109] Foster, *Modern Ireland*, p. 248.
[110] Cannon, *Parliamentary Reform*, p. 103.
[111] *Address to the Volunteers of Ireland*, Jebb II, pp. 523-24.
[112] JJ, 14 August 1783, in *Address to the Volunteers of Ireland*, Jebb II, p. 530.
[113] JJ to Archibald Hamilton Rowan, 5 March and 29 September 1785, *Autobiography of Archibald Hamilton Rowan*, pp. 128, 131.

genuine sense of the word' situation.[114] Colonel Sharman wrote to Jebb thanking him for his advice, but observing that not all the suggestions of their 'illustrious and much respected correspondents' could be applied to the Irish situation.[115] Nevertheless, the Dungannon resolutions and the call for a national convention gave Jebb a 'glow of satisfaction beyond the power of language to describe'.[116] He thought it necessary for the SCI and Westminster Committee to make declarations in support of Dungannon to 'intimidate ministers from pursuing works of blood' – though he confessed that the government was unlikely to resort to coercive measures.[117] In October Jebb told Francis Dobbs that the Volunteers should focus on demanding universal suffrage, after which law and religious reforms would naturally result.[118]

Prior to the national convention Jebb addressed another letter to the Volunteers urging the 'Third Estate' to force reform upon a House of Commons dominated by the 'voice of the aristocracy and the inclinations of the crown'. Yet the substance of the letter was a plea for recognition of the civil and political rights of the Catholic majority. Jebb pointed to the liberal sentiments respecting religious liberty espoused by the Dungannon meeting, and the benefits accrued in America by religious toleration. He argued that if Catholic claims were ignored, then the government would take advantage of the resulting national division. If Catholics were left to live like slaves, Jebb warned, 'you will impair your own title to the blessings of liberty, and must expect to live, for generations, in little less than a state of actual hostility with the majority of your countrymen'. As noted in chapter 9, Jebb confidently assured the Volunteers that,

> when under the influence of mild and equal laws, human industry shall be generally excited and encouraged, and that monster intolerance, the bane of human happiness, shall be banished from the state, is it not reasonable to conclude, that religious prejudices also will give away, and truth extend her salutary empire over the minds of men, in proportion as the light of science, the constant concomitant of an enlarged intercourse with our species, shall prevail?

As the Catholic laity no longer acknowledged the Pope's right to overrule an oath of allegiance, there could be no valid objection to allowing them full political rights. Jebb suggested a conference with the leading Catholics to resolve differences, because if 'the maxims of past ages be adhered to, human sagacity can see no end; at least, no end that can be contemplated with pleasure'.[119] Yet apart from Protestant bigotry, such a conference was unlikely

---

[114] Cannon, *Parliamentary Reform*, p. 104.
[115] Colonel Sharman to JJ, 11 October 1783, Jebb II, 534n.
[116] JJ to Francis Dobbs, 5 October 1783, NLI Dobbs papers.
[117] JJ to John Cartwright, 2 October 1783, *Life of Cartwright*, p. 156.
[118] JJ to Francis Dobbs, 5 October 1783, NLI Dobbs papers.
[119] JJ, 25 October 1783, in *Address to the Volunteers of Ireland*, Jebb II, pp. 536, 540, 543-49.

because the leading Catholics were trying to sit on the fence between reformers and the government.

The National Convention assembled in Dublin on 10 November. It quickly resolved to omit discussion of Catholic suffrage from its deliberations – there had been no clear request from the Catholic Committee, and the idea lacked any powerful individual or institutional support. As a result the Irish Parliament easily dismissed the Convention's reform petition as a sectarian document.[120] Fanned by Dublin Castle, caution and conservatism spread among the Irish corporate bodies.

In response, radicals began to establish reform clubs in an effort to maintain their momentum.[121] By early 1784 Ann Jebb thought the idea of granting Catholics the vote was gaining ground.[122] Theophilus Lindsey decided that it was a good idea to split the ecclesiastical revenues in Ireland and give half to the Catholic Church and the Dissenters.[123] In the early months of his prime ministership, William Pitt had suggested that a moderate parliamentary reform in Ireland would take the sting out of the Volunteer movement, and allow a government-controlled militia to be formed. Yet the Irish lord lieutenant, the Duke of Rutland, greeted this attitude with horror. Pitt gradually gave in to the more reactionary stance of Dublin Castle, and completely dropped the idea when his own moderate reform proposals were defeated in the British Parliament.[124]

In the summer of 1784 Lord Charlemont told the Belfast Volunteers that political rights should not be extended to Catholics. The radicals found themselves outflanked and outnumbered. As a result, debate at the poorly attended National Congress in October was languid and irresolute.[125] Archibald Hamilton Rowan (1751-1834), a delegate (and Jebb's former student while at Queen's College, Cambridge), was disappointed that the majority were not in favour of electoral reform.[126] Rowan's disappointment is all the more revealing in light of his difference of opinion with Jebb on the issue of Catholic rights.[127] In November 1784 Jebb told Henry Joy in Belfast that he wanted to see a federal union between Ireland and Britain, but only if both parliaments were elected upon a reformed franchise.[128] But the wind was clearly going out of the sails of

---

[120] Thomas Bartlett, *The Fall and Rise of the Irish Nation: the Catholic Question 1690-1830* (Dublin, 1992), p. 107.

[121] *Dublin Evening Post*, 20 November 1784, cited in Hill, *Patriots to Unionists*, p. 181. Over a year later Jebb congratulated Henry Joy on the establishment of a 'Reform Club' in Belfast. JJ to Henry Joy, 18 May 1785, LHL Joy papers.

[122] AJ to John Cartwright, 24 March 1784, *Memoir of Ann Jebb*, p. 22.

[123] Theophilus Lindsey to William Turner, 18 October 1783, DWL Lindsey-Turner correspondence.

[124] McDowell, *Ireland in the Age of Imperialism and Revolution*, p. 318-20.

[125] McDowell, *Irish Public Opinion*, chapter 6; James Kelly, 'The Parliamentary Reform Movement of the 1780s and the Catholic Question', *Archivium Hibernicum*, 43 (1988), pp. 97-8.

[126] Archibald Hamilton Rowan to Richard Joy, 24 October 1784, cited in McDowell, *Ireland in the Age of Imperialism and Revolution*, p. 324.

[127] *Autobiography of Archibald Hamilton Rowan*, p. 134.

[128] JJ to Henry Joy, 28 November 1784, 'Life of Jebb', p. 203.

reform.[129] Despite their military display and some colourful radical rhetoric, the Volunteers of Ireland proved to be loyal and law-abiding men.

Pitt turned his attention to establishing free trade across the Irish Sea, and ran into considerable opposition from British trade and manufacturing interests. Jebb applauded Pitt's commercial measures, but criticised his opposition to political reform in Ireland.[130] He continued to believe that an independent Ireland with a reformed Parliament would prove a solid ally of Britain, because of 'kindred-blood, a similarity of pursuits, and ancient habits of intercourse'.[131] But he complained of what he saw as Pitt's duplicity, and the efforts of the British government to reduce Ireland to 'servile dependence'.[132]

DECLINE AND DEATH

In June 1784 Jebb reflected the sense of national recovery associated with Pitt's administration when he observed that 'prejudices are everywhere rapidly giving way'. Rather than the comfortable political apathy that ensued, he was initially hopeful that there would be a slow revival of interest in parliamentary reform.[133] This hope arose in part from the parliamentary debate over John Sawbridge's motion of 16 June that a committee be appointed to examine the state of representation. While the motion was defeated by a majority of seventy-four votes led by Lord North, Pitt spoke in its favour.

The hopes of the reformers revived somewhat, but a sense of their marginal position in British politics is vividly illustrated by John Wilkes. In a private letter to his daughter two days after the defeat of Sawbridge's motion, he wrote:

> Yesterday, my dearest Polly, was sacred to the powers of dullness, and the anniversary meeting of the Quintuple Alliance, when I was obliged to eat stale fish, and swallow foul port, with Sir Cecil Wray, Mr Martin the banker, Dr Jebb, &c. to promote the grand reform of parliament. I was forced into the chair, and was so far happy to be highly applauded, both for a long speech, and my conduct as president through an arduous day. I have not however authenticated to the public any account of the day's proceeding, nor given to the press the various new-fangled toasts, which were the amusement of the hour, and should perish with it.[134]

Jebb hoped that the Celtic regions would take the lead on reform. On 20 July 1784 he addressed *A Letter to the Secretary of the Society for Constitutional*

---

[129] Jebb observed that the British government talked of the 'dying embers of sedition' in Ireland. JJ to John Forbes, 8 January 1785, NLI F.S. Bourke collection.

[130] JJ to Henry Joy, 26 January and 18 May 1785, LHL Joy papers.

[131] 'Trebatius' [JJ], 22 August 1785, Jebb III, p. 390.

[132] JJ to John Forbes, 22 November 1785, NLI F.S. Bourke collection.

[133] JJ to [?], 'Life of Jebb', p. 201.

[134] John Wilkes to Polly Wilkes, 18 June 1784, *Letters of John Wilkes to his Daughter, 1774-96* (John Almon ed., 1804), III, p. 41.

Information, in which he urged Englishmen to arm themselves, agitate for parliamentary reform, and pointed to the patriotic support for 'free parliaments' among the 'gallant people' of Scotland.[135] In late 1784 Jebb was elected as a member of the Association committee for Carnarvon.[136]

In early December 1784 Jebb's 'heart sank' when Wyvill told him that Pitt was going to introduce a reform bill that did not include repeal of the Septennial Act. His response was to suggest formation of a new 'party of the people', drawn from members of the Lords and Commons. Hopeful that a revival of public interest in reform was under way, Jebb told Cartwright that a meeting at the Shakespeare Tavern had been 'full of energy. I wish you had been there'.[137] A week later Wyvill told the SCI that Pitt had promised to introduce the question of parliamentary reform in the next session.[138] Jebb was suspicious ('I look with watchfulness for what is to be done about short parliaments') and set about warning friends not to support the Pitt-Wyvill plan if either the Septennial Act or the franchise were to be left untouched.[139] A meeting on 21 January was enthusiastic for 'substantial reform', and resolved against supporting Pitt's plan. He hoped 'for the honour of human nature that Mr Pitt is serious so far as he goes', but reflected that even if the Prime Minister were sincere, 'the majority of the Cabinet ... would over-rule the few friends we may possibly have in Power, and stop the affair for ever'.[140]

While Wyvill failed to win the support of the metropolitan radicals, Pitt was equally unsuccessful (to the extent that he tried) in gaining the approval of his political allies. One MP remarked on the prime minister being 'encumbered or enamoured with – I am not sure which – this Yorkshire reform'.[141] The House listened in respectful silence when Pitt tabled the bill in mid-April, and then, following numerous eloquent speeches ridiculing the proposal, left the Prime Minister with a minority of only 74 votes.

Wyvill made one last-ditch effort the save the cause. On 7 May 1785 he assembled a meeting of the Associated Counties at the Thatched-House Tavern to rally support for Pitt's reform proposals. On the preceding day he unsuccessfully pleaded with Jebb in person to attend the meeting. When this failed, he penned a last-minute appeal in which his frustration is evident. Having 'perhaps somewhat too bluntly' explained his position to Jebb in person, Wyvill

---

[135] 'A Letter to the Secretary of the Society for Constitutional Information' (July 1784), Jebb III, pp. 362-64. See SCI, *Constitutional Tracts*, II, pp. 59-62. In January 1785 Jebb noted that 'they are going on with vigour in Scotland', and that reformers were planing to draft a bill to be presented in parliament. JJ to John Forbes, 8 January 1785, NLI F.S. Bourke collection.

[136] JJ to the Committee of the County of Carnarvon, 19 November 1784, 'Life of Jebb', pp. 204-07.

[137] JJ to John Cartwright, 13 December 1784, *Life of Cartwright*, p. 159.

[138] 17 December 1784, PRO SCI Minutes II:91.

[139] JJ to John Cartwright, 18 December 1784, *Life of Cartwright*, p. 161; JJ to [?], [December 1784?], 'Life of Jebb', pp. 209-11.

[140] JJ to Henry Joy, 26 January 1785, LHL Joy papers.

[141] Daniel Pultney to Duke of Rutland, 19 April 1785, cited in Christie, *Wilkes, Wyvill and Reform*, p. 215.

urged him to attend the meeting in order to further discuss the reform proposals.[142] But Jebb would not allow himself to be placed in a minority at a meeting that endorsed Pitt's reform proposals. While he saw merit in the extension of suffrage to copyholders and a redistribution of some borough places to the counties, he thought 'something foreign to the main question, if not inimical to the real interests of the people, is intended, which may be revealed in its day'. Even on the face of it, Jebb thought Pitt's plan inadequate: many boroughs such as Bury, Yarmouth, Cambridge and Buckingham needed an extension of the franchise. Also, he claimed that the outcome of the reforms would be slow to come into effect, and in the mean-time the country could be ruined and the people 'totally enslaved'. Jebb pointed to Pitt's silence during the annual vote on Sawbridge's motion for annual parliaments, and his policy in Ireland (where restraints on the press and the right to bear arms had been introduced), and argued that that only 'the active energy of the people' could effect a substantial reform of the parliament.[143]

Along with Thomas Paine, Christopher Wyvill attended a general audit dinner for the SCI on 11 May and presented the case for moderate reform. A week later Jebb complained to a friend in Ireland that the cause of parliamentary reform in England was under threat: 'the zeal with which some of our ablest and worthy characters endeavour to form an union of the people around the banner of the minister will do us irreparable mischief, unless the delusion be soon discovered, and the friends of the People duly informed.' At the SCI dinner Jebb had strongly but unsuccessfully opposed a toast to 'the Principles of Mr Pitt', and sourly observed that 'propositions of a similar nature were proposed for *future* discussion at our Quintuple meeting ... where the *virtuous* sincerity and *practical* wisdom of the minister are held forth'. Jebb thought that Pitt and the King's Irish policy revealed the 'native deformity' of their principles.[144] He told Henry Joy in Belfast that 'efforts, strong efforts are exerted to engage our Constitutional Society in an approbation of Mr Pitt's plan'. He opposed this because 'Pitt is evidently the minister of the Crown', declaring that 'with my consent that best of Causes shall never be committed to the hands of a man, who has manifested so marked a disregard to the general Interest of Liberty'.[145]

At a general meeting on 3 June a supporter of the Pitt-Wyvill plan moved that the SCI should give its approval.[146] This led to a heated debate in which Jebb advocated publication and circulation of the proposals, but 'warmly' opposed any vote of support. According to Jebb he was accused by some of being 'an enemy to the cause'. 'I am censured', he complained, 'as meaning to overthrow a question, in support of which I have sacrificed my fortune, health, and peace of mind, ... but I will not swerve from principle, let them say what

---

[142] Christopher Wyvill to JJ, 6 May 1785, NYRO Wyvill mss.
[143] JJ to Christopher Wyvill, 7 May 1785, Jebb III, pp. 377-83; NYRO Wyvill mss; Jebb published the letter in the *Public Advertiser*, 26 May 1785.
[144] JJ to John Forbes, 18 May 1785, NLI F.S. Bourke collection.
[145] JJ to Henry Joy, 18 May 1785, LHL Joy papers.
[146] PRO SCI Minutes II, pp. 111-14.

they please'.[147] Thomas Day expressed the sentiments of those who were frustrated by Jebb's hard line stance:

> To expect that the minister of a great, and above all a corrupted state like this, should calmly and deliberately demolish the whole frame of government for the sake of making an experiment, is betraying a lamentable ignorance of human nature. I am not myself such a child as either to expect or wish that all government should stand still in such a wonderfully complicated system of society as our own, in order that two or three reformers may try their skill in greasing the wheels.[148]

Two thousand copies of Wyvill's pamphlet were printed, to which the Society added some generally critical comments.[149]

Amidst dissension and recrimination the cause of parliamentary reform was laid to rest until its resurrection during the French Revolution. Searching for someone to blame, Jebb publicly condemned Pitt's attempt at parliamentary reform as a 'solemn farce',[150] and privately complained that 'Mr Pitt has hurt our Cause by meddling with it'.[151] Until its revival in the 1790s, the SCI was reduced to voicing support for law reform, abolition of the slave trade, and cheering on Irish and Scottish political agitation.[152]

In his final years Jebb was plagued by illness. In the spring of 1784 he was sick and confined to his bed for several weeks with 'an inflamatory complaint, which formed an abscess in his groin'. He retired to Buxton for the summer but returned without any great improvement in his health.[153] In August 1785 Abigail Adams thought the 'poor man looks as if he was not long intended as an ornament to Science or Learning – his health is very poor'.[154] Jebb retired to the country for most of October, but again returned to London with his health little improved. Lindsey reported that in addition to a liver complaint, Jebb 'has various complaints, the relics of a putrid fever caught from a patient years ago, and never got rid of'.[155]

During the final months of ill-health leading up to his death on 2 March 1786, Jebb passed his time studying the Saxon language and reading Anglo-Saxon and English history, with an eye to examining the penal code and 'particular points of liberty'.[156] He bemoaned the 'general apathy' of his fellow

---

[147] 'Life of Jebb', p. 214; JJ to Archibald Hamilton Rowan, 29 September 1785, *Autobiography of Archibald Hamilton Rowan*, p. 130.
[148] Letter by Thomas Day, 5 September 1785, cited in James Keir, *An Account of the Life and Writings of Thomas Day* (1791), p. 66.
[149] SCI, *Constitutional Tracts*, II, pp. 47-52.
[150] 'Trebatius' [JJ], 22 August 1785, Jebb III, pp. 394.
[151] JJ to Henry Joy, [September 1785?], LHL Joy papers.
[152] Black, *Association*, pp. 203-05.
[153] 'Life of Jebb', p. 200.
[154] Abigail Adams jr to John Q. Adams, 13 September 1785, MHS Adams papers.
[155] Theophilus Lindsey to William Tayleur, 20 October 1785, JRL Lindsey-Tayleur correspondence.
[156] 'Life of Jebb', p. 216.

countrymen with respect to political reform.[157] Reading of developments in Ireland, he railed against his countrymen: 'ruin is pouring in upon us by a thousand channels; despotism approaches with alarming strides; we listen to the seducing tales of the partisans of power'. He criticised the widespread attack on the Irish, and argued that only a 'cordial spirit of good-will, nourished by reciprocal acts of kindness' would secure commerce between Britain, Ireland and America. With his health declining Jebb lamented that his voice was feeble and his pen 'destitute of that energy which is required to call the expiring virtue of my countrymen to a knowledge of their rights'.[158] He was becoming increasingly despondent at the lack of interest in reform:

> The present state of the commonality of England is indeed deplorable. We are exposed without friend or patron, like a helpless prey, to the depredations of ministers of state.... We are deprived of our right to arms, by iniquitous game laws; ... of the right of suffrage, at the same time that the long continuance of septennial parliaments has almost obliterated the remembrance of our former powers of control.[159]

Jebb's final months, however, were not entirely unhappy. As noted in chapter 8, in August and September he enjoyed the company of John Adams, the recently appointed ambassador to Britain (and future second president of the United States). Adams had first met Jebb during a quick visit to London in November 1783.[160] From the start he had a high esteem for Jebb, whom he thought 'one of the best Citizens of the little Commonwealth of the just upon Earth'.[161] Theophilus Lindsey also met Adams and thought him 'a grave but agreeable character'.[162] Along with his wife and daughter (both named Abigail), Adams was snubbed by the British elite. While they enjoyed the social and artistic scene, the Adams family frowned upon the decadence of the aristocracy. Abigail wrote home to America that 'I am ... so old fashioned as to prefer the society of Dr Price, Dr Jebb and a few others like them to the midnight Gamblers and titled Gamesters;'[163] and she seems to have derived much comfort from the company of Ann Jebb.[164] After John Adams and Jebb had discussed the issue of providing salaries for public offices, Adams wrote that 'I wish to continue our disquisitions concerning the American Constitutions, because I

---

[157] 'Trebatius' [JJ], 2 August 1785, Jebb III, p. 386.

[158] 'Trebatius' [JJ], 22 August 1785, Jebb III, pp. 390, 393.

[159] 'A Letter to the Secretary of the Society for Constitutional Information' (1785), Jebb III, pp. 395-402, at 396.

[160] Smith, *John Adams*, pp. 581-84; Jebb presented Adams with some SCI pamphlets. JJ to John Adams, 27 November 1783, MHS Adams Papers. At this time John Disney records that he 'supped at the London Coffee House Club, when Messers Adams and Jay were there'. Disney, 'Diary', 13 November 1783.

[161] John Adams to Mr Stockdale, 31 January 1784, MHS Adams papers.

[162] McLachlan, *Letters of Lindsey*, p. 86.

[163] Abigail Adams snr., 15 September 1785, cited in Smith, *John Adams*, p. 184.

[164] Upon leaving England she repeatedly conveyed her affectionate regards to Ann Jebb: Abigail Adams to Thomas Brand Hollis, Portsmouth 5 April 1788 and New York 6 September 1788, MHS Adams papers.

think many things require amendment, and I hope for Lights and aids from you in maturing them.'[165] Unfortunately Jebb's ill health and death soon terminated these discussions.

Throughout his life Jebb had spent much time associating with like-minded people. The pages of John Disney's diary reveal the frequency with which Rational Dissenters and their friends met and dined together. Thanks to the young Abigail Adams we can glimpse this aspect of Jebb's life. She has left an account of a dinner at Jebb's house that was also attended by Richard Brocklesby, two Irishmen, and a young man who was possibly Samuel Romilly. Unfortunately the dinner does not seem to have gone off quite as well as the Jebbs would have hoped. A 'flaming son of St Patrick' dominated the conversation, Abigail told her brother:

> he had got his dinner from somewhere else – and when we went to table had nothing to do but talk, and so improved his faculty of speech that he stunned the rest of the company. Such prejudices against the French nation I never heard – the country, its government, laws, manners, customs, &c. were attacked by him without reason, prudence or good sense. He was very violent upon the American War also. He approved the independence of America because it could not be avoided by this country, but attributed to the fault of their generals that we were not conquered. He would have granted the independence first and then have attacked the French. He could bear to see America independent, but could not support it that France should be at peace. Every Englishman and Irishman too, I suppose, thinks he has a right to condemn or oppose measures adopted by the rulers, as they seem fit in his eyes – my Lord North, Mr Fox, &c. were condemned ...there was nothing that did not receive his disapprobation in the line of politicks. When your father was speaking, or appeared as if going to speak, he was all attention. I feared he was going to make pappa warm, by his [--] of our country and at the same time giving his wise opinions respecting the War.

After this rather awkward start, things seem to have settled down somewhat as the others cleared their food and found their tongues. Abigail found herself seated next to the young man who was probably Samuel Romilly, and was initially delighted that he had visited her beloved France. Yet as they began to converse it became clear that he

> viewed everything I found with an eye of prejudice. Paris was not so fine a city as London, the French ladies he was sure could not be agreeable in the eyes of the English, and in all he found a preference for this country. ... before I sat down to table I had conceived an opinion that this gentleman was a native of France, but had been long in this country. From his name, complexion, and manners I was led to judge thus, and I

165 John Adams to JJ, 26 September 1785, MHS Adams papers.

> thought myself perfectly safe in the preference I gave to that country. But I soon found I had a wrong idea, for he was verily English. Both the Dr and Mrs Jebb spoke highly in praise of his abilities, good sense, judgement, &c.[166]

While young Abigail longed to return to France, her parents felt entirely at home indulging in vigorous political discussion with the enlightened and patriotic Jebbs.

ANN JEBB AND THE FRENCH REVOLUTION

Unfortunately Jebb died just over three years before the outbreak of the French Revolution. But Ann Jebb survived her husband until 1812 and maintained a lively interest in politics. She was consoled with remembrance of John's 'talents and virtues' and 'invariably spoke of him, though still without repining, in language of the deepest regret'.[167] She continued to entertain friends despite illness up until her death. In the course of conversation Ann would often refer to the authority of her late husband, pointing to his bust that stood beside her on a table.[168] While largely confined to her house in Halfmoon Street in Piccadilly for the last decade of her life, old friends such as John Disney and his daughter regularly visited.[169] Among Ann's most frequent visitors were Thomas Jervis (1748-1833), who succeeded Andrew Kippis as minister at the Unitarian chapel in Westminster (1796-1808), and the novelist and travel writer Anne Plumptre.[170] The latter was an author and enthusiastic Jacobin who in 1795 addressed her literary agent in London as 'Dear Citizen' and expressed an admiration for John Thelwall.[171]

Ann was unimpressed with the political gymnastics performed by both Pitt and Fox during the Regency Crisis. 'I have been very poorly', she wrote to Cartwright, 'and am almost worn out by reading long speeches, without finding a single argument to make me alter my sentiments; but a great deal of foreign matter, illiberal language, and a want of honesty in both sides of the House.'[172] She was also disappointed when Pitt turned his back on the Dissenters and opposed abolition of the Test Act. Yet she had the satisfaction of witnessing Fox's Libel Act and extension of the franchise to Irish Catholics.

Along with many other Britons, Ann Jebb enthusiastically welcomed the French Revolution. She was 'thankful that I am living to see a dispensation to bind tyrants in chains, to reform the sanguinary laws, and to let the oppressed go free'. After reading of the Festival of Federation, she declared that Louis XVI should think himself 'superior to all the kings and emperors who ever tyrannised

---

[166] Abigail Adams jr. to John Q. Adams, 13 September 1785, MHS Adams papers.

[167] Meadley, *Memoir of Ann Jebb*, p. 24.

[168] Meadley, *Memoir of Ann Jebb*, pp. 53-4.

[169] John Disney to Mary Hayes, 31 January 1793, DWL Mss. 24.93.3.

[170] Meadley, *Memoir of Ann Jebb*, p. 49; *DNB*.

[171] C.B. Jewson, *The Jacobin City: a portrait of Norwich in its reaction to the French Revolution, 1788-1802* (1975), p. 90.

[172] AJ to John Cartwright, [?] February 1789, *Memoir of Ann Jebb*, pp. 26-27.

over mankind'.[173] While concerned by the aristocratic presence in the National Assembly, Ann remained confident that the majority would 'complete the glorious work'. 'You see', she told Brand Hollis, 'the fire is spreading everywhere. I tell you the world is a good world, as the Doctor used to say, and the people who find fault with it should mend themselves. There is a time for everything; if the French had reformed sooner, the reformation would have been less complete.'[174]

When France went to war against its monarchical European neighbours in 1792, she argued against Britain's involvement in two short pamphlets. In response to a loyalist broadside,[175] Ann argued that 'the swinish multitude are not destitute of humanity: do not make them mad, and they can feel, as sensibly, at least, as Mr Burke', and declared that if the necessary reforms had not been resisted then there would have been no conflict.[176] Writing five days after the execution of Louis XVI, Ann blamed those who encouraged him to oppose the Revolution rather than submit to popular sovereignty. She pleaded against entering into another war when Britain was only recently recovered from the disastrous American conflict. 'Surely ... the shedding *rivers of blood,* in revenge for the blood of *one man*, will be no proof of our *superior justice*, nor will the making of *thousands of weeping widows* and *helpless orphans*, give us reason to boast our *superior humanity*'.[177]

Charles James Fox regained Ann's respect through this support for the French Revolution, abolition of the slave trade, religious toleration and parliamentary reform. When Pitt died in January 1806, Ann observed that Fox and the 'ministry of talents' would be constrained by the need to conclude an unfavourable peace with Napoleon and raise taxes in preparation for more war. 'Mr Pitt did not live long enough to convince the City or the people sufficiently, that that he was driving the nation to a precipice; and left just in time to avoid the odium of the strong measures, which must be resorted to.'[178] But her hopes of peace waned with Fox's ill health and his death later in the year.

The factional instability in high politics following the death of Pitt in 1806 was accompanied by some revived interest in the cause of parliamentary reform. The divisions that were evident among the reformers, however, disappointed Ann Jebb. While she saw 'violent friends of liberty' emerging from the lower classes, Ann remained a supporter of the Foxites: 'Some people seem to wish for a new party: – but where are we to get them? Who can point out to us where these wonder working men are to be found, who can do the work of thirty years in a single session? Rome was not built in a day.'[179]

---

[173] AJ to Thomas Brand Hollis, 24 July 1790, *Memoir of Ann Jebb*, p. 29.
[174] AJ to Thomas Brand Hollis, 31 August 1790, *Memoir of Ann Jebb*, p. 30.
[175] [Rev William Jones of Nayland], *One Penny-Worth of Truth from Thomas Bull to his brother John Bull* (1792); this was initially answered by [----], *John Bull's Answer to Thomas Bull's Pennyworth of Truth* (13 December 1792).
[176] AJ, *Two Pennyworth of Truth for a Penny*, p. 11; *Memoir of Ann Jebb*, pp. 32-33.
[177] AJ, *Two Pennyworth More of Truth for a Penny*, p. 15.
[178] AJ to John Disney, 23 January & 20 February 1806, *Memoir of Ann Jebb*, pp. 37-38.
[179] AJ to John Disney, 10 June 1807, *Memoir of Ann Jebb*, p. 41.

She continued to support some of the Whigs, and was particularly impressed with Samuel Romilly's commitment to penal reform.[180] Ann Jebb remained an opponent to the war against Napoleon, even refusing to approve of Wellington's campaign on the Iberian Peninsula.[181] She passed away on 20 January 1812. Frail, sickly and relatively housebound, to the last Ann Jebb observed and commented upon political developments with a mind shaped by the religious, philosophical and political debates of the first half of George III's reign.

[180] Meadley, *Memoir of Ann Jebb*, p. 45.
[181] Meadley, *Memoir of Ann Jebb*, pp. 42-45.

Conclusion

Because Jebb did not compose a timeless political tract his friend John Cartwright has overshadowed his important role in the development of radical politics.[1] This study has sought to correct this neglect. There were over six hundred subscribers for John Disney's *The Works: Theological, Medical, Political and Miscellaneous of John Jebb, MD. FRS., with a Life of the Author* (1787). At the Revolution Society commemorative dinner in 1788 a toast to 'the immortal memory of Hampden, Pym, Russell, and Sydney' was followed with one to 'the memory of Andrew Marvell, Milton, Locke, the late Mr Hollis, and the late Dr John Jebb'.[2] The leading role Jebb played in the reform movement in the early 1780s was recognised by both friend and foe. If it can be said that Richard Price was the 'first and original Left-Wing Intellectual'[3] in British history, Jebb was one of the first 'left-wing' activists.

Herbert Butterfield once argued that Britain came close to revolution in 1780.[4] This view has since been discredited. Despite the strong language used by Jebb and his fellow radicals, they remained middle-class reformers committed to the rule of law. Nevertheless, their vision of a British constitution in which the House of Commons represented the common people rather than propertied and corporate interests had radical implications – something borne out by the reaction of mainstream Whigs such as Burke and Rockingham. At the end of 1779 Jebb had suggested that the parliament should be reformed in order

---

[1] For example, in his recent important study of *The British Isles and the War of American Independence,* Stephen Conway makes several references to Cartwright but does not mention Jebb.

[2] *An Abstract of the History and Proceedings of the Revolution Society in London, to which is annexed a copy of the Bill of Rights* (1789), p. 4.

[3] Pocock, 'Radical Criticisms of the Whig Order', p. 48.

[4] Butterfield, *George III, Lord North, and the People*.

to free the House of Commons from crown and aristocratic manipulation and allow it to accurately represent the will of 'the people'. But few in Britain's governing classes shared his desire for radical reform. When William Pitt drew up a moderate reform bill, Jebb angrily observed that his rejection of 'the principle of universal suffrage, shews that he either understands not or denies the existence of [the people's] primary rights'.[5] In a private letter Jebb expressed a hope that the example of the Irish Volunteers would 'shake the Aristocracy to its centre', after which 'the tyranny of the Church must give way', and there would be nothing left to 'obstruct complete success'.[6] Jebb envisioned a profound moral and political 'reformation' that would have encouraged religious pluralism and placed greater political and social power in the hands of the 'middling sort'.

Jebb's commitment to a radical political platform was rooted in a combination of scientific empiricism, Socinianism, philosophical determinism and radical Whig politics. Of particular importance was David Hartley's attempt to combine a determinist philosophy and the notion of universal salvation with a powerful call for moral and religious reform. Jebb's religious and philosophical disposition allowed him confidently to support demands for reform with a mix of historical, natural rights and utilitarian arguments – his intellectual confidence and inclination for radical ideas moved forward under the influence of his social and political experience. At Cambridge he worked to reform some aspects of what was later termed 'Old Corruption'. The fierce opposition Jebb encountered provided an education in the politics of institutional inertia. Such first hand experience of the difficulties attending institutional reform set him apart from many fellow Rational Dissenters such as Price, Priestley and Lindsey, and may partly explain his more active interest in politics.

Following his death Jebb's friends praised his candour and unrelenting efforts to realise high ideals. In answer to Burke's denigration of the members of the Society for Constitutional Information, Benjamin Bousfield declared that the example of the late Dr Jebb 'should shield them from detraction', as a man 'whose labours, and whose learning were dedicated to the service, the freedom, and the happiness of mankind. His benevolent disposition was neither bound by space nor time'.[7] To the moderate reformer and political realist Christopher Wyvill, Jebb 'was a man of great abilities, of extensive learning; eloquent in his writing and in debate; amiable for his candour and benevolence; exemplary for his piety, and the strict morality of his private life; and in his public conduct he maintained Truth with the intrepidity of a Martyr; and pursued the General Good with the ardour of an Enthusiast'.[8] The general opinion of both friend and opponent was that Jebb would have been satisfied with nothing short of heaven-on-earth – which is exactly what he was working toward. At the age of fifty, however, a life of earnest agitation was ended by persistent ill health. Perhaps Jebb should have listened to the advice Henry Taylor proffered Ann: 'I wish the

[5] JJ to Henry Joy, 18 May 1785, LHL Joy papers.
[6] JJ to Henry Joy, [1785?], LHL Joy papers.
[7] Bousfield, *Observations on the Right Hon. Edmund Burke's Pamphlet*, p. 96.
[8] *Wyvill Papers*, IV, p. 521n.

Dr loved nonsense as well as I do. It would take off all the ill consequence of his thinking and acting with so little relaxation. Your souls are only fit for Spiritual Bodies; they will wear out such as are made of flesh and blood too soon.'[9]

Historians have disagreed fiercely in recent decades as to how we should characterise eighteenth-century Britain.[10] Was it a conservative and deferential society, dominated by aristocracy and Church? Or is it more accurately depicted as a dynamic society, with a burgeoning middle-class, and in which established institutions were on the back foot, having to adapt in the face of continual social, economic, intellectual and political change and challenge? While this debate will continue to rage, it is clear that any understanding of the period must take into account both perspectives. Eighteenth-century England was a society with its roots firmly planted in the past – governed by a wealthy landed class who copied continental fashions. Parliament was composed of the representatives of various corporate 'interests' (landed, mercantile and institutional). While providing a classical education for some of the ruling class, Oxford and Cambridge acted as seminaries for a Church of England that preached submission to established authority. And a brutal criminal code guarded property against the desires or desperation of the propertyless. Yet it is also clear that within this old society there were stresses and strains, disaffection and dissent. In the second half of the century in particular, traditional institutions, beliefs and practices had to adapt to enlightened, evangelical and popular criticism. The degree to which the character of Britain's governing institutions and ideology were challenged will remain the subject of debate, yet challenges were clearly mounted by the likes of John and Ann Jebb.

This study informs our understanding of eighteenth-century Britain in a number of ways. Jebb highlights the importance of heterodox theology as a source of political radicalism. As with his fellow traveller Joseph Priestley, however, Jebb's heterodoxy needs to be seen as encompassed within a more general 'rational dissent' that drew intellectual confidence from David Hartley's optimistic Enlightenment philosophy that combined determinism, materialism and Christianity. Jebb supports a depiction of the old order being undermined by a broad range of dissent characterised as 'an ecumenical expression of the drive to criticise, question and subvert'.[11] Writing in relation to the advancement of medical knowledge, Jebb neatly expressed this critical attitude: 'the interests of truth have nothing to apprehend from the keenness of investigation, and the utmost severity of human judgement.'[12]

At the same time, this study has added to our growing appreciation of the strong support that existed for the establishment in Church and State. Only a small number of particularly earnest heterodox clergy resigned from the Church

---

[9] Henry Taylor to AJ, [1785?], CUL Taylor papers.

[10] For an overview see Jeremy Black, *Eighteenth-Century Britain, 1688-1783* (Basingstoke, 2001), pp. 1-11.

[11] Porter, *Enlightenment*, p. 480. See also, Wilfrid Prest, *Albion Ascendant: English history 1660-1815* (Oxford, 1998), pp. 143-46.

[12] *Select Cases of the Disorder commonly termed the Paralysis of the Lower Extremities*, Jebb II, p. 441.

for reasons of conscience rather than persecution. While High Churchmen found the paths to preferment open again under George III, in general loyalty and moderate orthodoxy were rewarded. Thus, while many saw the need for education reform at Cambridge, Jebb's proposals for annual examinations were ultimately defeated because his restless heterodoxy and rationalism provoked determined opposition from some powerful defenders of the status quo. Having said this, Jebb's education reforms came very close to being accepted, and the virulence of the opposition that confronted him in the Church and at Cambridge indicates that his ideas and actions were considered to be a real threat. Colin Haydon's note of caution on reviewing the burgeoning literature on eighteenth-century Anglicanism needs to be heeded: 'there may, perhaps, now be a danger in playing down the very real problems which beset the Church of England and, indeed, organised religion in general'.[13]

Jebb highlights the growth of individualism and 'liberal' values in the late Enlightenment. Roy Porter has pointed to the 'pervasive individualism' of the British Enlightenment, in which the hallmark of thinking 'lay in casting progress as a matter of individual improvement or (as with hospitals, schools and charities) as the work of voluntary associations'.[14] Jebb began his life under the Whig Ascendancy, expecting to follow his father into a comfortable career in that corporate pillar of the established order, the Church of England. Had he managed to become the Professor of Arabic at Cambridge in 1768, what, we might reflect, would have been the result? Would he have lost himself in scholarly studies? Or would a secure position, combined with an increasing familiarity with the Koran and another cultural perspective, have strengthened his determination to reform the University, Church and State? His opponents seem to have envisioned that the outcome would be something like the latter. Having failed to gain the patronage of the University, however, by the 1780s Jebb had become a full participant in a rapidly expanding civil society and consumer economy in London – building up a customer base for his medical practice, supporting his friend's Unitarian church, organising political associations in taverns and coffee-houses, independently proposing a model for the construction of prisons and contributing to the burgeoning newspaper and pamphlet market. In the last ten years of his life Jebb's focus shifted away from study of the Scriptures, and his 'rational piety' was increasingly expressed through work as a doctor and agitation for political reform. By his death in 1786 Jebb's everyday life was a manifestation of dissent from many of the 'Old Regime' aspects of eighteenth-century Britain.

Substantial parliamentary reform was not enacted until nearly fifty years after Jebb's death, and that was only the first stage of a process in which the Parliament eventually became fully representative. But if the eighteenth-century reformers failed to see Parliament adopt their proposals, they succeeded in developing ideas and establishing organisations that formed the basis of the nineteenth-century reform movement. Jebb's time was a period of great demographic change and an increasing flow of information through newspapers

[13] Haydon, *Anti-Catholicism*, p. 257.
[14] Porter, *Enlightenment*, p. 482.

and pamphlets. The pamphlets of the Society for Constitutional Information and the declarations of the Association movement played an important role in the expansion of the political nation, the growing importance of public opinion and increasing debate over the nature of the constitution. 'What has become evident, right into the twentieth century', according to Patrick Joyce, 'is just how central a role the constitution played in the generation of political identity and conflict'. In particular, 'early nineteenth-century radicalism and Chartism were suffused in the language of the ancient constitution'.[15] In the context of the Enlightenment and the American Revolution, Jebb helped to revive, develop and promote this influential tradition of radical interpretations of the British constitution. While he saw little in the way of reforms enacted during his lifetime, Jebb nevertheless made an important contribution to the development of politics in modern Britain and some of its colonies.

---

[15] Patrick Joyce, *Democratic Subjects: the self and the social in nineteenth-century England* (Cambridge, 1994), p. 193.

Bibliography

PRIMARY SOURCES

Manuscripts

British Library (BL)

Add. Mss.

Hardwicke papers Add. Mss. 35,351-35,632.

Newcastle papers Add. Mss. 32,731-33,053.

Cole 'Diary'

William Cole, 'Diary 1766-70', Add. Mss. 5835.

Cole 'Journal'

William Cole, 'Journal of My Journey to Paris 1765', Add. Mss. 5835.

Cole mss.

William Cole, 'Alphabetical Collections for an Athenae Cantabrigienses', Add. Mss. 5862-5885, 5954-55.

Fox papers

The papers of Charles James Fox (15 microform reels). BL Add. Mss. 47,559-47,581 and Holland House papers Ad. Mss. 51,457-51,475 (Harvester Microform, Sussex, 1984).

Jebb family papers

Add. Mss. 6,696; 32,979; 35,755; 35,678; 36,305.

Westminster Committee Minutes

Add. Mss. 38595.

Cambridge University Library (CUL)

Taylor papers

Letters from the Reverend Henry Taylor to Mrs Ann Jebb, 1772-85, Add. Mss. 7901.3.

Doctor Williams Library, London (DWL)

Blackburne correspondence

Letters of Archdeacon Francis Blackburne to Theophilus Lindsey 1756-75 (includes some miscellaneous correspondence by John Jebb, Thomas Blackburne, etc.), mss. 12.52.

Disney mss.

'A Collection of Letters and Essays on the Subject of Religious Liberty published in the Newspapers 1771-74' (compiled by John Disney), mss. 87.1-6.

Illustrated Life of Priestley

J.T. Rutt, *The Illustrated Life and Correspondence of Joseph Priestley*, mss. 12.79.

Jebb mss.

John Jebb manuscripts (6 volumes): 'Interleaved Greek New Testament' (vols. 1-5) and 'Lectures and Miscellaneous Notes' (vol. 6), mss. 24.168-73.

Joseph Johnson letters

Copies of letters by Joseph Johnson, mss. 12.58.

Letters of Lardner &c.

Letters of Nathaniel Lardner, Joseph Priestley, Francis Blackburne, Gilbert Wakefield and J. Toulmin, mss. 12.45.

Lindsey letters

Letters to Theophilus Lindsey, mss. 12.56.

Lindsey-Turner correspondence

Letters of Theophilus Lindsey and others to William Turner (1714-94) and William Turner (1761-1859), mss. 12.44.

'Memoir of John Disney'

'Memoir of John Disney' (incomplete and author unknown), mss. 28.165.

Millar papers

Robert Millar Papers, mss. 12.46.

Purves-Fyshe Palmer correspondence

Letters between James Purves and Thomas Fyshe Palmer 1785-87, mss. 24.80.

Stanus papers

Papers of B.T. Stanus, mss. 24.54.

Wodrow-Kenrick correspondence

Correspondence between James Wodrow (1731-1810) and Samuel Kenrick (1728-1811), mss. 24.157.

Gloucestershire Record Office (GRO)

Sharp Diary

Extracts from the Diaries of Granville Sharp 1772-1813.

Sharp papers

Correspondence of Granville Sharp.

Harvard University Library (HUL)

Miscellaneous Jebb letters

Two Letters by Jebb to unidentified correspondents.

John Ryland's Library, Manchester (JRL)

Lindsey - Tayleur correspondence
Autograph Letters of Theophilus Lindsey to William Tayleur 1775-89.
Tayleur letters
Letters of William Tayleur and miscellaneous theological notes.

Linen Hall Library, Belfast (LHL)

Joy papers
Letters from John Jebb and others to Henry Joy.

Massachusetts Historical Society (MHS)

Adams papers
Correspondence of John Adams and his family.

National Library of Ireland (NLI)

Bourke collection
Letters by John and Ann Jebb to John Forbes in the F.S. Bourke collection, mss. 10,713.3.
Dobbs papers
Letters to Francis Dobbs from John Cartwright and John Jebb, Dobbs papers mss. 2251.

North Yorkshire Record Office (NYRO)

Wyvill mss.
The Papers of Christopher Wyvill.

Privately held

Disney, 'Diary'
John Disney, 'Diary 1783-84', in the possession of D.O. Thomas, Emeritus Professor of Philosophy, University of Wales, Aberystwyth.

Public Record Office, London (PRO)

SCI Minutes
Minutes of the Society for Constitutional Information, Books 1-3 Treasury Solicitor II/1133, II/961, II/962.

Printed Primary Sources

Place of publication is London unless otherwise indicated.

Chronological List of Publications by John and Ann Jebb

Thorpe, R., Wollaston, G. and Jebb, J., *Excerpta quaedam e Newtoni Principiis philosophiae naturalis, cum notis variorum* (Cambridge, 1765).

Jebb, John, *A Short Account of Theological Lectures now reading at Cambridge, to which is added a New Harmony of the Gospels* (1770, 2nd ed. 1772).

_____ *'Circular Letter' of the Feathers Tavern Petition* (1771).

_____ *Letters on the Subject of Subscription to the liturgy and thirty-nine articles of the Church of England* (1772).

_____ *Letter to Sir William Meredith* (1772).

_____ *The Excellency of the Spirit of Benevolence, a sermon preached before the University of Cambridge on Monday, December 28, 1772* (1773).

_____ *Remarks upon the Present Mode of Education in the University of Cambridge: to which is added a proposal for its improvement* (April 1773; 4th ed., January 1774).

_____ *A Proposal for the Establishment of Public Examinations in the University of Cambridge, with occasional remarks* (1774).

Jebb, Ann, *A Letter to the Author of an Observation on the Design of Establishing Annual Examinations at Cambridge* (Cambridge, November 1774).

Jebb, John, *A Short State of the Reasons for a Late Resignation* (October 1775).

_____ *An Address to the Members of the Senate of Cambridge* (Cambridge, March 1775; 2nd ed. December 1775).

_____ 'A Postscript by Dr Jebb to the Author of a Letter &c', attached to Theophilus Lindsey, *Two Dissertations* (April 1778).

_____ *Address to the Freeholders of Middlesex, on Monday 20th December* (December 1779; 4th ed. May 1782).

_____ *Report of the Westminster Committee* (May 1780).

_____ *A Letter to Sir Robert Bernard, Chairman of the Huntingdonshire Committee* (1781).

_____ *Select Cases of the Disorder commonly termed the Paralysis of the Lower Extremities* (1782).

_____ *Letters Addressed to the Volunteers of Ireland, on the subject of parliamentary reform* (1784).

_____ *A Sketch of the Plan of the Society for Promoting the Knowledge of the Scriptures* (1783).

_____ *A Letter to the Secretary of the Society for Constitutional Information* (July 1784).

_____ *Thoughts on the Construction and Polity of Prisons* (Capel Lofft ed., 1785).

_____ *The Works: Theological, Medical, Political and Miscellaneous of John Jebb, MD. FRS., with a Life of the Author* (3 vols., John Disney ed., 1787).

Jebb, Ann, *Two Pennyworth of Truth for a Penny; or, a true state of Facts; with an Apology for Tom Bull, in a Letter to Brother John* (13 December 1792).

_____ *Two Pennyworth of More of Truth for a Penny; being a Second Letter from – Bull to Brother John* (26 January 1793).

Newspapers and Magazines

Annual Register
General Evening Post
Gentleman's Magazine
Lloyd's Evening Post
London Chronicle
London Evening Post
London Packet
Middlesex Journal
Monthly Review
St James's Chronicle
Volunteer's Journal or *Irish Herald* (Dublin, 1783-86)
Whitehall Evening Post

Tracts, Pamphlets, Memoirs and Collected Works

An Abstract of the History and Proceedings of the Revolution Society in London, to which is annexed a copy of the Bill of Rights (1789).

The Adams Family Correspondence (L.H. Butterfield ed., 6 vols., Cambridge, Mass., 1963-93.

Adams, John, *The Diary and Autobiography of John Adams* (L.H. Butterfield ed., 4 vols., Cambridge, Mass., 1961).

Anson, William ed., *Autobiography and Political Correspondence of Augustus Henry, 3rd Duke of Grafton* (1898).

Balguy Thomas, *A Charge Delivered to the Clergy of the Archdeaconry of Winchester in the year 1772* (1772).

_____ *A Sermon Preached at Lambeth Chapel* (1769).

_____ *A Sermon preached in Lambeth Chapel, on the consecration of the Right Reverend Richard Hurd and the Right Reverend John Moore* (1775).

Bartlett, Thomas, *Memoirs of Bishop Joseph Butler (1692-1768)* (1839).

Beccaria, Cesare, *Of Crimes and Punishments* (Jane Grigson trans., Marsilio, N. Y., 1996).

Belsham, Thomas, *Memoirs of the Late Theophilus Lindsey* (2nd ed., 1820).

Bentham, Edward, *Reflections upon the Study of Divinity* (Oxford, 1771).

Blackall, Samuel, *A Letter to Dr Hallifax upon the subject of his Three Discourses preached before the University of Cambridge* (Cambridge, 2nd ed., 1782 [1772]).

Blackburne, Francis, *The Confessional: or a full and free inquiry into the Right, Utility, Edification, and Success of establishing systematical confessions of faith and doctrine in Protestant churches* (1766, 2nd ed. 1767, 3rd ed, 1770).

_____ *Memoirs of Thomas Hollis* (2 vols., 1780).

_____ *The Works Theological and Miscellaneous* (Francis Blackburne ed., 7 vols., Cambridge, 1805).

_____ ed., *A Collection of Letters and Essays in Favour of Public Liberty, 1764-70* (3 vols., 1774).

Blackstone, William, *Commentaries on the Laws of England* (6 vols., Oxford, 1765-69).

Bolingbroke, Lord, *Historical Writings* (Isaac Kramnick ed., Chicago, 1972).

Boswell, James, *Boswell in Search of a Wife, 1766-69* (Frank Brady and Frederick A. Pottle eds., 1957).

_____ *Life of Samuel Johnson* (G.B. Hill ed., Oxford, 1934).

Bousfield, Benjamin, *Observations on the Right Hon. Edmund Burke's Pamphlet, On the Subject of the French Revolution* (Dublin, 1791) in Gregory Clayes ed., *Political Writings of the 1790s* (8 vols., 1995).

Brown, John, *Estimate of the Manners of the Times* (1757).

Burgh, James, *Crito, or, essays on various subjects* (2nd ed.1767).

_____ *Britain's Remembrancer, or the danger not over* (1746).

_____ *Political Disquisitions* (3 vols., 1774-75).

Burke, Edmund, *Reflections on the Revolution in France* (Conor Cruise O'Brien ed., Harmondsworth, 1968 [1790]).

_____ *Thoughts on the Cause of the Present Discontents* (1770).

_____ *The Writings and Speeches of Edmund Burke* (Paul Langford ed., Oxford, 1981).

Butler, Joseph, *Analogy of Religion and Nature* (1736).

Cappe, Catherine, *Memoirs of the Life of Catherine Cappe, by herself* (1822).

_____ *A Small Tribute of Respect to the Memory of Mrs Lindsey* (York, 1812).

Cartwright, F.D., ed., *The Life and Correspondence of Major Cartwright* (1826).

Cartwright, John, *An Address to the Public from the Society for Constitutional Information* (April, 1780).

_____ *Declaration of Those Rights of the Commonality of Great Britain without Which They Cannot Be Free* (1780).

_____ *Give Us Our Rights!* (1782).

_____ *Internal Evidence; or, an inquiry how far truth and the Christian religion have been consulted by the author of 'Thoughts on Parliamentary Reform'* (1784).

_____ *Legislative Rights of the Commonality Vindicated, or Take Your Choice* (1776, 2nd ed. 1780).

_____ *The People's Barrier against Undue Influence and Corruption: or, the Commons House of Parliament according to the Constitution* (1780).

Claeys, Gregory ed., *Political Writings of the 1790s* (8 vols., 1995).

Clarke, Samuel, *Discourse on the Being and Attributes of God, the Obligations of Natural Religion, and the truth and certainty of the Christian Revelation* (1732).

_____ *The Scripture-Doctrine of the Trinity* (1712).

_____ *The Verity and Truth of Natural and Revealed Religion* (1705).

Clayton, Robert, *Essay on Spirit ... with some remarks on the Athanasian and Nicene Creeds* (Dublin, 1751).

_____ *Vindication of the Old and New Testament* (Dublin, 1757).

Cole, William, *A Journal of My Journey to Paris in the Year 1765* (F.G. Stokes ed., 1931).

A Collection of Letters which have been Addressed to the Volunteers of Ireland, on the subject of Parliamentary Reform by the Earl of Effingham &c. (1783).

Cooper, C.H., *Annals of Cambridge* (5 vols, 1842-1908).

Crane, Verner, *Benjamin Franklin's Letters to the Press 1758-75* (1950).

Dawes, Manassah, *An Essay on Crimes and Punishments; with a view of and commentary upon Beccaria, Rousseau, Voltaire, Montesquieu, Fielding and Blackstone* (1782).

Day, Thomas, *The History of Sanford and Merton* (1783-89).

_____ *A Letter on the Slavery of the Negroes* (1776).

_____ *Reflections Upon the Present State of England, and the Independence of America* (1782).

Dickinson, John, *Letters from a Farmer in Pennsylvania* (Philadelphia, 1768)

Disney, John, *Animadversions on the Conduct of Dr Rutherford in the Controversy which has followed the Publication of the Confessional* (1768).
_____ *The Duty of Circumspection in Licensing Public Ale-houses* (1776).
_____ *The Progressive Improvement of Civil Liberty: a sermon preached at the Essex Street on the anniversary of the Revolution of 1688, November 4, 1792* (1792).
_____ *Memoirs of Thomas Brand-Hollis* (1808).
_____ *A Short Memoir of the Late William Hopkins* (1787).
_____ *A Short Memoir of Michael Dodson* (1800).
_____ *A Short View of the Controversies Occasioned by the Confessional* (1773).
Dyer, George, *History of the University and Colleges of Cambridge* (2 vols., 1814).
_____ *Memoirs of the Life and Writings of Robert Robinson* (1796).
Dury, John ed., *Critics of the Bible: 1724-1873* (Cambridge, 1989).
Farmer, Hugh, *Dissertation on Miracles* (1771).
_____ *An Inquiry into the Nature and Design of Christ's Temptation in the Wilderness* (1761).
Findlay, Robert, *A Letter to the Rev Mr Jebb with relation to his Declared Sentiments about the Unlawfulness of all Religious Addresses to Christ Jesus* (1778).
_____ *Remarks on Mr Lindsey's Dissertation upon Praying to Christ; with a Second Letter to Mr Jebb* (1781).
Firebrace, John, *A Further Defence of the Present Scheme of Petitioning Parliament* (1771).
_____ *A Letter to Rev James Ibbetson, occasioned by a third edition of his Plea* (1771).
_____ *The Plea of the Petitioners, Stated and Vindicated from the misrepresentations contained in a late Charge delivered by Dr Balguy* (1773).
Forster, Nathaniel, *An Essay on Establishments in Religion, with Remarks on the Confessional* (August, 1767).
_____ *The Establishment of the Church of England defended upon the Principles of Religious Liberty* (1770).
Fortesque, Sir J., ed., *The Correspondence of George the Third from 1760 to December 1783* (6 vols., 1973).
Franklin, Benjamin, *Benjamin Franklin's Letters to the Press 1758-75* (Verner Crane ed., Chapel Hill, N.C., 1950).
_____ *The Papers of Benjamin Franklin* (W.B. Willcox ed., New Haven, Conn., 1978).
Grafton, Augustus Henry, Duke of, *Autobiography and Political Correspondence* (1898).
Gordon, John, *The Causes and Consequences of evil speaking against the Government considered* (1771).
Hallifax, Samuel, *A Sermon Preached before the Honourable House of Commons ... on Monday, January 30, 1769* (Cambridge, 1769).
_____ *Three Sermons preached before the University of Cambridge, Occasioned by an Attempt to Abolish Subscription to the XXXIX Articles of Religion* (Cambridge, 1772).
_____ *Two Sermons delivered before the University in 1768, in Praise of Benefactors* (Cambridge, 1768).
Hamilton Rowan, Archibald, *The Autobiography of Archibald Hamilton Rowan* (Dublin, 1840).
Hare, Francis, *The Difficulties and Discouragement which attend the Study of the Scriptures* (1736).
Hartley, David, *Observations on Man, his frame, his duty, and his expectations* (David Hartely jr. ed., 1791 [1749]).
[Hartley, J.], *History of the Westminster Election* (2nd ed., 1785).
Harwood, Edward, *Of the Socinian Scheme* (2nd ed., 1783).

Henley, Samuel, *The Distinct Claims of Government and Religion, considered in a sermon preached before the Honourable House of Burgesses, at Williamsburg in Virginia, March 1, 1772* (Cambridge, 1772).

Hoadly, Benjamin, *The Nature of the Kingdom, or Church of Christ* (1717).

_____ *The Objections Against the Repeal of the Test and Corporation Acts Considered* (1739).

_____ *The Original Institution of Civil Government, discuss'd* (1710).

_____ *A preserve against the Principles of the Non-Jurors* (1716).

_____ *The Rational Christian's Assistant to the Worthy Receiving of the Lord's Supper* (John Disney ed., 1774).

Hodgson, R., *The Life of Beilby Porteus, late Bishop of London* (5th ed., 1811).

Holbach, Paul Henri Thiry baron'd, *The System of Nature* (Robert D. Richardson ed., New York, 1984).

Horne, George, *The Works of George Horne* (William Jones ed., 1809).

Howard, John, *The State of the Prisons in England and Wales, with preliminary observations, and an account of some foreign prisons and hospitals* (1929 [1777-80]).

Hulme, Obidiah, *An Historical Essay on the English Constitution* (1771).

Hume, David, *Political Writings* (Knud Haakonssen ed., Cambridge, 1994).

Hurd, Bishop Richard, *The Early Letters of Bishop Richard Hurd: 1739-1762* (Sarah Brewer ed., 1995).

_____ *The Works of Bishop Richard Hurd* (8 vols., 1811).

Jacobsen, David L., *The English Libertarian Heritage: from the writings of John Trenchard and Thomas Gordon* (Indianapolis, 1965).

Johnson, Samuel, *Poetry and Prose* (Mona Wilson ed., 1957).

Jones, John, *Free and Candid Disquisitions relating to the Church of England* (1749).

Jones, William, *The Theological and Miscellaneous Works* (6 vols., 1826).

Jones, William (of Nayland), *One Penny-Worth of Truth from Thomas Bull to his brother John Bull* (1792).

Jones, Sir William, *The Letters of Sir William Jones* (Garland Cannon ed., 2 vols., Oxford, 1970).

_____ *On the Legal Mode of Suppressing Riots* (1781).

_____ *The Principles of Government in a Dialogue between a Scholar and a Peasant* (1782).

Jortin, John, *Remarks on Ecclesiastical History* (1751-54).

Kier, J., *An Account of the Life and Writings of Thomas Day* (1791).

King, William, *An Essay on the Origin of evil* (Edmund Law ed., 3rd ed., 1739).

Kramnick, Isaac, ed., *The Portable Enlightenment Reader* (Harmondsworth, 1995).

Kippis, Andrew, *A Vindication of the Protestant Dissenting Ministers* (1773).

Lardner, Nathaniel, *The Credibility of Gospel History* (1727-57).

Law, Edmund, *Considerations on the Propriety of Requiring a Subscription to Articles of Faith* (Cambridge, 2nd ed., 1774).

_____ *Considerations on the State of the World with regard to the Theory of Religion* (1745, 6th ed. 1774, 8th ed. 1820).

_____ *A Defence of Mr Locke's Opinion concerning Personal Identity* (Cambridge, 1769).

_____ *Reflections on the Life and Character of Christ; with an essay on the nature and end of death under the Christian covenant* (T. Lindsey ed., 1803).

Lindsey, Theophilus, *Apology on Resigning the Vicarage of Catterick, Yorkshire* (1774).

_____ *The Catechist: or, an inquiry into the doctrine of the Scriptures, concerning the only true God and object of religious worship* (1781).

_____ *A Farewell Address to the Parishioners of Catterick* (1774).

_____ *A Sermon preached at the opening of the Chapel in Essex House, Essex St, in the Strand, on Sunday April 17, 1774. To which is added a summary account of the Reformed Liturgy, on the plan of the late Dr Samuel Clarke* (1774).
_____ *Two Dissertations* (April 1778).
Locke, John, *Epistola de Tolerantia: a letter on toleration* (Raymond Klibansky ed., J.W. Gough trans., Oxford, 1968).
_____ *Essay Concerning Human Understanding* (A.D. Woozley ed., 1964).
_____ *Locke: Political Essays* (Mark Goldie ed., Cambridge, 1997).
_____ *A Paraphrase and Notes on the Epistles of St Paul* (Arthur W. Wainwright ed., Oxford, 1987 [1707]).
_____ *Some Thoughts Concerning Education* (John W. and Jean S. Yolton eds., 1989).
_____ *The Reasonableness of Christianity* (I.T. Ramsey ed., 1958 [1705]).
_____ *Two Treatises of Government* (Peter Laslett ed., Cambridge, 1960).
Lofft, Capel, *An Inquiry into the Legality and Expediency of increasing the Royal Navy by Subscription for building County Ships. Being the correspondence on the subject between Arthur Young and Capel Lofft* (1783).
_____ *Observations on Mrs Macaulay's History of England; (lately published) from the Revolution to the resignation of Sir Robert Walpole, in a letter addressed to that lady* (1778).
_____ *On the Revival of the Cause of Reform in the Representation of the Commons House of Parliament* (1809).
Lucretius, *On the Nature of the Universe* (Harmondsworth, 1951).
Maclaurin, Colin, *The Philosophy of Isaac Newton* (1748).
Maty, Paul Henry, *An History of the Instances of Exclusion from the Royal Society* (1784).
Meadley, G.M., *Memoir of Mrs Jebb* (1812).
_____ *Memoirs of William Paley* (1809).
Montesquieu, Baron, *The Spirit of the Laws* (Anne M. Cohler trans., Cambridge, 1989).
Mill, John Stuart, *Autobiography* (Jack Stillinger ed., Oxford, 1971 [1873]).
Milner, Mary, *The Life of Isaac Milner* (1842).
Nichols, John, *Literary Anecdotes of the Eighteenth Century* (9 vols., 1813).
Neiman, Fraser, 'The Letters of William Gilpin to Samuel Henley', *Huntington Library Quaterly* 35 (1971-72), pp. 159-69.
Neville, Sylas, *The Diary of Sylas Neville 1767-1788* (Basil Cozens Hardy ed., Oxford, 1950).
Newton, Isaac, *Newton's Philosophy of Nature: selections from his writings* (H.S. Thayer ed., New York, 1953).
Paley, William, 'Life of Edmund Law', affixed to Edmund Law, *Considerations on the State of the World with regard to the Theory of Religion* (8th ed., 1820).
_____ *The Works of William Paley: with additional sermons, and a corrected account of the life and writings of the author* (Victor Nuovo ed., Bristol, 1998 [1830]).
Peckard, Peter, *Subscription; or, historical extracts humbly inscribed to the Bishops and to the Petitioners showing the impropriety of their petition* (1776).
Pitt, William the Younger, *The Speeches of the Right Honourable William Pitt* (3 vols., 1817).
Pott, Percival, *Remarks on that kind of Palsy of the Lower Limbs which is frequently found to accompany a Curvature of the Spine* (1779).
Powell, William Samuel, *A Defence of the Observations on the first chapter of a book called Miscellanea Analytica* (Cambridge, 1760).
_____ *A Defence of the Subscriptions required in the Church of England* (Cambridge, 1772 [1757]).
_____ *Heads of a Course of Lectures in Experimental Philosophy* (1746).

_____ *An Observation on the Design of Establishing Annual Examinations at Cambridge* (1774).

_____ *Observations on the first chapter of a book called Miscellanea Analytica* (Cambridge, 1760).

Price, Richard, *The Correspondence of Richard Price* (3 vols., W. Bernard Peach and D.O. Thomas eds., Chapel Hill, N.C. and Cardiff, Wales, 1983-94).

_____ *Four Dissertations* (1767).

_____ *Observations on the Nature of Civil Liberty, the Principles of Government, and the Justice and Policy of War with America* (1776).

_____ *Price: Political Writings* (D.O. Thomas ed., Cambridge, 1991).

Priestley, Joseph, *The Autobiography of Joseph Priestley* (Jack Lindsey ed., Bath, 1970).

_____ *Priestley: Political Writings* (Peter Miller ed., Cambridge, 1993).

_____ *The Theological and Miscellaneous Works of Joseph Priestley* (J.T. Rutt ed., 25 vols., 1832).

Pringle, John, *Observations on the Nature and Cure of Hospital and Jayl-fevers* (1750).

Randolph, Thomas, *An Answer to a Pamphlet, entitled Considerations on the Propriety of Requiring a Subscription to Articles of Faith* (Oxford, 1774).

_____ *Reasonableness of Requiring Subscription to Articles of Religion from Persons to be Admitted to Holy Orders* (Oxford, 1771).

_____ *A Vindication of the Worship of the Son and the Holy Ghost against the exceptions of Mr Theophilus Lindsey* (Oxford, 1775).

Robinson, Robert, *A Plea for the Divinity of our Lord Jesus Christ: in a pastoral letter addressed to a congregation of Protestant Dissenters at Cambridge* (1776).

_____ *A Political Catechism* (1783).

Romilly, Samuel, *The Life of Sir Samuel Romilly*, with a 'Journal' of their travels in France by John Baynes attached as an appendix (1842).

Scott, John, *The Life of Reverend Thomas Scott* (1823).

Seward, Anna, *The Letters of Anna Seward* (6 vols., Edinburgh, 1811).

Sharp, Granville, *A Declaration of the People's Natural Right to a Share in the Legislature* (1774).

_____ *An Essay on Slavery* (Burlington, 1773; reprinted London, 1776).

Shepard, Richard, *The Requisition of Subscription to the 39 Articles of the Church of England not Inconsistent with Christian Liberty* (1771).

Society for Constitutional Information, *An Abridgement of that eminent Patriot Mr John Trenchard's History of Standing Armies, with an incomparable Preface upon Government* (1780).

_____ *An Address to the Public* (1780).

_____ *A Second Address to the Public* (1782).

Spears, Robert, *A Record of Unitarian Worthies* (1876).

Stephens, John A. ed., 'The Correspondence of Benjamin Rush and Granville Sharp 1773-1809', *Journal of American Studies* 1 (1967), pp. 1-38.

Sterne, Laurence, *The Life and Opinions of Tristram Shandy* (Graham Petrie ed., Harmondsworth, 1967 [1759-67]).

Swift, Jonathan, *Correspondence* (6 vols., 1911-13).

Sykes, Arthur A., *An Essay on the Nature, Design and Origin of Sacrifices* (1748).

Taylor, Henry, *The Apology of Benjamin Ben Mordecai to his Friends for Embracing Christianity* (2nd ed., 1784).

_____ *Confusion worse Confounded; Rout upon Rout; or, the Bishop of G-----r's echo from heaven examined and exposed* (1772).

Temple, Anthony, *A Letter to the Rev John Jebb M.A. Occasioned by his Short State of the Reasons for a Late Resignation* (1776).

_____ *A Sermon preached at the Visitation held at Richmond in Yorkshire* (1766).

Tew, Edward, *Resignation No Proof: A Letter to Mr Jebb, with occasional remarks on his Spirit of Protestantism* (Cambridge, 1776).

Thale, Mary, ed., *Selections from the Papers of the London Corresponding Society 1792-99* (Cambridge, 1983).

Thorpe, Robert, Wollaston, George, and Jebb John, *Excerpta quadaem e Newtoni Principiis philosophie naturalis, cum notis varoirum* (Cambridge, 1965).

Tindal, Matthew, *Christianity as Old as the Creation* (1730).

Tooke, John Horne, *The Memoirs of John Tooke* (A. Stephens ed., 2 vols., 1813).

Towers, Joseph, *Biographia Britannica* (5 vols., 1778-93).

_____ *Observations on the Rights and Duty of Juries in trials for libels* (1784).

_____ *A Vindication of the Political Principles of Mr Locke, in Answer to the Objections of Dr Tucker* (1782).

Towers, Joseph Lomas, *Illustrations of Prophecy* (1796).

Tucker, Josiah, *A Treatise Concerning Civil Government* (1781).

Unitarian Society, *Tracts, printed and published by the Unitarian Society for promoting Christian Knowledge and the Practice of Virtue* (13 vols., 1791-1802).

Vaughan, E.T., *Life of the Rev Thomas Robinson, late vicar of St Mary's, Leicester* (1816).

Voltaire, *Letters on England* (L. Tancock trans., Harmondsworth, 1980 [1733]).

Wakefield, Gilbert, *Memoirs of the Life of Gilbert Wakefield* (2 vols., 1804).

Walpole, Horace, *The Yale Edition of Horace Walpole's Correspondence* (W.S. Lewis ed., 48 vols., New Haven, 1937-83).

Warburton, William, *The Alliance between Church and State* (1736).

Waring, Edward, *A Letter to Dr Powell ... in Answer to his Observatons on the first chapter of a book called Miscellanea Analytica, and his defence of those Observations* (Cambridge, 1760).

Watson, Charles and Pritchett, James P., *Plans etc. and Description of the Pauper Lunatic Asylum* (York, 1819).

Watson, Richard, *Anecdotes of the Life of Richard Watson, Bishop of Landaff* (2nd ed., 1818).

_____ *Miscellaneous Tracts: on religious, political and agricultural subjects* (2 vols., 1815).

Wilkes, John, *The Letters of John Wikes to his Daughter, 1774-96* (John Almon ed., 1804).

_____ *The North Briton* (2 vols., 1769-71).

Williams, David, *Letters on Political Liberty* (3rd ed., 1789).

Wilson, John, *A Vindication of the Miscellanea Analytica in answer to a late pamphlet entitled Observations&c* (Cambridge, 1760).

[-----], *John Bull's Answer to Thomas Bull's Pennyworth of Truth* (13 December 1792).

Wollaston, Francis, *An Address to the Clergy of the Church of England in particular, and to all Christians in general* (1772).

Wyvill, Christopher, *Political Papers, Chiefly Respecting the Attempt of the County of York and Other Considerable Districts ... to Effect a Reformation of the Parliament of Great Britain* (6 vols., York, 1794-1806).

_____ *Thoughts on our Articles of Religion with Respect to their supposed Utility to the State* (3rd ed., 1773).

SECONDARY SOURCES

Place of publication is London unless otherwise indicated.

Albee, Ernest, *A History of English Utilitarianism* (New York, 1962 [1902]).
Allen, Richard C., *David Hartley on Human Nature* (New York, 1999).
Anderson, R.G.A. and Laurence, Christopher eds., *Science, Medicine and Dissent: Joseph Priestley (1733-1804)* (1987).
Andrew, Donna T., 'Popular Culture and Public Debate: London 1780', *The Historical Journal,* 39 (1996), pp. 405-23.
Anstey, Roger, *The Atlantic Slave Trade and British Abolition* (1975).
Appleby, Joyce, *Liberalism and Republicanism in the Historical Imagination* (Cambridge, Mass., 1992).
Ashcraft, Richard, 'Faith and knowledge in Locke's philosophy', in John Yolton ed., *John Locke: problems and perspectives* (Cambridge, 1969), pp. 194-223.
_____ 'Latitudinarianism and Toleration: historical myth versus political history', in Richard Kroll et al. eds., *Philosophy, Science, and Religion in England 1640-1700* (Cambridge, 1992).
_____ 'John Locke, Religious Dissent and the Origins of Liberalism', in Gordon J. Schochet ed., *Restoration, Ideology, and Revolution* (Washington, D.C., 1990), pp. 149-68.
_____ ed., *John Locke: critical assessments* (1991).
Aston, Nigel, 'Horne and Heterodoxy: the defence of Anglican beliefs in the late Enlightenment', *English Historical Review,* 108 (1993), pp. 895-919.
_____ 'Infidelity Ancient and Modern: George Horne reads Edward Gibbon', *Albion,* 27 (1995), pp. 561-82.
_____ 'The Limits of Latitudinarianism: English reactions to Bishop Clayton's *An Essay on Spirit*', *Journal of Ecclesiastical History*, 49 (1998), pp. 407-33.
Attwater, A., *Pembroke College Cambridge: a short history* (Cambridge, 1936).
Bailyn, Bernard, *The Ideological Origins of the American Revolution* (Cambridge, Mass., 1967).
Baker, Hershall Clay, *The Wars of Truth* (Cambridge, Mass., 1952).
Barlow, Richard Burgess, *Citizenship and Conscience: a study in the theory and practice of religious toleration in England during the eighteenth century* (Philadelphia, 1962).
Bartlett, Thomas, *The Fall and Rise of the Irish Nation: the Catholic Question 1690-1830* (Dublin, 1992).
Baylen, J.O. and Grossman, N.J., eds., *A Biographical Dictionary of Modern British Radicals: volume 1, 1770-1830* (Salem, N. H., 1979).
Beattie, J.M., *Crime and the Courts in England: 1660-1800* (Princeton, 1986).
Becker, Carl, *The Declaration of Independence: a study in the history of political ideas* (New York, 1942 [1922]).
_____ *The Heavenly City of the Eighteenth-Century Philosophers* (New Haven, Conn., 1932).
Beer, J.B., *Coleridge the Visionary* (New York, 1959).
Birken, William, 'The Dissenting Tradition in English Medicine of the Seventeenth and Eighteenth Centuries', *Medical History,* 39 (1995), pp. 197-218.
Black, Eugene Charlton, *The Association: British extraparliamentary political organization 1769-1793* (Cambridge, Mass., 1963).
Black, Jeremy, *Eighteenth-Century Britain, 1688-1783* (Basingstoke, 2001).
_____ 'Eighteenth-Century English Politics: recent work and current problems', *Albion,* 25 (1993), pp. 419-41.
_____ *The English Press in the Eighteenth Century* (1987).

_____ *The Politics of Britain 1688-1800* (Manchester, 1993).
_____ ed., *British Politics and Society from Walpole to Pitt, 1742-1789* (1990).
Bonwick, Colin, 'English Dissenters and the American Revolution', in H.C. Allen and Roger Thompson eds., *Contrast and Connection: bicentennial essays in Anglo-American history* (1976), pp. 88-112.
_____ *English Radicals and the American Revolution* (Chapel Hill, N.C., 1977).
Bossy, John, *The English Catholic Community, 1570-1850* (1975).
Bower, George Spencer, *Hartley and James Mill* (1881).
Bradley, James E., 'The Anglican Pulpit, the Social Order, and the Resurgence of Toryism during the American Revolution', *Albion*, 21 (1989), pp. 361-388.
_____ *Popular Politics and the American Revolution in England: petitions, the crown and public opinion* (Cambridge, 1986).
_____ 'Religion and Reform at the Polls: Nonconformity in Cambridge politics', *Journal of British Studies*, 20 (1984), pp. 55-78.
_____ *Religion, Revolution and English Radicalism: nonconformity in eighteenth-century politics and society* (Cambridge, 1990).
_____ 'Whigs and Nonconformists: "slumbering radicalism" in English politics, 1739-89', *Eighteenth Century Studies*, 9 (1775-76), pp. 1-27.
Brain, T.J., 'Richard Watson and the Debate on Toleration in the Late Eighteenth Century', *The Price-Priestley Newsletter*, 2 (1978), pp. 4-26.
_____ 'Some Aspects of the Life and Works of Richard Watson, Bishop of Llandaff, 1737-1816' (unpublished University of Wales PhD. thesis, 1982).
Brauer, George C., *The Education of a Gentleman: theories of gentlemanly education in England, 1660-1775* (New York, 1959).
Brewer, John, 'English Radicalism in the Age of George III', in Pocock, *Three British Revolutions: 1641,1688, 1776*, pp. 323-67.
_____ *The Sinews of Power: war, money and the English state 1688-1783* (1989).
_____ 'The Wilkites and the Law, 1763-74: a study of radical notions of governance', in John Brewer and J. Styles, *An Ungovernable People* (1980).
Brinkley, Richard, 'A Liberal Churchman: Edmund Law (1703-87)', *E&D*, 6 (1987), pp. 6-11.
Brogue, David and Bennett, James, *History of the Dissenters from the Revolution to the Year 1808* (4 vols., 1808).
Brooke, John Hedley, *Science and Religion: some historical perspectives* (Cambridge, 1991).
Brown, Susan E., 'Rational Creatures and Free Citizens: the language of politics in the eighteenth-century debate on women', *Historical Papers* (Canadian Historical Association, 1988), pp. 35-47.
Brown, S.J., *The Press in Ireland: a survey and guide* (Dublin, 1937).
Browne, Alice, *The Eighteenth-Century Feminist Mind* (Brighton, 1987).
Browning, Reed, *The Duke of Newcastle* (New Haven, Conn., 1975).
_____ *Political and Constitutional Ideas of the Court Whigs* (Baton Rouge, La.,1982).
Bynum, W.F. and Porter, Roy, *William Hunter and the Eighteenth-Century Medical World* (Cambridge, 1985).
Butterfield, Herbert, *George III, Lord North, and the People, 1779-1780* (1949).
_____ 'The Yorkshire Association and the Crisis of 1779-80', *Transactions of the Royal Historical Society*, 29 (1947), pp. 69-91.
Cannon, John, *The Fox-North Coalition: crisis of the constitution, 1782-84* (Cambridge, 1969).
_____ *Parliamentary Reform, 1640-1832* (Cambridge, 1973).
_____ ed., *The Whig Ascendancy* (1981).
Canovan, Margaret, 'Paternalistic Liberalism: Joseph Priestley on rank and inequality', *E&D*,

2 (1983), pp. 23-38.

_____ 'Two Concepts of Liberty: eighteenth-century style', *Price-Priestley Newsletter,* 2 (1978), pp. 27-43.

Champion, J.A.I., *The Pillars of Priestcraft Shaken: the Church of England and its enemies, 1660-1730* (Cambridge, 1992).

Christie, Ian R., *Crisis of Empire: Great Britain and the American Colonies 1754-1783* (1966).

_____ *The End of North's Ministry, 1780-1782* (1958).

_____ *Myth and Reality in Late Eighteenth-Century British Politics* (1970).

_____ *Wars and Revolutions: Britain 1760-1815* (1982).

_____ *Wilkes, Wyvill and Reform: the parliamentary reform movement in British politics, 1760-1785* (1962).

_____ 'The Yorkshire Association, 1780-84: a study in political organisation', *Historical Journal,* 3 (1960), pp. 144-61.

Claeys, Gregory, 'The French Revolution Debate and British Political Thought', *History of Political Thought,* 11 (1990), pp. 59-80.

_____ 'Republicanism versus Commercial Society: Paine, Burke and the French Revolution Debate', *History of European Ideas,* 11 (1990), pp. 313-24.

_____ *Thomas Paine: social and political thought* (Boston, 1989).

Clark, J.C.D., 'Eighteenth-Century Social History', *The Historical Journal,* 27 (1984), pp. 773-88.

_____ 'England's Ancien Regime as a Confessional State', *Albion,* 21 (1989), pp. 450-74.

_____ *English Society, 1688-1832* (Cambridge, 1985).

_____ 'On Hitting the Buffers: the historiography of England's ancien regime. A response', *Past and Present,* 117 (1987), pp. 195-207.

_____ *The Language of Liberty 1660-1832: political discourse and social dynamics in the Anglo-American world* (Cambridge, 1994).

_____ *Revolution and Rebellion: state and society in England in the seventeenth and eighteenth centuries* (Cambridge, 1986).

Clarke, M.L., *Paley: evidences for the man* (1974).

Cobb, Sanford H., *The Rise of Religious Liberty in America* (New York, 1968).

Cockburn, J.S., 'Punishment and Brutalization in the English Enlightenment', *Law and History Review,* 12 (1994), pp. 155-79.

Colley, Linda, *Britons: forging the nation, 1707-1837* (1992).

_____ 'Eighteenth-Century English Radicalism before Wilkes', *Transactions of the Royal Historical Society,* 5th Series, 31 (1981), pp. 1-19.

_____ *In Defiance of Oligarchy: the Tory Party 1714-60* (Cambridge, 1982).

_____ 'Radical Patriotism in Eighteenth-Century England', in Raphael Samuel, *Patriotism: the making and the unmaking of British national identity* (1989), I, pp. 169-87.

_____ 'Whose nation? Class and national consciousness in Britain 1750-1830', *Past and Present,* 113 (1986), pp. 97-117.

Cone, Carl B., *The English Jacobins: reformers in late eighteenth-century England* (New York, 1968).

Connolly, S.J., 'Late Eighteenth-Century Irish Politics', *Parliamentary History,* 13 (1994), pp. 227-35.

Conway, Stephen, *The British Isles and the War of American Independence* (Oxford, 2000).

Countryman, Edward O., *The American Revolution* (Harmondsworth, 1985).

Cragg, G.R., *From Puritanism to the Age of Reason* (Cambridge, 1950).

Crane, R.S., *The Idea of the Humanities* (Chicago, 1967).

Crane, Verner W., 'The Club of Honest Whigs: friends of science and liberty', *William and Mary Quarterly*, 23 (1966), pp. 210-33.

Crosland, Maurice, 'The Image of Science as Threat: Burke versus Priestley and the "Philosophic Revolution"', *British Journal for the History of Science*, 20 (1987), pp. 277-307.

Cunningham, Andrew and French, Roger eds., *The Medical Enlightenment of the Eighteenth Century* (Cambridge, 1990).

Cunningham, Hugh, 'The Language of Patriotism, 1750-1914', *History Workshop*, 12 (1981), pp. 8-33.

Curtis, L.P., *Anglican Moods of the Eighteenth Century* (New Haven, Conn., 1966).

Dann, Otto and Dinwiddy, John eds., *Nationalism in the Age of the French Revolution* (1988).

Davie, Donald, *Dissentient Voice: the Ward-Phillips lectures for 1980 with some related pieces* (New York, 1982).

Davis, Horton, *Worship and Theology in England from Watts and Wesley to Maurice 1690-1850* (Princeton, N.J., 1961).

Davis, Michael T. ed., *Radicalism and Revolution in Britain, 1775-1848* (2000).

Davis, Paul C., 'The Debate on Eternal Punishment in Late Seventeenth-Century and Eighteenth-Century Literature', *Eighteenth-Century Studies*, 4 (1970-71), pp. 257-76.

Davis, Richard W., *Dissent in Politics, 1780-1830: the political life of William Smith MP* (1971).

_____ 'The Politics of the Confessional State, 1760-1832', *Parliamentary History*, 9 (1990), pp. 38-49.

DeLacy, Margaret, 'Influenza Research and the Medical Profession in Eighteenth-Century Britain', *Albion*, 25 (1993), pp. 37-66.

_____ *Prison Reform in Lancashire, 1700-1850: a study in local administration* (Manchester, 1986).

Delkeskamp, Corinna, 'Medicine, Science and Moral Philosophy: David Hartley's attempt at a reconciliation', *Journal of Medicine and Philosophy*, 2 (1977), pp. 162-76.

Derry, John, *English Politics and the American Revolution* (1976).

Dickinson, H.T., 'Benjamin Hoadly', *History Today*, 25 (1975), pp. 348-55.

_____ '"The Friends of America": British sympathy with the American Revolution', in Michael T. Davis, *Radicalism and Revolution in Britain*, pp. 1-29.

_____ *Liberty and Property: political ideology in eighteenth-century Britain* (1977).

_____ *The Politics of the People in Eighteenth-Century Britain* (New York, 1994).

_____ 'Whiggism in the Eighteenth Century', in Cannon, *Whig Ascendancy*, pp. 28-44.

_____ ed., *Britain and the American Revolution* (Harlow, Essex, 1998).

Dinwiddy, John, 'England', in Dann and Dinwiddy, *Nationalism in the Age of the French Revolution*, pp. 53-70.

Ditchfield, G.M., 'Anti-Trinitarianism and Toleration in Late Eighteenth-Century British Politics: the Unitarian petition of 1792', *Journal of Ecclesiastical History*, 42 (1991), pp. 39-67.

_____ 'Ecclesiastical Policy under Lord North', in Walsh, Haydon and Taylor, *The Church of England c.1649-c.1833*, pp. 228-46.

_____ 'English Rational Dissent and Philanthropy, c.1760-c.1810', in Hugh Cunningham and Joanna Innes eds., *Charity, Philanthropy and Reform from the 1690s to 1850* (1998), pp. 193-207.

_____ 'Some Aspects of Unitarianism and Radicalism 1760-1810' (unpublished Cambridge PhD. thesis, 1968).

_____ 'The Revd. William Chambers, D.D. (c.1724-77), *E&D*, 4 (1985), pp. 3-12.

_____ 'The Subscription Issue in British Parliamentary Politics, 1772-79', *Parliamentary History,* 7 (1988), pp. 45-80.

_____ 'Three Unpublished Letters of Joseph Priestley', *E&D*, 2 (1983), pp. 101-06.

_____ and Keith-Lucas, Bryan eds., *A Kentish Parson: selections from the private papers of the Revd. Joseph Price, Vicar of Brabourne, 1767-86* (Kent County Council, 1991).

Dobbs, Betty Jo Teeter and Jacob, Margaret C., *Newton and the Culture of Newtonianism* (New Jersey, 1995).

Dobson, Jessie, 'Percivall Pott', *Annals of the Royal College of Surgeons of England,* 50 (1972), pp. 54-65.

Doig, A. et. al. eds., *William Cullen and the Eighteenth-Century Medical World* (Edinburgh, 1993).

Donnelly, F.K., 'Joseph Towers and the Collapse of Rational Dissent', *E&D,* 6 (1987), pp. 31-38.

Drinkwater-Lunn, David, 'John Cartwright, Political Education, and English Radicalism, 1774-94' (unpublished Oxford DPhil. thesis, 1970).

Duffy, Edward, *Rousseau in England: the context for Shelley's critique of the Enlightenment* (Los Angeles, 1979).

Dunn, John, *Locke* (Oxford, 1984).

_____ 'The Politics of Locke in England and America in the Eighteenth Century', in Yolton ed., *John Locke: problems and perspectives*, pp. 56-62.

Dunthorne, Hugh, 'Beccaria and Britain', in Kenneth O. Morgan and David W. Howell eds., *Crime, Protest and Police in Modern British Society: essays in memory of David J.V. Jones* (Cardiff, 1999).

Dworetz, Steven N., *The Unvarnished Doctrine: Locke, liberalism and the American Revolution* (Chapel Hill, N.C., 1990).

Dybikowski, James, *On Burning Ground: an examination of the ideas, projects and life of David Williams* (Studies of Voltaire and the Eighteenth Century, no. 307, Oxford, 1993).

_____ 'David Williams and the Eighteenth-Century Distinction between Civil and Political Liberty', *E&D,* 3 (1984), pp. 15-39.

_____ 'Review of Peter N. Miller, *Joseph Priestley: political writings*', *E&D*, 15 (1996), pp. 117-27.

_____ 'Samuel Clarke: Special Issue – Editorial', *E&D*, 16 (1997), pp. 1-2.

Eastwood, David, 'Patriotism and the English State in the 1790s', in Philp, *French Revolution and British Popular Politics*, pp. 146-68.

Eckersley, Rachel, 'John Cartwright: radical reformer and Unitarian?' *Transactions of the Unitarian Historical Society,* 22 (1999), pp. 37-53.

Ehrman, Bart, *The Orthodox Corruption of Scripture: the effect of early Christological controversies on the text of the New Testament* (Oxford, 1993).

Elofson, W.M., *The Rockingham Connection and the Second Founding of the Whig Party, 1768-1773* (Montreal, 1996).

Evans, A.W., *Warburton and the Warburtonians: a study of some eighteenth-century controversies* (Oxford, 1932).

Evans, Robin, *The Fabrication of Virtue: English prison architecture, 1750-1840* (Cambridge, 1982).

Ferguson, James P., *The Philosophy of Dr Samuel Clarke* (New York, 1974).

Fiering, Norman S., 'Irresistible Compassion: an aspect of eighteenth-century sympathy and humanitarianism', *JHI,* 37 (1976), pp. 195-218.

Fitzpatrick, Martin, 'Enlightenment in Britain', in Iain McCalman ed., *The Oxford Companion to the Age of Revolutions and Romanticism* (Oxford, 1999), pp. 299-311.

_____ 'Heretical Religion and Radical Politics', in Hellmuth, *Transformation of Political Culture*, pp. 341-71.

_____ 'Joseph Priestley and the Millennium', in Anderson and Lawrence, *Science, Medicine and Dissent*, pp. 29-37.

_____ 'Latitudinarianism at the Parting of the Ways', in Walsh, Haydon and Taylor, *The Church of England c.1649-c.1833*, pp. 209-227.

_____ 'Patriotism and Patriotisms: Richard Price and the early reception of the French Revolution in England', *Studies of Voltaire and the Eighteenth Century,* 335 (1995), pp. 211-29.

_____ 'Science and Society in the Enlightenment', *E&D,* 4 (1985), pp. 83-103.

_____ '"Through the Glass of History": the nature and purpose of historical knowledge in the thought of Joseph Priestley', *E&D,* 17 (1998), pp. 172-209.

_____ 'Toleration and Truth', *E&D*, 1 (1982), pp. 3-31.

_____ and Dybikowski, James, 'David Williams, John Jebb and Liturgical Reform', *E&D,* 9 (1990), pp. 106-13.

Foreman, Amanda, *Georgiana, Dutchess of Devonshire* (Hammersmith, 1998).

Forster, R.F., *Modern Ireland 1600-1972* (Harmondsworth, 1989).

Fromigari, Lia, 'Language and Society in the Late Eighteenth Century', *JHI,* 35 (1974), pp. 275-93.

Fruchtman, Jack, 'Late Latitudinarianism: the case of David Hartley', *E&D,* 11 (1992), pp. 3-22

_____ 'Politics and the Apocalypse: the republic and the millennium in late eighteenth-century English political thought', *Studies in Eighteenth-Century Culture,* 10 (1981), pp. 153-64.

Garrett, Clark, *Respectable Folly: millenarians and the French Revolution in France and England* (1975).

Gascoigne, John, 'Anglican Latitudinarianism and Political Radicalism in the Late Eighteenth Century', *History*, 71 (1986), pp. 22-38.

_____ 'Anglican Latitudinarianism, Rational Dissent and Political Radicalism in the Late Eighteenth Century', in Haakonssen, *Enlightenment and Religion*, pp. 224-26.

_____ 'From Bentley to the Victorians: the rise and fall of Newtonian natural theology', *Science in Context,* 2 (1988), pp. 219-56.

_____ *Cambridge in the Age of Enlightenment: science, religion and politics from the Restoration to the French Revolution* (Cambridge, 1989).

_____ 'Church and State Allied: the failure of parliamentary reform of the English universities', in L. Beier, David Cannadine and J. Rosenheim eds., *The First Modern Society* (Cambridge, 1989), pp. 401-29.

_____ *Joseph Banks and the English Enlightenment: useful knowledge and polite culture* (Cambridge, 1994).

_____ 'Mathematics and Meritocracy: the emergence of the Cambridge mathematical tripos', *Social Studies of Science,* 14 (1984), pp. 547-84.

_____ 'Science, Religion and the Foundations of Morality in Enlightenment Britain', *E&D,* 17 (1998), pp. 83-103.

Gatrell, V.A.C., *The Hanging Tree: execution and the English people, 1770-1868* (Oxford, 1994)

Gay, Peter, *The Enlightenment: an interpretation* (2 vols., 1967-70).

George, Dorothy, *English Political Caricature to 1792: a study in opinion and propaganda* (Oxford, 1959).

_____ 'Fox's Martyrs: the General election of 1784', *Transactions of the Royal Historical Society,* 4th series, 21 (1939), pp. 133-68.

Goldie, Mark, 'The Roots of True Whiggism 1688-94', *History of Political Thought,* 1

(1980), pp. 196-236.
Gordon, Alexander, *Heads of Unitarian History* (1895).
Gould, Eliga H., *The Persistence of Empire: British political culture in the age of the American Revolution* (Chapel Hill, N.C., 2000).
Graham, Jenny, 'Revolutionary Philosopher: the political ideas of Joseph Priestley (1733-1804)', Part I, *E&D*, 8 (1989), pp. 44-68.
Grainger, J.H., *Patriotisms: Britain 1900-1939* (1986).
Gray, Arthur and Brittain, Frederick, *A History of Jesus College Cambridge* (1979).
Gray, John, 'Matter and Freedom in the Thought of Samuel Clarke', *JHI*, 24 (1963), pp. 85-105.
Green, Donald, 'Latitudinarianism and Sensibility: the genealogy of the "man of feeling" reconsidered', *Modern Philology*, 75 (1977).
Green, Jack P., 'Why did they Rebel?', *Times Literary Supplement*, 10 June 1994.
Green, Thomas, *Verdict According to Conscience: perspectives on the English criminal trial jury, 1200-1800* (Chicago, 1985)
Gregory, Jeremy, 'The Eighteenth-Century Reformation: the pastoral task of Anglican clergy after 1689', in Walsh, Haydon and Taylor, *The Church of England c.1649-c.1833*, pp. 67-85.
Guy, Williams, *The Age of Agony: the art of healing 1700-1800* (1975).
Haakonssen, Knud, *Natural Law and Moral Philosophy: from Grotius to the Scottish Enlightenment* (Cambridge, 1996).
_____ ed., *Enlightenment and Religion: Rational Dissent in eighteenth-century Britain* (Cambridge, 1996).
Haakonssen, Lizabeth, *Medicine and Morals in the Enlightenment, John Gregory, Thomas Percival and Benjamin Rush* (Amsterdam, 1997).
Halevy, Elie, *The Growth of Philosophic Radicalism* (1928).
Hall, Catherine, *White, Male and Middle Class: explorations in feminism and history* (Cambridge, 1995).
Hampsher-Monk, Iain, 'British Radicalism and the Anti-Jacobins', in *The Cambridge History of Political Thought: the Enlightenment and Revolution* (forthcoming).
Hampson, Norman, *The Enlightenment: an evaluation of its assumptions, attitudes and values* (Harmondsworth, 1982 [1968]).
_____ 'The Enlightenment in France', in Roy Porter and Mikulas Teich, *The Enlightenment in National Context* (Cambridge, 1981), pp. 41-53.
Haraszti, Zoltan, 'John Adams Flays a Philosophe: Annotations on Condorcet's *Progress of the Human Mind*', *William and Mary Quarterly*, 7 (1950), pp. 323-54.
Harrison, J.F.C., *The Second Coming: popular millenarianism 1780-1850* (1979).
Harrison, Peter, *'Religion' and the Religions in the English Enlightenment* (Cambridge, 1990).
Hawkins, T.L., *Science and the Enlightenment* (Cambridge, 1985).
Hay, Clara H., *James Burgh: spokesman for reform in Hanoverian England* (Washington, D.C., 1979).
_____ 'The Making of a Radical: the case of James Burgh', *Journal of British Studies*, 18 (1979), pp. 90-117.
Hay, Douglas, et. al., *Albion's Fatal Tree: crime and society in eighteenth-century England* (Harmondsworth, 1975).
Haydon, Colin, *Anti-Catholicism in Eighteenth-Century England, c. 1714-80* (Manchester, 1993).
_____ 'The Gordon Riots in the English Provinces', *Historical Research*, 63 (1990), pp. 354-59.

Hazard, Paul, *European Thought in the Eighteenth Century* (Harmondsworth, 1965 [1946]).
Heberden, Ernest, *William Heberden: physician of the Age of Reason* (1989).
Hellmuth, Eckhart, ed., *The Transformation of Political Culture: England and Germany in the late eighteenth century* (Oxford, 1990).
Henriques, Ursula, *Religious Toleration in England 1787-1833* (1961).
Hepworth, B., *Robert Lowth* (Boston, 1978).
Hibbert, Christopher, *King Mob* (1959).
Hill, Brian, *The Early Parties and Politics in Britain, 1688-1832* (1996).
Hill, Bridget and Christopher, 'Catherine Macaulay and the Seventeenth Century', *The Welsh History Review*, 3 (1967), pp. 381-402.
Hill, Christopher, *Milton and the English Revolution* (1977).
_____ 'The Norman Yoke', in *Puritanism and Revolution: studies in interpretation of the English Revolution in the seventeenth century* (New York, 1958)
Hill, Jaqueline, *From Patriots to Unionists: Dublin civic politics and Irish Protestant patriotism, 1660-1840* (Oxford, 1997).
Hilton, Boyd, *The Age of Atonement: the influence of evangelicalism on social and economic thought, 1795-1865* (Oxford, 1988).
Hirschman, Albert O., *The Passions and the Interests: political arguments for capitalism before its triumph* (Princeton, 1977).
Hobhouse, Christopher, *Fox* (1934).
Hoecker, James J., 'Joseph Priestley and the Reification of Religion', *Price-Priestley Newsletter*, 2 (1978), pp. 44-75.
_____ 'Joseph Priestley and Utilitarianism in the Age of Reason', *E&D*, 3 (1984), pp. 55-64.
_____ 'Joseph Priestley as a Historian of the Idea of Progress', *Price-Priestley Newsletter*, 3 (1979), pp. 29-40.
Hole, Robert, *Pulpits, Politics, and Public Order in England 1760-1832* (Cambridge, 1989).
Holt, R.V., *The Unitarian Contribution to Social Progress* (1952).
Hughes, Graham Werden, *'With Freedom Fired': the story of Robert Robinson, Cambridge nonconformist* (1955).
Ignatieff, Michael, *A Just Measure of Pain: the penitentiary in the industrial revolution, 1750-1850* (New York, 1978).
Illich, Ivan, *Limits to Medicine: the expropriation of health* (Harmondsworth, 1976).
Innes, Joanna, 'Politics and Morals: the reformation of manners movement in later eighteenth-century England', in Hellmuth, *Transformation of Political Culture*, pp. 57-118.
Isaac, Rhys, *The Transformation of Virginia, 1740-90* (Chapel Hill, N.C., 1982).
Jacob, Margaret C., *The Radical Enlightenment* (1981).
_____ and Dobbs, B.J.T., *Newton and the Culture of Newtonianism* (Atlantic Highlands, N.J., 1995).
_____ and Jacob, James R. ed., *The Origins of Anglo-American Radicalism* (1984).
Jarrett, Derek, *The Begetters of Revolution* (1973).
_____ 'The Myth of "Patriotism" in Eighteenth-Century English Politics', *Britain and the Netherlands*, 5 (1975), pp. 120-40.
Jewson, C.B., *The Jacobin City: a portrait of Norwich in its reaction to the French Revolution, 1788-1802* (1975).
Jones, E. Alfred, 'Two Professors of William and Mary College', *William and Mary Quarterly*, 26 (1918), pp. 221-31.
Jones, J.R. ed., *Liberty Secured? Britain before and after 1688* (Stanford, Calif., 1992).

Joyce, Patrick, *Democratic Subjects: the self and the social in nineteenth-century England* (Cambridge, 1994).

Kelly, James, 'The Parliamentary Reform Movement of the 1780s and the Catholic Question', *Archivium Hibernicum,* 43 (1988), pp. 97-8.

Kelly, Paul, 'Radicalism and Public Opinion in the General Election of 1784', *Bulletin of the Institute for Historical Research,* 45 (1972), pp. 73-88.

Kenyon, J.P., *Revolution Principles: the politics of party 1689-1720* (Cambridge, 1977).

Kirk, Linda, 'The Matter of Enlightenment', *The Historical Journal,* 43 (2000), pp. 1129-43.

Knight, Frida, *University Rebel: the life of William Frend 1757-1841* (1971).

Knox, Thomas R., 'Popular Politics and Provincial Radicalism: Newcastle Upon Tyne, 1769-1785', *Albion,* 11 (1979), pp. 224-41.

Kramnick, Isaac, 'Religion and Radicalism: English political theory in the age of Revolutions', *Political Theory,* 5 (1977), pp. 505-34.

_____ *Republicanism and Bourgeois Radicalism: political ideology in late eighteenth-century England and America* (Ithaca, N.Y., 1990).

Laboucheix, Henri, *Richard Price as Moral Philosopher and Political Theorist* (Studies of Voltaire and the Eighteenth Century, Oxford, 1982).

Langford, Paul, 'The English Clergy and the American Revolution,' in Hellmuth, *Transformation of Political Culture,* pp. 275-308.

_____ 'Old Whigs, Old Tories, and the American Revolution', *Journal of Imperial and Commonwealth History,* 8 (1980), pp. 106-30.

_____ *A Polite and Commercial People: England 1727-1783* (Oxford, 1989).

_____ *Public Life and the Propertied Englishman, 1689-1798* (Oxford, 1991).

_____ 'Thomas Day and the Politics of Sentiment', in R.F. Holland and G. Rizvi eds., *Perspectives on Imperialism and Decolonisation* (1984), pp. 57-79.

Lawrence, Christopher, 'Priestley in Tahiti: the medical interests of a Dissenting chemist', in Anderson, *Science, Medicine and Dissent,* pp. 1-10.

Lawson, John and Silver, Harold, *A Social History of Education in England* (1973).

Lecky, W.E.H., *A History of England in the Eighteenth Century* (1892).

_____ *A History of Ireland in the Eighteenth Century* (abridged by L.P. Curtis, 1972 [1892]).

Lincoln, Anthony, *Some Political and Social Ideas of English Dissent 1763-1800* (Cambridge, 1938).

Lindberg, David C. and Numbers, Ronald L. eds., *God and Nature: historical essays on the encounter between Christianity and science* (Berkeley, 1986).

Linebaugh, Peter, *The London Hanged: crime and civil society in the Eighteenth Century* (Harmondsworth, 1991)

Lottes, Gunter, 'Radicalism, Revolution and Political Culture: an Anglo-French comparison', in Philp, *The French Revolution and British Popular Politics,* pp. 78-98.

MacCoby, S., ed., *The English Radical Tradition, 1763-1914* (1952).

MacMichael, William, *Lives of British Physicians* (1830).

MacNevin, Thomas, *The History of the Volunteers of 1782* (Dublin, 1845).

Maier, Pauline, *From Resistance to Revolution: colonial radicals and the development of opposition to Britain, 1765-1776* (New York, 1973).

Mather, F.C., *High Church Prophet: Bishop Samuel Horsley (1733-1806) and the Caroline tradition in the later Georgian Church* (Oxford, 1992).

May, Henry F., *The Enlightenment in America* (Oxford, 1976).

McCalman, Ian, 'Mad Lord George and Madame La Motte: riot and sexuality in the Genesis of Burke's *Reflections on the Revolution in France*', *Journal of British Studies,* 35 (1996), pp 343-67.

McConville, Sean, *A History of English Prison Administration: vol. 1, 1750-1877* (1981).

McDowell, R.B., *Ireland in the Age of Imperialism and Revolution, 1760-1801* (Oxford, 1979).

_____ *Irish Public Opinion 1750-1800* (1944).

_____ and Webb, D.A., *Trinity College Dublin 1592-1952: an academic history* (Cambridge, 1982).

McGirr, E.M., 'Politics, Society and Medicine in the Eighteenth Century', *Scottish Medical Journal,* 36 (1991), pp. 119-21.

McKendrick, Neil, Brewer, John and Plumb, J.H., *The Birth of a Consumer Society: the commercialisation of eighteenth-century England* (1982).

McLachlan, H. John, 'Correspondence of Theophilus Lindsey with William Turner of Wakefield and his son (1771-1803)', *Transactions of the Unitarian Historical Society,* 18 (1985), pp. 152-64.

_____ *Essays and Addresses* (Manchester, 1950).

_____ *Letters of Theophilus Lindsey* (Manchester, 1920).

_____ 'Mary Priestley: a woman of character', in Schwartz and McEvoy, *Motion Toward Perfection,* pp. 251-64.

_____ 'More Letters of Theophilus Lindsey', *Transactions of the Unitarian Historical Society,* 3 (1923-26), pp. 361-77.

Medd, Patrick, *Romilly: a life of Sir Samuel Romilly, lawyer and reformer* (1968).

Miller, Peter N., *Defining the Common Good* (Cambridge, 1994).

_____ '"Freethinking" and "Freedom of Thought" in Eighteenth-Century Britain', *Historical Journal,* 36 (1993), pp. 599-617.

Mitchell, L.G., *Charles James Fox* (Oxford, 1992).

Molivas, Gregory, 'Richard Price, the Debate on Free Will, and Natural Rights', *JHI,* 58 (1997), pp. 105-23.

Money, John, *Experience and Identity: Birmingham and the West Midlands, 1760-1800* (Manchester, 1977).

_____ 'Provincialism and the English "Ancien Regime": Samuel Pipe-Wolferstan and "the confessional state", 1776-1820', *Albion,* 21 (1989), pp. 389-425.

Morris, Norval and Rothman, David J., *Oxford History of the Prison: the practice of punishment in Western Society* (Oxford, 1995).

Muggeridge, Malcom, 'The Great Liberal Death Wish', in Russell Kirk ed., *The Portable Conservative Reader* (Harmondsworth, 1982).

Mulligan, Lotte, '"Reason", "Right Reason", and "Revelation" in mid-seventeenth-century England', in Brian Vickers ed., *Occult and Scientific Mentalities in the Renaissance* (1984), pp. 103-23.

_____ 'Robert Boyle, "Right Reason", and the Meaning of Metaphor', *JHI,* 55 (1995), pp. 235-57.

Munk, William, *Roll of the Royal College of Physicians of London: vol. 2, 1701-1800* (1878).

Nagle, Benjamin C., *The Monthly Review First Series 1749-89: index of contributors and articles* (Oxford, 1934).

Namier, Louis, *The Structure of Politics at the Accession of George III* (1957).

Neiman, Fraser, 'The Letters of William Gilpin to Samuel Henley', *Huntington Library Quarterly,* 35 (1971-72), pp. 159-69.

Newman, Gerald, *The Rise of English Nationalism: a cultural history,* (1987).

Nockles, P.B., *The Oxford Movement in Context: Anglican High Churchmanship, 1760-1857* (Cambridge, 1994).

Oberg, Barbara Bowen, 'David Hartley and the Association of Ideas', *JHI,* 37 (1976), pp. 441-53.

O'Brien, Conor Cruse, *The Great Melody: a thematic biography of Edmund Burke* (1992).

O'Gorman, Frank, 'Fifty Years After Namier: the eighteenth century in British historical writing', *The Eighteenth Century,* 20 (1979), pp. 99-120.

_____ *The Long Eighteenth Century: British politics and social history, 1688-1832* (1997).

_____ 'The Unreformed Electorate of Hanoverian England: the mid-eighteenth century to the Reform Act of 1832', *Social History,* 11 (1986), pp. 33-52.

_____ *Voters, Patrons and Parties: the unreformed electorate of Hanoverian England, 1734-1832* (Oxford, 1989).

Oldham, James, *The Mansfield Manuscripts; and the growth of English Law in the eighteenth century* (Chapel Hill, N.C., 1992).

Olson, Alison G., *The Radical Duke: the career and correspondence of Charles Lennox, Third Duke of Richmond* (Oxford, 1961).

Olson, Richard G., 'Tory-High Church Opposition to Science and Scientism in the Eighteenth Century: the works of John Arbuthnot, Jonathan Swift, and Samuel Johnson', in J.G. Burke ed., *The Uses of Science in the Age of Newton* (Berkeley, 1983), pp. 171-203.

Osler, Margaret J., 'John Locke and the Changing Ideal of Scientific Knowledge', *JHI,* 31 (1970), pp. 3-16.

Page, Anthony, 'Enlightenment and a "Second Reformation": the Religion and Philosophy of John Jebb (1736-86)', *E&D,* 17 (1998), pp. 48-82.

_____ '"Liberty has an asylum": John Jebb, British Radicalism and the American Revolution', *History,* 87:286 (2002), pp. 204-26.

Pailin, David A., 'Rational Religion in England from Herbert of Cherbury to William Paley', in Sheridan Gilly and W.J. Sheils eds., *The History of Religion in Britain: practice and belief from pre-Roman times to the present* (Oxford, 1994), 211-33.

Palmer, R.R., *The Age of Democratic Revolution: a political history of Europe and America, 1760-1800: volume 1, The Challenge* (Princeton, N.J., 1959).

Parssinen, T.M., 'Association, Convention, and Anti-Parliament in British Radical Politics 1771-1848', *English Historical Review,* 88 (1973), pp. 504-33.

Passmore, J.A., *The Perfectibility of Man* (1970).

_____ ed., *Priestley's Writings on Philosophy, Science and Politics* (1965).

Peach, W. Bernard, 'Human Nature and the Foundation of Ethics', *E&D,* 4 (1985), pp. 13-34.

Pearl, Kenneth, 'John Jebb, a British Radical in the Age of the American Revolution' (unpublished PhD. thesis, City University of New York, 1998).

_____ 'The Society for Constitutional Information and the Publication of a Radical Agenda', *Consortium on Revolutionary Europe 1750-1850: Selected Papers* (1995), pp. 77-85.

Peters, Marie, 'The *Monitor* on the Constitution, 1755-1765: new light on the ideological origins of English radicalism', *English Historical Review,* 86 (1971), pp. 706-27.

Phillips, John A., *Electoral Behaviour in Unreformed England: plumpers, splitters, and straights* (Princeton, N.J., 1982).

_____ 'Popular Politics in Unreformed England', *Journal of Modern History,* 52 (1980), pp. 599-625.

Phillips, N.C., 'Country against Court: Christopher Wyvill, a Yorkshire champion', *Yorkshire Archaeological Journal,* 40 (1962), pp. 588-603.

Philp, Mark, 'Burke and Paine: texts in context', *E&D,* 9 (1990), pp. 93-105.

_____ 'The Fragmented Ideology of Reform', in Philp, *The French Revolution and British Popular Politics*, pp. 50-77.

_____ *Godwin's Political Justice* (1986).

_____ *Paine* (Oxford, 1989).

_____ 'Rational Religion and Political Radicalism in the 1790s', *E&D*, 4 (1985), pp. 35-46.

_____ ed., *The French Revolution and British Popular Politics* (Cambridge, 1991).

Pittock, Murry G.H., *Inventing and Resisting Britain: cultural identities in Britain and Ireland, 1685-1789* (1997).

Planngesis, Yannis, *Matter and Spirit in Joseph Priestley's Philosophical Thought* (1991).

Plumb, J.H., *The Growth of Political Stability* (Harmondsworth, 1969 [1967]).

Pocock, J.G.A., *The Ancient Constitution and the Feudal Law: a study in English historical thought in the seventeenth century* (Cambridge, 1957).

_____ 'Burke and the Ancient Constitution - a problem in the history of ideas', *The Historical Journal*, 3 (1960), pp. 125-43.

_____ 'Conservative Enlightenment and Democratic Revolutions: the American and French cases in British perspective', *Government and Opposition*, 24 (1989), pp. 81-105.

_____ 'History and Sovereignty: the historiographical response to Europeanization in two British Cultures', *Journal of British Studies*, 31 (1992), pp. 358-89.

_____ 'Machiavelli, Harrington, and English Political Ideologies in the Eighteenth Century', *William and Mary Quarterly*, 22 (1965), pp. 549-83.

_____ *The Machiavellian Moment: Florentine political thought and the Atlantic republican tradition* (Princeton, N.J., 1975).

_____ '*The Machiavellian Moment* Revisited: a study in history and ideology', *Journal of Modern History*, 53 (1981), pp. 49-72.

_____ 'Radical Criticisms of the Whig Order in the Age between Revolutions', in Margaret C. and James R. Jacob, *The Origins of Anglo-American Radicalism* (1984), pp. 35-59.

_____ *Virtue, Commerce and History: essays on political thought and history, chiefly in the eighteenth century* (Cambridge, 1985).

_____ ed., *Three British Revolutions: 1641, 1688, 1776* (Baltimore, 1979).

_____ ed., *The Varieties of British Political Thought 1500-1800* (Cambridge, 1993).

Popkin, R.H., 'Joseph Priestley's Criticism of David Hume's Philosophy', *Journal of the History of Philosophy*, 15 (1977), pp. 437-47.

Porter, Dorothy and Roy, *Patient's Progress: doctors and doctoring in eighteenth-century England* (Cambridge, 1989).

Porter, Roy, *Disease, Medicine and Society in England, 1550-1860* (1987).

_____ *English Society in the Eighteenth Century* (Harmondsworth, 1982).

_____ *Enlightenment: Britain and the creation of the modern world* (2000).

_____ 'The Enlightenment in England', in Roy Porter and Mikulas Teich, *The Enlightenment in National Context* (Cambridge, 1981), pp. 1-18.

_____ *Gibbon: making history* (1988).

_____ *The Greatest Benefit of Mankind: a medical history of humanity from antiquity to the present* (1997).

_____ 'Medical Lecturing in Georgian London', *British Journal of the History of Science*, 28 (1995), pp. 91-99.

_____ 'Science, Provincial Culture and Public Opinion in Enlightenment England', *British Journal for Eighteenth-Century Studies*, 3 (1980), pp. 20-46.

_____ 'Was there a Medical Enlightenment in Eighteenth-Century England?' *British Journal for Eighteenth-Century Studies*, 5 (1982), pp. 49-63.

_____ 'William Hunter: a surgeon and a gentleman', in W.F. Bynum and Roy Porter eds., *William Hunter and the Eighteenth-Century Medical World* (Cambridge, 1985), pp. 7-34.
_____ ed., *Patients and Practitioners: lay perceptions of medicine in pre-industrial society* (Cambridge, 1985).
Potter, Harry, *Hanging in Judgement: religion and the death penalty in England from the Bloody Code to abolition* (1993).
Prest, Wilfrid, *Albion Ascendant: English history 1660-1815* (Oxford, 1998).
_____ 'Law, Lawyers and Rational Dissent', in Haakonssen, *Enlightenment and Religion*, pp. 169-92.
Qvist, George, *John Hunter 1728-1790* (1981).
Rail, Tony, and Thomas, Beryl, 'Joseph Priestley's Journal while at Daventry Academy, 1754', *E&D,* 13 (1994), pp. 49-53.
Rashid, Salim, '"He startled ... as if he saw a spectre": Tucker's Proposal for American Independence', *JHI,* 43 (1982), pp. 437- 60.
Ravitch, Mark M., 'Invective in Surgery: William Hunter versus Monro Primus, Monro Secundus, and Percival Pott', *Bulletin of the New York Academy of Medicine,* 50 (1974), pp. 796-815.
Rawls, John, *A Theory of Justice* (1971).
Redwood, John, *Reason, Ridicule and Religion: the age of Enlightenment in England, 1660-1750* (1976).
Reedy, Gerard, *The Bible and Reason: Anglicans and Scripture in late seventeenth-century England* (Philadelphia, 1985).
Rees, Ronald, 'Under the Weather: climate and disease 1700-1900', *History Today,* 46 (January 1996), pp. 35-41.
Reventlow, Henning Graft, *The Authority of the Bible and the Rise of the Modern World* (1984).
Richey, Russell E., 'The Origins of British Radicalism: the changing rational for dissent', *Eighteenth-Century Studies,* 7 (1973-74), pp. 179-92.
Robbins, Caroline, *The Eighteenth-Century Commonwealthman: studies in the transmission, development and circumstance of English liberal thought from the Restoration of Charles II until the war with the Thirteen Colonies* (Cambridge, Mass., 1959).
_____ 'The Strenuous Whig: Thomas Hollis of Lincoln's Inn', *William and Mary Quarterly,* 7 (1950), pp. 406-53.
Rogers, G.A.J., 'The Empiricism of Locke and Newton', in S.C. Brown ed., *Philosophers of the Enlightenment* (Royal Institute of Philosophy Lectures, 12, 1977-78).
_____ ed., *Locke's Philosophy: content and context* (Oxford, 1994).
Rogers, N.A.M., *The Insatiable Earl: a life of John Montagu, 4th Earl of Sandwich* (1993).
Rolleston, Humphry, 'Medical Friendships, Clubs, and Societies', *Annals of Medical History* (1930), pp. 249-66.
Rothblat, Sheldon, 'The Student Subculture and the Examination System in Early Nineteenth-Century Oxbridge', in Lawrence Stone ed., *The University in Society* (1974), I, pp. 247-303.
Rousseau, G.S., *The Languages of Psyche: mind and body in Enlightenment thought* (Berkeley, 1990).
Rowden, Aldred W., *The Primates of the First Four Georges* (1916).
Royle, Edward, and Walvin, James, *English Radicals and Reformers 1760-1848* (1982).
Rude, George, *Wilkes and Liberty* (1983 [1962]).
Rupp, Ernest Gordon, *Religion in England, 1688-1791* (Oxford, 1986).
Ruston, Alan, 'A Servant's View of Joseph Priestley', *E&D,* 8 (1989), pp. 115-19.

Sack, James J., *From Jacobite to Conservative: reaction and orthodoxy in Britain, 1760-1832* (Cambridge, 1993).

Sainsbury, John *Disaffected Patriots: London supporters of revolutionary America 1769-1782* (Kingston, Ont., 1987).

Saunders, Alan, 'The State as Highwayman: from candour to rights', in Haakonssen, *Enlightenment and Religion*, pp. 241-71.

Schaffer, Simon, 'Natural Philosophy and Public Spectacle in the Eighteenth Century', *History of Science,* 21 (1983), pp. 1-43.

Schofield, Robert E., *The Enlightenment of Joseph Priestley: a study of his life and work from 1733-73* (University Park, Pennsylvania, 1998).

Scholtz, Gregory F., 'Anglicanism in the Age of Johnson: the doctrine of conditional salvation', *Eighteenth-Century Studies,* 22 (1988-89), pp. 182-207.

Schwartz, A. Truman, 'Priestley's Materialism: the consistent connection', Schwartz and McEvoy, *Motion toward Perfection,* pp. 109-28.

_____ and McEvoy, John G., eds., *Motion toward Perfection: the achievement of Joseph Priestley* (Boston, 1990).

Searby, Peter, *A History of the University of Cambridge: volume III, 1750-1870* (Cambridge, 1997).

Seed, John, 'Gentlemen Dissenters: the social and political meanings of Rational Dissent in the 1770s and 1780s', *Historical Journal,* 28 (1985), pp. 299-325.

_____ '"A set of men powerful enough in many things": Rational Dissent and Political Opposition in England, 1770-1790', in Haakonssen, *Enlightenment and Religion,* pp. 140-68.

Sell, Alan P.F., *John Locke and the Eighteenth-Century Divines* (Cardiff, 1997).

_____ 'Samuel Clarke on the Existence of God', *E&D*, 3 (1984), pp. 65-75.

Sharp, R., 'New Perspectives on the High Church Tradition', in G. Rowell ed., *Tradition Renewed* (1986), pp. 4-23.

Shelton, George, *Dean Tucker and Eighteenth-Century Economic and Political Thought* (1981).

Shennan, J.H., *Liberty and Order in Early Modern Europe: the subject and the state, 1650-1800* (1986).

Skinner, Quentin, 'Meaning and Understanding in the History of Ideas', *History and Theory,* 8 (1969), pp. 3-53.

_____ 'The Principles and Practice of Opposition: the case of Bolingbroke versus Walpole', in Neil McKendrick ed., *Historical Perspectives: studies in English thought and society in honour of J.H. Plumb* (1974).

Smith, Page, *John Adams* (New York, 1962).

Smith, R.J., *The Gothic Bequest: medieval institutions in British thought 1688-1863* (Cambridge, 1987).

Smith, Wilfred Cantwell, *The Meaning and End of Religion: a new approach to the religious traditions of mankind* (New York, 1963).

Snobelen, Stephen, 'Caution, Conscience and the Newtonian Reformation: the public and private heresies of Newton, Clarke and Whiston', *E&D,* 16 (1997), pp. 151-84.

Sosin, Jack M., 'A Proposal in the Pre-Revolutionary Decade for Establishing Anglican Bishops in the Colonies', *Journal of Ecclesiastical History,* 13 (1962), pp. 76-84.

Spadafora, David, *The Idea of Progress in the Eighteenth Century* (Princeton, N.Y., 1990).

Spears, Robert, *A Record of Unitarian Worthies* (1876).

Speck, W.A. et al., '1688 and all that', *British Journal for Eighteenth-Century Studies,* 15 (1992), pp. 131-49.

_____ *Stability and Strife: England 1714-1760* (1977).
_____ 'Whigs and Tories dim their glories: English political parties under the first two Georges', in Cannon, *Whig Ascendancy,* pp. 51-70.
_____ 'Will the Real 18th Century Stand Up?' *The Historical Journal,* 34 (1991), pp. 203-06.
Spurr, John, '"Rational Religion" in Restoration England', *JHI,* 49 (1988), pp. 563-85.
Stephen, Leslie, *History of English Thought in the Eighteenth Century* (Crane Brinton ed., New York, 1962 [1876]).
Stephens, John, 'Edmund Law and his Circle at Cambridge: some philosophical activity of the 1730s', in G.A.J. Rogers and Sylvana Tomaselli eds., *The Philosophical Canon in the 17th and 18th Centuries. Essays in Honour of John W. Yolton* (Rochester, New York, 1996), pp. 163–73.
'An Unrecorded Letter from Theophilus Lindsey to William Tayleur', *Price-Priestley Newsletter,* 4 (1980), pp. 65-68.
Stevenson, John, *Popular Disturbances in England 1700-1870* (1979).
Stewart, Larry, 'Samuel Clarke, Newtonianism and the Factions of Post-Revolutionary England', *JHI,* 42 (1981), pp. 53-72.
Stone, Lawrence, *The Past and Present Revisited* (1987).
_____ ed., *The University in Society: vol. I Oxford and Cambridge* (Princeton, N.J., 1974).
Strauss, E., *Irish Nationalism and British Democracy* (1951).
Stromberg, R.N., *Religious Liberalism in Eighteenth-Century England* (Oxford, 1954).
Sutherland, Lucy, 'Edmund Burke and the Relations between Members of Parliament and their Constituents', *Studies of Burke and his Time,* 10 (1968), pp. 1005-21.
Sykes, Norman, *Church and State in England in the Eighteenth Century* (Cambridge, 1934).
Tapper, Alan, 'The Beginnings of Priestley's Materialism', *E&D,* 1 (1982), pp. 73-81.
_____ 'Priestley's Metaphysics' (unpublished University of Western Australia PhD. thesis, 1987).
Thale, Mary, 'Women in London Debating Societies in 1780', *Gender and History,* 7 (1995), pp. 5-24.
Thomas, D.O., 'Benjamin Hoadly: the ethics of sincerity', *E&D,* 15 (1996), pp. 71-88.
_____ 'Francis Maseres, Richard Price, and the Industrious Poor', *E&D,* 4 (1985), pp. 67-82.
_____ *The Honest Mind: the thought and work of Richard Price* (Oxford, 1977).
_____ 'Progress, Liberty and Utility: the political philosophy of Joseph Priestley', in Anderson, *Science, Medicine and Dissent*, pp. 73-79.
_____ 'Richard Ashcraft on Locke's *Two Treatises*', *E&D,* 14 (1995), pp. 128-54.
Thomas, Keith, *Religion and the Decline of Magic* (Harmondsworth, 1973).
Thomas, P.D.G., *Lord North* (1976).
Thompson, E.P., 'Eighteenth-Century English Society: class struggle without class?', *Social History,* 3 (1978), pp. 133-65.
_____ *The Making of the English Working Class* (1963).
Trengrove, Leonard, 'Newton's Theological Views', *Annals of Science,* 22 (1966), pp. 277-94.
Trevelyan, G.M., *English Social History* (1944).
Trigg, W.B. ed., 'The Correspondence of David Hartley and Rev John Lister', *Transactions of the Hallifax Antiquarian Society* (1938), pp. 231-78.
Tuck, Richard, *Natural Rights Theories: their origin and development* (Cambridge, 1979).
Turner, William, *Lives of Eminent Unitarians* (2 vols., 1843).
Tyson, G.P., *Joseph Johnson: a liberal publisher* (Iowa City, 1979).

Van Leeuen, Henry G., *The Problem of Certainty in English Thought: 1630-1690* (The Hague, 1963).

Venturi, Franco, *Italy and the Enlightenment* (New York, 1972).

_____ *Utopia and Reform in the Enlightenment* (Cambridge, 1971).

Vernon, James ed., *Re-Reading the Constitution: new narratives in the political history of England's long nineteenth century* (Cambridge, 1996).

Virgin, Peter, *The Church in an Age of Negligence: ecclesiastical structure and problems of Church reform 1700-1840* (Cambridge, 1989).

Wallis, P.J. and R.V., *Eighteenth-Century Medics: subscriptions, licences, apprenticeships* (2nd ed., Phibb, Newcastle Upon Tyne, 1988).

Walsh, John, Haydon, Colin and Taylor, Stephen eds., *The Church of England, c.1689-c.1833: from toleration to Tractarianism* (Cambridge, 1993).

Walvin, James, *England, Slaves and Freedom 1776-1838* (1986).

Ward, W.R., *Georgian Oxford: university politics in the eighteenth century* (Oxford, 1958).

Waterman, A.M.C., 'A Cambridge "Via Media" in Late Georgian Anglicanism', *Journal of Ecclesiastical History*, 42 (1991), pp. 419-36.

Watts, Michael, *The Dissenters: from the Reformation to the French Revolution* (Oxford, 1978).

Watts, Ruth, *Gender, Power and the Unitarians in England 1760-1860* (1998).

_____ 'Joseph Priestley and Education', *E&D*, 2 (1983), pp. 83-100.

Webb, R.K., 'The Crisis in Authority: early nineteenth century British thought', *Albion*, 24 (1992), pp. 1-16.

_____ 'The Emergence of Rational Dissent', in Haakonssen, *Enlightenment and Religion*, pp. 12-41.

_____ 'The Faith of Nineteenth-Century Unitarians: a curious incident', in Richard J. Helmstadter and Bernard Lightman eds., *Victorian Faith in Crisis: essays on continuity and change in nineteenth-century religious belief* (1990).

_____ *Harriet Martineau* (New York, 1960).

_____ 'Miracles in English Unitarian Thought', in Mark S. Micale and Robert L Dietle eds., *Enlightenment Passion and Modernity: historical essays in European thought and culture* (Stanford, California, 2000), pp.113-130.

_____ *Modern England: from the eighteenth century to the present*, (2nd ed., 1980).

_____ 'Perspectives on David Hartley', *E&D*, 17 (1998), pp. 17-47.

_____ 'Rational Piety', in Haakonssen, *Enlightenment and Religion*, pp. 287-311.

Westfall, Richard, *The Life of Isaac Newton* (Cambridge, 1993).

Whitney, R.D.J., *David Williams: the anvil and the hammer* (Cardiff, 1986).

Wicker, William, 'Helvetius and Holbach', in F.J.C. Hearnshaw ed., *Social and Political Ideas of Some Great French Thinkers of the Age of Reason* (1930).

Wilde, C.B., 'Hutchinsonianism, Natural Philosophy and Religious Controversy in Eighteenth-Century Britain', *History of Science*, 18 (1980), pp. 1-24.

Willen, Diane, 'Godley Women in Early Modern England: Puritanism and Gender', *Journal of Ecclesiastical History*, 43 (1992), pp. 561-80.

Willey, Basil, *The Eighteenth-Century Background* (Harmondsworth, 1972 [1940]).

Williams, E.N., *The Eighteenth-Century Constitution* (Cambridge, 1960).

Williamson, Audrey, *Wilkes, 'a friend to liberty'* (1974).

Wilson, Kathleen, 'Inventing Revolution: 1688 and eighteenth century popular politics', *Journal of British Studies*, 28 (1989).

_____ *The Sense of the People: politics, culture and imperialism in England, 1715-1785* (Cambridge, 1995).

_____ 'Urban Culture and Political Activism in Hanoverian England', in Hellmuth, *Transformation of Political Culture*, pp. 165-84.

Winstanley, D.A., *Unreformed Cambridge* (Cambridge, 1935).

Withey, Lynne E., 'Catharine Macaulay and the Uses of History: ancient rights, perfectionism, and propaganda', *Journal of British Studies,* 16 (1976), pp. 59-83.

Wood, Neal, 'The Baconian Character of Locke's *Essay'*, *Studies in the History and Philosophy of Science,* 6 (1975), pp. 42-84.

Woods, John A., 'The Correspondence of Benjamin Rush and Granville Sharp 1773-1809', *Journal of American Studies,* 1 (1967), pp. 1-29.

Wordsworth, Christopher, *Scholae Academicae: university studies in the eighteenth century* (1910).

_____ *Social Life at the English Universities in the Eighteenth Century* (1874).

Yolton, John, *Thinking Matter: materialism in eighteenth-century Britain* (Minneapolis, 1983).

_____ ed., *The Blackwell Companion to the Enlightenment* (Oxford, 1992).

York, Neil Longley, *Neither Kingdom nor Nation: the Irish quest for constitutional rights, 1698-1800* (Washington, D.C., 1994).

Young, B.W., *Religion and Enlightenment in Eighteenth-Century England: theological debate from Locke to Burke* (Oxford, 1998).

_____ '"Scepticism in Excess": Gibbon and eighteenth-century Christianity', *Historical Journal,* 41 (1998), pp. 179-99.

_____ 'The "Soul-Sleeping System": politics and heresy in eighteenth-century England', *Journal of Ecclesiastical History,* 45 (1994), pp. 64-81.

Young, David, 'Despotism and the Road to Freedom: Beccaria and Eighteenth-Century Lombardy', *Studies in Eighteenth-Century Culture,* 13 (1984), pp. 271-79.

Young, David, *F.D. Maurice and Unitarianism* (Oxford, 1992).

Young, Francis, *The Making of the Creeds* (1991).

Zebrowski, Martha K., 'The Corruption of Politics and the Dignity of Human Nature: the critical and constructive radicalism of James Burgh', *E&D,* 10 (1991), pp. 78-103.

_____ 'Richard Price: British Platonist of the eighteenth century', *JHI,* 55 (1994), pp. 17-35.

Index

About the Author

ANTHONY PAGE is a Lecturer in European History at the Launceston campus of the University of Tasmania.